24.75

Karen K Day
839-14th St
SF, CA 94114
Phone (415) 552-0969

UCSF-
X ~~2028~~ 1181
on
666-2252

K Day
ADM for Nursing
University
Hospital
(617) 2475480

Hospital Materiel Management

Charles E. Housley, F.A.C.H.A.

Aspen Systems Corporation
Germantown, Maryland
1978

Library of Congress Cataloging in Publication Data

Housley, Charles E.
Hospital materiel management.

Includes index.
1. Hospitals—Materials management. I. Title.
[DNLM: 1. Materials management, Hospital. WX150.3 H842h]
RA971.33.H68 658.7 78–14526
ISBN 0-89443–046–7

Library of Congress Catalog Card Number: 78–14526
ISBN: 0-89443–046–7

Printed in the United States of America

1 2 3 4 5

Table of Contents

Preface .... **ix**

Acknowledgments .... **xi**

Chapter 1—The Case for Materiel Management **1**

Chapter 2—Planning and Implementing Materiel Management **9**
An Administrative Understanding 10
Selection of the Materiel Manager 10
Establishment of Objectives 12
An Organizational Format 13
Key Personnel Conference 19
Recruiting and Developing Personnel 19

Chapter 3—The Making of the Materiel Manager **21**
Who Is This Materiel Manager? 23
The Managerial Profile of the Materiel Manager 24

Chapter 4—Job Descriptions for Key Departmental Positions **31**
Position Description for the Materiel Manager 32
Position Description for Assistant Director of Materiel Management or Director of Purchased Services 36
Position Description for the Chief Pharmacist 40
Position Description for the Supply, Process, and Distribution Supervisor 44
Position Description for the Exchange Cart Coordinator 46

Position Description for the Cart Attendant 52
Position Description for the Receiving Clerk 55
Position Description for the Processing Supervisor 57

Chapter 5—Pertinent Policies and Procedures Set the Pace for Progress .. 63
An Organizational Format for Policy and Procedure Determination 64

Chapter 6—The Act of Purchasing Should be Simple and Results Oriented 109
A Simple System Must be Planned and Initiated 109
Don't Forget the Fundamentals 112
The Necessity for Centralized Purchasing 115
Hospitals Should Share Prices 117

Chapter 7—All About the Product Standardization Process 121
Planning for Effectiveness 121
Administrative Support Through Policy Delineation 122
Committee Representation 126
Objectives, Scope, and Mission of the Standardization Committee 129
Fundamental Policies and Guidelines for the Standardization Committee 130
Interface of the Standardization Committee with Other Committees 135
Product Evaluation Procedure 135

Chapter 8—Distributing the Goods the Right Way 163
Requisition System 164
Par Level Transfer System 165
Exchange Carts 166
Materiel Manager's Role 167
Automated vs. Manual 167
Summary 168

Chapter 9—A Supply Cart System: Highlights of a Ten-Year Study 169
A Pilot Program is Recommended 170
Form Follows Function 172
Depletion—Repletion Cycle of Distribution 175
A Patient Charge Mechanism Is Built In 176
Ten Years Later 178
Functions of the Total Supply Cart 181

Chapter 10—Inventory Reduction Is a Financial Must **187**
A Different Philosophy 187
What Actually Constitutes Inventory 188
What Is a Responsible Per-Bed Inventory 190
Some Disturbing Characteristics of Supply Inventories 191
Plan to Reduce Unnecessary Inventories 193

Chapter 11—Stockless Purchasing Makes Dollars and Sense **197**

Chapter 12—Creating a Buyer's Market **203**
The Great Fallacies of Hospital Purchasing 203
Methodology for Initiating Contract Purchasing 207
Advantages of Contract Purchasing 207
Anatomy of the Prime Supplier Concept 208

Chapter 13—Suppliers Can Provide Much More Than Price **213**

Chapter 14—Capital Equipment Acquisition Considerations **217**
Hospital Policy for Capital Equipment Acquisition 217
Negotiation Considerations 219

Chapter 15—Effective Reporting Provides Administrative Support **223**
Monthly Reports 223
Quarterly Reports 225
Semiannual Reports 226
Annual Reports 226

Chapter 16—Working with the Hospital Committee Structure **229**

Chapter 17—The Materiel Manager's Role in the Budgetary Process **235**

Chapter 18—The Pharmacist as a Materiel Manager **241**
The Hospital-Trained Materiel Manager 241
The Industry-Trained Materiel Manager 242
The Pharmacist as Materiel Manager 243

Chapter 19—Consumer Evaluation of the Materiel Efforts **245**

Chapter 20—Telling the Story of Materiel Management **251**
Telling the Materiel Management Staff 252
Telling Nursing and Other Consumer Departments 253
Telling the Medical Staff 254
Telling the Sales Representatives 255

Chapter 21—The Many Ways to Contain Costs Through Effective Materiel Management 259

Reducing Official Inventory 259
Reducing Unofficial Inventory 260
Amalgamating Supply, Process, and Distribution Functions and Areas 261
Eliminating Excess Personnel in the Materiel Areas 261
Using Consignment as an Alternative to Purchasing 262
Stockless Purchasing 262
Product Standardization 262
Buying Special Items Locally 262
Indirect or Wholesale Drug Purchasing 263
Negotiating Term Instead of Full Service Contracts 264
Controlling Forms 264
Purchasing Copying Machines 266
Sharing Infrequently Used Supplies with Other Hospitals . . 266
Limiting the Number of Supplies in the Central Stores Area 266
Developing a Drug Formulary 267
Reducing the Frequency of Linen Changes 267
Prime Supplier Concept 268
Group Purchasing 268
Requesting Instant Credit on Overcharges by the Vendors . . 268
Centralizing Purchasing 269
Hand Writing Purchase Orders 269
Using FAX Equipment for Purchase Data Transmission 269
Consolidating Rebates, Discounts and Allowances into the Invoiced Price 269
Tough But Ethical Negotiation 270
Industrial Engineering Applications 270
Reviewing and Studying All Purchase Alternatives 270
Supply Utilization Studies 271
Eliminating All Bulk Warehousing 272
Establishing Effective Limits for All Supplies Based on an Economic Order 272
Better Utilization of the Vendors 272
Evaluating New Products at the Vendor's Expense 273
Employee Orientation 273
Time and Motion Studies of All Supply Functions 273
Continuous Patient Charge Review 274
Inhouse Biomedical Engineering Expertise 274

Effective Preventive Maintenance Programs 274
An Assets Management Program 274
Appropriate Product Substitution 275
Value Analysis 275
Results-Oriented Product Inservice Programs 275
Pay for Capital Equipment Purchases Only After Installation and Hospital Approval 276
Simplifying the Purchase Process 276
Questioning All Computer Applications in the Materiel Areas for Cost Effectiveness 276
Sharing Services 277
Questioning All Automated Efforts in the Materiel Areas for Cost Effectiveness 277
Negotiating for Longer Equipment Warranties 277
Supply Cost Emphasis and Awareness Program 278
Return for Credit Policy 278
Using Hot Air Hand Dryers Instead of Paper Towels 278
Using All of a Product Before Replacing It 279
In Some Cases, Lower the Standards of Quality 279
Question All Patient Convenience Products 279

Chapter 22—Excuses, Excuses, Excuses 283
Excuse Number 1—Materiel Management Is Too Expensive . 283
Excuse Number 2—My Administrator Won't Support Me .. 283
Excuse Number 3—Materiel Management Means More Personnel 284
Excuse Number 4—My Hospital Is Too Small for Materiel Management 284
Excuse Number 5—Materiel Management Is a Fad that Will Soon Pass 284
Excuse Number 6—Materiel Management Is Too Complex . 285
Excuse Number 7—My Hospital Is Too Large and Complicated 285
Excuse Number 8—My Hospital Is Too Old for This New Concept 285
Excuse Number 9—Materiel Management Takes Too Long to Implement 285
Excuse Number 10—My Hospital Is Different 285
Excuse Number 11—Materiel Management Takes Specially Trained Personnel 286
Excuse Number 12—I've Got Bigger Problems, Materiel Management Is the Least of My Worries 286

Chapter 23—Case Reports of Materiel Management Implementation 287
Case Report 1—Development of the Materiel Management Concept 287
Case Report 2—The Total Supply Cart Exchange Program .. 290
Case Report 3—A Group Purchasing Dilemma 292
Case Report 4—Board of Trustees and Potential Conflict of Interest 294
Case Report 5—The Small Hospital Situation 296
Case Report 6—The Standardization Committee 297
Case Report 7—Central Sterile Supply 299
Case Report 8—Internal Control 301
Case Report 9—Selecting the Materiel Manager 303
Case Report 10—Product and Equipment Specifications 305
Case Report 11—Problems with Group Purchasing 308
Case Report 12—The Perpetual Inventory 310
Case Report 13—Organizational Structure 313
Case Report 14—Centralization of Purchasing 316
Case Report 15—Decentralized Materiel Management 319
Case Report 16—Stockless Purchasing 321
Case Report 17—Patient Charges 324
Case Report 18—The Prime Supplier Concept 326
Case Report 19—Evaluation of the Materiel Efforts 329
Case Report 20—Supply Cost Reimbursement 332
Case Report 21—Administrative Reports 334
Case Report 22—Centralized Warehousing 337
Case Report 23—Cost Containment Efforts 339
Case Report 24—Prudent Purchaser Considerations 342
Case Report 25—The Profit-Making Hospital 345

Glossary 349

Index 355

Preface

Materiel management is a philosophy whose time has finally arrived. However, this philosophy must be translated into practice, and as is the case with many ideas, there are obstacles to its development and initiation. Hospitals certainly have their share of members of the Discouragement Society, and encouragement for the promotion of good materiel management practices is often lacking—from top management to the materiel manager and purchasing agent. If the materiel manager looks for excuses for not implementing materiel management, he or she will most certainly find them. However, the time for voluntary action and effort to meet the materiel obligations of the health care institution has arrived. It is a tremendous challenge which requires persistence and determination. The materiel manager must be willing to bear the cross in order to wear the crown.

This book represents a progressive and provocative plan for the management of the materiel aspects of today's hospitals. It is not just another book on purchasing. It represents a total approach to materiel management which is practical, effective, and oriented toward results. Hospital materiel management represents the trend of the future. The "turned-on" materiel manager will keep his/her goals and options very flexible. If a particular program is not accepted by top management, an alternative plan should be available. The materiel manager should never get into a situation that has no alternatives. In other words, the materiel programs should be kept dynamic so that managerial stagnation is not allowed to arise.

Hospitals must do something in the area of materiel management before it is done for them. A position of malignant concern should be taken rather than one of benign neglect. Remember, in reference to materiel management, when all is said and done, there is more said than done. Will you accept the challenge? The next move is yours.

Acknowledgments

I would like to express my gratitude and appreciation to the administration and staff of Saint Anthony Hospital, Columbus, Ohio. Without them, this work would not have been possible. They not only supported me, they also participated in the pilot programs and projects which made many of the ideas in this volume come to life as practical and efficient procedures.

Especially, I owe a great debt of gratitude to a real health care professional, Mr. Charles A. Turner, administrator of Saint Anthony Hospital. It was through his concern, encouragement, and support for me that I was able to develop and implement the total concept of materiel management at a results-oriented level.

Also, I would like to express my sincere thanks to my secretary, Mrs. Trevia Diebel, for her untiring efforts in typing, copying, and proofing the original manuscript.

Chapter 1

The Case for Materiel Management

Throughout this book the words "materiel management" are used instead of "material management" or "materials management," the latter of which is probably the most frequently used phrase of the three in the United States. Webster defines the word "material" as "of or relating to the production and distribution of economic goods and the social relationships of owners and laborers." "Materiel" is defined as "equipment, apparatus and supplies used by an organization or institution." It is very apparent that the latter is the more appropriate definition. Furthermore, the Canadian Hospital Association has decided to use the word "materiel" to relate to hospital supplies and equipment. The author believes "materiel" should be used universally to refer to hospital supplies and equipment.

In the industrial world the term "materiel management" is not uncommon, and the industrial manager of materiel has a definite position and field of endeavor. Additionally, the military has used it for many years to denote the area of supply logistics. However, it is a different story with hospitals. In the past, too much emphasis was placed on just having supplies on hand, without regard for the method, volume, or use. There was too much emphasis on simply finding the elusive best price. Recently, though, there has been increasing interest in the effective and efficient utilization of supplies and equipment within the hospital. Administrators realize the definite need to scrutinize the entire acquisition-utilization-disposition cycle and decrease or maintain costs in this highly inflationary area. Hence, many hospitals have just flirted with the concept of materiel management. In many cases, this has translated into a name change in the purchasing function, with the same familiar inefficiencies and fragmentations in authority and responsibilities remaining.

A pertinent question at this juncture is "what exactly is materiel management as it relates to the modern hospital?" It is the management and control of goods, services, and equipment from acquisition to disposition, encompassing the following areas:

- writing and adhering to product specifications;
- procuring all supplies and services through centralized purchasing;
- receiving and accounting for all supplies;
- stocking supplies for "adequate" periods of time only;
- studying and reviewing utilization of the materiel;
- developing and adhering to policies and procedures for product utilization;
- standardizing and evaluating all products and services;
- processing and reprocessing reusable supplies and materiel;
- distributing all goods and services;
- controlling "unofficial" inventories;
- assuming accountability for capital equipment;
- reviewing and servicing patient care equipment;
- controlling printing and all printed matter, including xerography;
- reviewing and evaluating patient charges; and
- disposing efficiently of the waste products of the goods and services purchased.

Materiel management can best be described as a concept or philosophy that is religiously applied to the materiel process on a consistent basis. It is a continuum along which many important supply functions take place under the disciplined supervision of the materiel manager (Figure 1–1). If developed and implemented properly, the idea of total materiel management represents control of "anything that moves and is not alive."

Much has been written about the concept of materiel management from the fundamental principles and the various methods of implementation to associated problems. However, the fundamental question must be answered: What will it do for me and my hospital that the more conventional programs have failed to do? Today, when new ideas are not adopted simply because they are new, someone must be willing to test them in the performance arena. Materiel management is one such idea that has been shown to be an effective and practical management tool for several hospitals in the United States and Canada. Accordingly, if materiel management is supported by top management and the total concept effectively implemented, then a number of advantages can be expected.

One of the first and foremost byproducts of initiating the total materiel management concept is centralization of the authority and responsibility for all supply, process, and distribution functions. This is generally accompanied

Figure 1-1 The Continuum of Supply Functions Supervised by the Materiel Manager

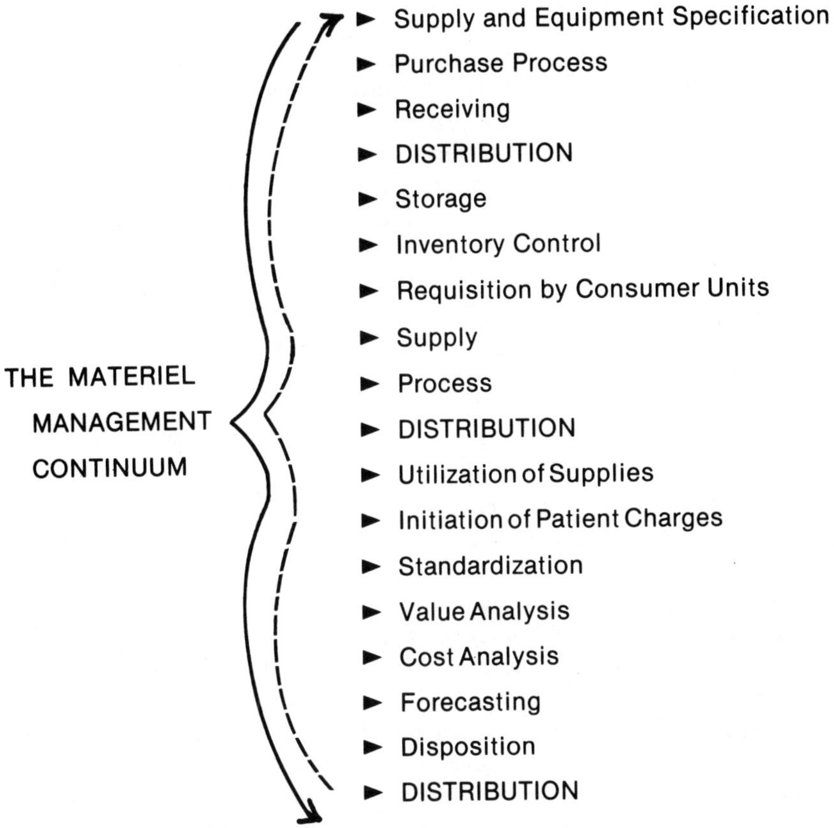

by at least the realization that the major divisions of materiel management should all be located in one area of the building. It is hoped that hospital managers, architects, and designers are learning not to decentralize the materiel functions by locating, for example, the pharmacy on the first floor, the C.S.R. on the second floor, and the central stores in the basement. All areas dealing directly with supply, process, and distribution of goods and services should, instead, be designed to function together for the sake of efficiency.

Another result of materiel management implementation is a reduction in the number of employees involved in similar functions. Effective materiel management unifies the efforts of all those involved, eliminating expensive duplication of tasks, time, and effort. For example, if the central sterile room

(C.S.R.) and central stores are amalgamated into one unified area, both areas can then be accessible for the same number of hours per day without adding more employees. This is a prime example of cost containment in an area that is prone to be labor intensive.

Moreover, there are many similar tasks performed in the central stores, C.S.R. and pharmacy that duplicate supplies and labor. For example, distribution for all three areas can be performed by the same employees. While C.S.R. has always duplicated the supply function, its objective should be process, not supply. It exists because central stores was kept open only during the day shift, five days per week in institutions in which many departments, especially nursing, must operate continuously. As a result, the nurses began to deal with this discrepancy by instituting central sterile rooms. Unfortunately, in many cases the C.S.R. was staffed by high salaried professional personnel. It is hoped that materiel management will not only reduce the number of personnel performing these functions, but also will result in the functions being performed at the most appropriate level (Figure 1–2).

Most hospitals are in need of additional space for patient care and storage. However, building costs are averaging about $70 to $80 per square foot. At this rate, space should be utilized primarily for patient care services, with storage space kept at an absolute minimum. Under good materiel practices, a hospital should need about 1,000 to 1,500 square feet of central storage space per 100 beds. Moreover, it should function with rapid supply turnover, stockless purchasing and minimum inventories. What this actually means is that reduced demand for storage produces enhanced space capabilities for the revenue-producing patient care areas. With the elimination of such storage areas, inventories are reduced to a more reasonable level and the demand for expensive built-in storage areas is removed from plans to build or expand facilities. The experience has been that many hospitals on an average can account for at least a $100,000 reduction in supply inventories with the implementation of the total materiel management concept!

The costs of the total supply-related areas can be most deceiving. It has often been quoted that 55 to 65 percent of the hospital expense budget is for personnel, as compared to 18 to 25 percent for supplies. It would seem, then, that hospital management should concentrate cost containment and management efforts in the area of personnel. However, these figures do not reveal that up to 46 percent of the hospital expense budget centers around materiel management (Figure 1–3). Moreover, materiel costs are rising at a rate of one and one-half times that of personnel.

Development of the total materiel management concept has other advantageous spinoffs. It puts the responsibility of this function solely in the hands of the trained and capable materiel manager and relieves the nursing staff of supply, process and distribution functions. Paperwork for the materiel

Figure 1-2 Organization of a Department of Materiel Management

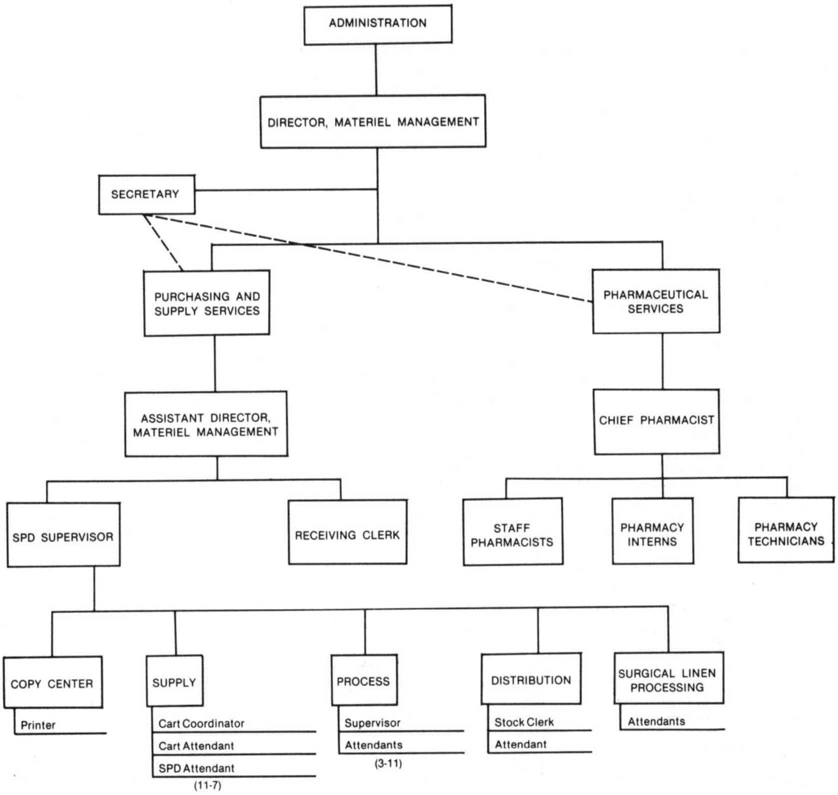

management department is greatly reduced and becomes more meaningful as the departments are freed from the tedious tasks of ordering, stocking, and controlling supplies. Finally, the process of implementing materiel management concepts and principles seems to become contagious as the institution begins to benefit from centralized purchasing and standardization.

Materiel management is not some mysterious rite that has been imposed upon the hospital and materiel manager. It is as natural and fundamental as personnel or fiscal management and the advantages will be just as rewarding. This concept of managing and controlling supplies and services from acquisition to disposition should be encouraged and enforced by top management in today's hospitals.

Figure 1-3 Distribution of Hospital Expenses

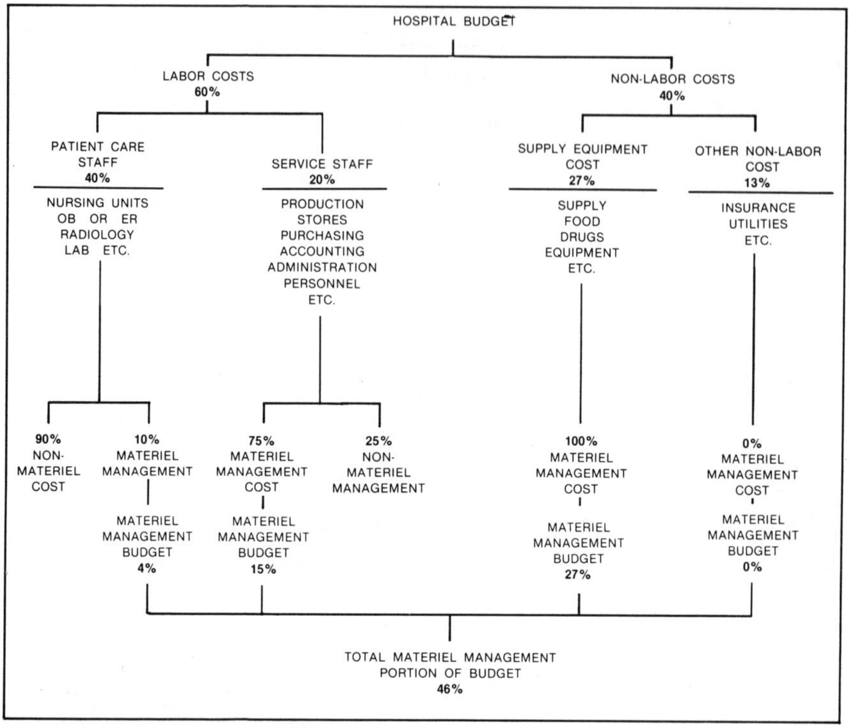

Source: AMSCO Fact Summary, SC-2533, March, 1977, Exhibit 3, p. 2. © AMSCO Systems. Reprinted with permission.

Figure 1-4 Major Functions of Materiel Management

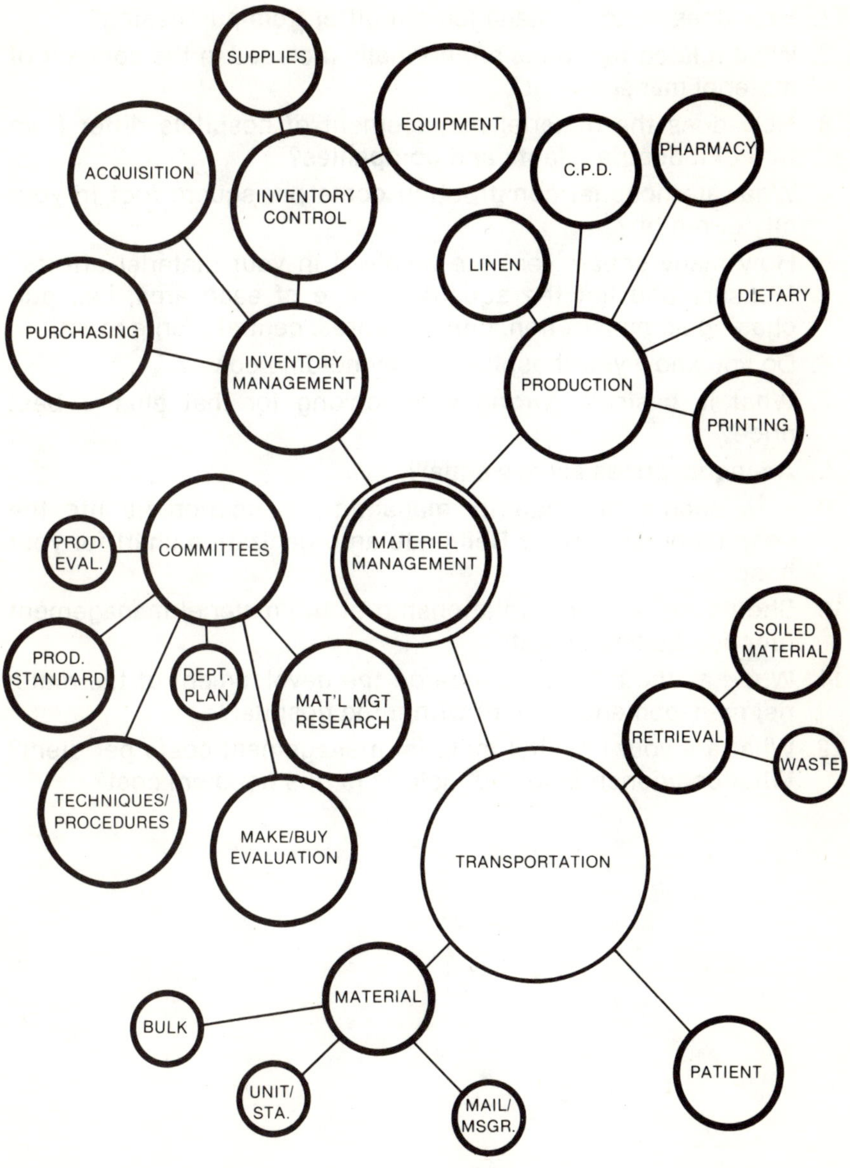

Source: AMSCO Fact Summary, SC-2533, March 1977, Exhibit 6, p. 4. © AMSCO Systems. Reprinted with permission.

Pertinent Points to Ponder

1. How does materiel management differ from purchasing?
2. What related functions are normally included in the concept of materiel management?
3. How does the materiel management of hospitals differ from that of industrial plants and companies?
4. What are hospital construction costs per square foot in your city or region?
5. How many square feet are involved in your materiel efforts? Measure and list the square footage of each area, i.e., purchasing administration, central stores, central sterile room.
6. Do you know your hospital supply holding costs?
7. What is basically wrong with looking for that elusive best price?
8. Are equal prices always equal?
9. How should the materiel management function fit into the hospital organization? Delineate an organization chart for your hospital.
10. Should the authority relationship of the materiel management function be line or staff?
11. Who has the most influence on the development of the materiel management concept within the hospital?
12. What are your hospital materiel management costs per diem? What components do you include in this per diem cost?

Chapter 2

Planning and Implementing Materiel Management*

One of the most frequently asked questions is "How can I initiate total materiel management in my hospital?" Often the questioner has been excited or intrigued about the idea after attending an educational seminar on the concept, then discouraged or bewildered after actually beginning implementation. It seems that for every advantage someone can come up with ten or more reasons why it won't work.

There are some fundamental precepts for the managers to keep in mind. First, there is no set starting place. Maybe materiel management would be easier to implement if there were a magical beginning and ending, but in truth the key is to begin somewhere, whether it be with centralized purchasing, product standardization, or any other of the myriad key materiel functions. Second, timing is important. For example, an excellent time for the materiel manager to present top management with a well-developed plan for performing a decentralized department's purchasing would be when that department head announces his retirement. Third, the concept of materiel management cannot be implemented within a short time, but may take three to five years to begin to see progress. Last, this complex concept must truly be a team concept from beginning to end. Moreover, there is a definite order and priority to the implementation process, and the following considerations should be addressed carefully for best results.

---

*Reprinted with the permission of DIMENSIONS in Health Service, Journal of the Canadian Hospital Association.

An Administrative Understanding

The most critical phase of planning and implementing materiel management is obtaining support and credibility for the program from top management. It is here that the total concept is either blessed or cursed. There are really two primary models of approach to this understanding. The most prevalent approach is where the decision is made to proceed toward materiel management using the current purchasing organization with expanded responsibilities as the basic springboard. This responsible and effective means of implementation, however, infers that the hospital has the necessary personnel, expertise, and administrative backing to accomplish this managerial feat.

Unfortunately, the person selected from within may not understand the organizational and managerial format of materiel management. It is at this point that one hears that management is not supportive or materiel management is not responsive and receptive. Many times a total materiel management program implemented from within seems fragmented and without intermediate and long-term goals. This could be that since hospital personnel are being used for the effort, the administration and materiel management are not going to the trouble to delineate objectives and establish priorities. Also, hospital personnel in line for promotions prompted by the proposed changes seem reluctant to criticize the plan lest the promotions be tabled.

The second approach model involves recruiting from outside the hospital. In this situation, top management gives more time to defining objectives, delineating organizational structure, and carefully establishing an effective job description for the new director. Conversely, well-trained materiel managers worth recruiting also have their perspective of what materiel management should encompass. They want to know what their title will be and to whom they will report. Administrative philosophy toward materiel management will be discussed at great length. Most effective materiel managers will have ideas about the total concept and will request authority to implement a certain structure. In other words, a materiel master plan will be defined before the manager is hired. Whichever method of selection is employed, it is imperative that the administration provide a supportive structure on which to build and grow.

Selection of the Materiel Manager

Another important decision is choosing the director of materiel management. Where does one start? In many cases, the person for the job is within the hospital organization, especially in the positions of director of purchasing, director of pharmacy, central supply supervisor, manager of central stores, and supply, process, and distribution supervisor. Their foremost qualification is their experience with supplies and the institution. Nonetheless, they may have no conceptual scheme of materiel management. Other potential sources for consideration are hospital supply buyers, sales representatives and warehouse managers, as well as industrial purchasing agents, marketing managers, and personnel and public relations directors.

Selecting a director of materiel management involves both recruiting and selection by the hospital and consideration of career development and acceptance by the materiel manager. In the recruiting and selection of a candidate for the director of materiel management, hospitals should consider several guidelines.

Managerial Potential

Of all the criteria for performance, managerial potential tops the list. The effective director of materiel of the future will be a manager of people, systems, policies, monies, regulations, and negotiations and must, therefore, possess superior management skills.

A Written Job Description

The job description should clearly spell out certain factors:

- Title of the position
- Title of the person to whom the manager is responsible
- Title of the persons for whom the manager is responsible
- Amount of supervision required
- Management skills necessary
- Nonmanagement duties
- Delineated list of all major tasks
- Educational requirement
- Experience requirements and equivalents
- Date and frequency of performance evaluations

The description should be flexible enough to allow appropriate changes and ideas from the new director.

Salary

The salary arrangements should be commensurate with potential and assigned responsibility. There also should be some means of recognition for performance based on objective administrative analysis. The potential for savings and cost containment is high and should be considered when selecting the materiel manager and establishing the salary. After all, top management must realize that the person they are recruiting is likely an effective manager elsewhere.

Demonstrated Ability

The one most important qualification is that the person considered for the job of materiel manager be able to present actual examples of accomplishment in his or her last position. The person should be able to quote such achievements as reducing official inventory from $500,000 to $250,000 in a three-year period, reducing personnel in the central supply area from eighteen to eight by combining the function with central stores, and obtaining better overall supply prices by initiating the prime supplier approach. Hospitals should look for demonstrated ability and success in the person's last position instead of toying with the ideals of experience and education.

Definition of Materiel Management

It is necessary that top management and materiel management agree as to exactly what functions or responsibilities will belong to materiel management. This will vary from hospital to hospital. It should be kept in mind that the management responsibilities of this area will certainly resemble those of an assistant administrator in many hospitals. The scope and authority of materiel management should be clearly delineated in writing to all appropriate people, especially to the candidates for the job of director of materiel management.

Establishment of Objectives

After the administrative philosophy has been established and the candidate selected, appropriate objectives should be defined collectively. Why should a department of materiel management be structured? What can it do that the purchasing department and related functions have not done? These and other questions should be answered by the statement of materiel management objectives. However, many hospitals which have initiated materiel management have not yet delineated their objectives. It should be an essential part of the planning and implementation phases. Most objectives will parallel this model set:

1. To manage and control the flow of supplies and equipment from acquisition to disposition.
2. To apply management methods to the supply, process, and distribution of products and equipment, i.e., value analysis, cost analysis, and product utilization studies.
3. To centralize all purchasing functions for control and cost effectiveness.
4. To provide the mechanism whereby improved patient care will prevail through product standardization and evaluation, with emphasis on quality of care and containment of costs.

5. To provide for unified supply, process, and distribution of goods and services under the same area and supervision.
6. To reduce costly inventories to cost-effective minimums.
7. To keep administration, department heads, and other appropriate parties informed of changes in equipment, products, and supply methods.
8. To meet or exceed all of the requirements of the prudent buyer concept.
9. To control the amounts of unofficial inventory (that which has been expensed and dispensed) by quarterly physical inventories and stockless purchasing.
10. To relieve nursing and other departments of all supply functions—inventory, requisitioning, recording, delivering, and processing supplies and equipment.
11. To provide all consumer departments with a total supply system in which the right supply is always available at the right place and time in the right quantities.
12. To purchase all supplies and equipment prudently with consideration for cost, service, and quality.
13. To improve vendor relations through centralized contacts and sales representative orientations to the hospital materiel management philosophy.
14. To reduce and contain all direct and indirect operating costs of the total materiel function.
15. To establish an effective property management program.

After the objectives have been agreed upon, they should be classified and put on a priority basis according to either immediate, short-term, intermediate, or long-term objectives (Figure 2-1).

An Organizational Format

An organizational structure can best be developed by asking the question, "What organizational format can best meet the delineated objectives?" Many hospitals include only the functions of purchasing, central stores, and central supply in their concept of materiel management. Others branch out to include all supply, process, and distribution functions, pharmacy, print shop, and linen distribution (Figure 2-2). Additionally, some hospitals have expanded the responsibility index of materiel management to include the morgue, laundry, housekeeping, trash collection, and even data processing. However, the functions to be included should be determined by each individual hospital.

Figure 2-1 Objectives of a Materiel Management Program

IMPLEMENTATION OF OBJECTIVES
TIMETABLE

MODEL GUIDELINES

Objectives	High Priority	Moderate Priority	Less Urgent	Persons Responsible For Action
1. To initiate total centralized purchasing for all departments				1-a. Administration b. Materiel Manager c. Department Heads
2. To provide for the centralization of all of the functions of supply, process and distribution under one area and supervision				2-a. Administration b. Materiel Manager c. Director of Maintenance d. C.S.R. Supervisor
3. Reduction of official inventories to cost effective minimums				3-a. Materiel Manager b. Central Stores Manager c. Director of Pharmaceutical Services d. Director of Dietary
4. Reduction of all unofficial inventories to two week maximums				4-a. Materiel Manager b. All department directors c. Head nurses
5. To provide a total supply cart exchange program for all applicable areas				5-a. Materiel Manager b. S.P.D. Supervisor c. All department directors d. Head nurses
	4 Months	8 Months	12 Months	

12 MONTH PERIOD

Evaluation or Study
Implement
Ongoing

Figure 2-1 continued

IMPLEMENTATION OF OBJECTIVES
TIMETABLE

MODEL GUIDELINES

Objectives	High Priority	Moderate Priority	Less Urgent	Persons Responsible For Action
6. To meet or exceed all of the requirements of the Prudent Buyer concept				6-a. Administration b. Materiel Manager c. Director of Purchased Services
7. To reduce paperwork in the purchase order process				7-a. Materiel Manager b. Director of Purchased Services c. Sales Representatives
8. To develop an effective standardization procedure				8-a. Administration b. Materiel Manager c. Director of Purchased Services d. All Standardization Committee Members
9. To explore the feasibility of the prime supplier approach to purchasing				9-a. Materiel Manager b. Director of Purchased Services c. Sales Representatives
10. To perform "stockless" purchasing				10-a Materiel Manager b. Director of Purchased Services
	4 Months	8 Months	12 Months	

12 MONTH PERIOD

Evaluation or Study

Implement

Ongoing

Figure 2-1 continued

IMPLEMENTATION OF OBJECTIVES
TIMETABLE

MODEL GUIDELINES

Objectives	High Priority	Moderate Priority	Less Urgent	Persons Responsible For Action
11. To reduce and contain all direct and indirect operating costs of the total material management functions				11-a. Materiel Manager b. Director of Purchased Services c. S.P.D. Supervisor d. Processing Supervisor e. Director of Pharmaceutical Services f. All applicable departments and units
12. To meet or exceed all accreditation standards that are applicable to the department				12-a. Materiel Manager b. Director of Purchased Services c. S.P.D. Supervisor d. Processing Supervisor e. Director of Pharmaceutical Services
13. To apply management methods to the supply process and distribution of products and equipment				13-a. Materiel Manager b. Director of Purchased Services c. S.P.D. Supervisor d. Director of Pharmaceutical Services
	4 Months	8 Months	12 Months	

12 MONTH PERIOD

Evaluation or Study
Implement
Ongoing

Figure 2-1 continued

IMPLEMENTATION OF OBJECTIVES
TIMETABLE

MODEL GUIDELINES

Objectives	High Priority	Moderate Priority	Less Urgent	Persons Responsible For Action
14. To establish an evaluation procedure for measuring materiel management effectiveness				14-a. Administration b. Materiel Manager c. Fiscal Officer
15. To establish a Property Management System				15-a. Administration b. Materiel Manager c. Fiscal Officer

4 Months 8 Months 12 Months
12 MONTH PERIOD

Evaluation or Study

Implement

Ongoing

Figure 2-2 Inter- and Intradepartmental Reporting and Authority Relationships Within the Hospital Organization

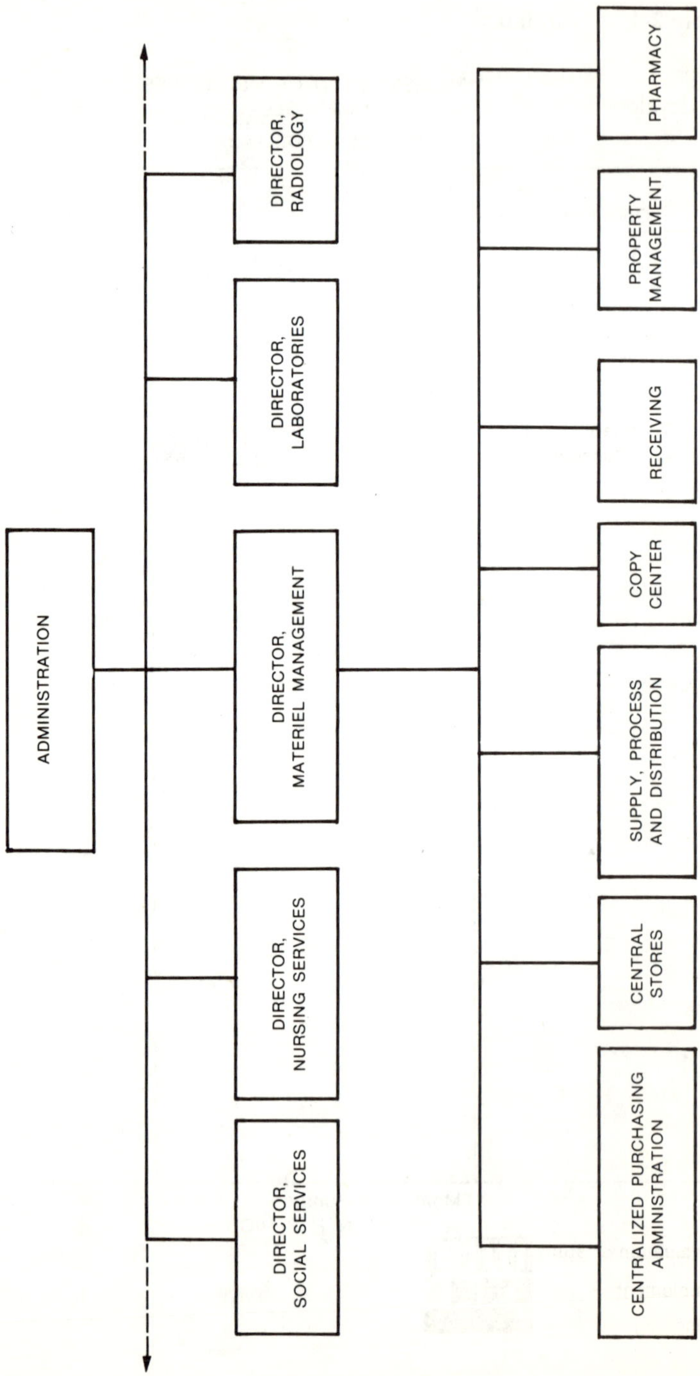

Key Personnel Conference

After all of the other criteria have been considered, a plan of attack must be developed, agreed upon, and put into a time sequence. This plan should be discussed at a key personnel conference scheduled by top management and including anyone who is either a consumer or a provider of supplies. This will provide credibility and support to the materiel management thrust. It will also be an effective means of communication in that all appropriate parties get the same information at the same time. After introduction of the philosophy by top management, the materiel manager should outline the entire plan, emphasizing all the advantages. Ideas should be solicited from the group, and the notion that materiel management is a group endeavor should be reiterated. Organizational relationships and new policies and procedures should be communicated.

When the program is first instituted, several orientation sessions must be held to familiarize all personnel to the total materiel management concept. Again, the positive attributes ought to be accentuated. A simple but thorough slide presentation based on actual hospital situational settings would be helpful, as would be written handouts which summarize the orientation session. Furthermore, each newly hired employee should be exposed to these sessions, as should groups of all employees at least every six months. A special orientation program structured just for materiel management personnel, stressing the service aspect and the importance of quality performance, should also be created.

Recruiting and Developing Personnel

Many hospitals hire an effective materiel manager and expect him or her to provide the necessary results. However, the materiel manager is only as effective as his personnel make him. Other key positions in the scheme are those of purchasing director and supply, process, and distribution supervisor. Preparation of personnel from the supervisory to the line level is imperative because the materiel management department must be operated by skilled, motivated, and knowledgeable personnel.

One way of insuring that this occurs is to periodically evaluate the performance of materiel management. This can best be done by reviewing the objectives and assessing whether or not they have been met. If they have been, top management and materiel management can delineate further objectives. If they have not, a new priority must be set. The materiel manager should make monthly progress reports to the administration, as well as provide semiannual performance evaluations.

Pertinent Points to Ponder

1. What is your administrator's view of the importance and functions of materiel management?
2. As a materiel manager, to whom do you report and for whom are you responsible?
3. What do you consider to be the first steps in the proper implementation of materiel management?
4. What are your objectives for materiel management and are they written?
5. What single characteristic is the most important in the selection of an effective materiel manager?
6. To whom should the materiel manager report and what are some other effective alternative reporting routes?
7. On what criteria should the materiel manager be evaluated and how often?
8. How often should the objectives and the materiel master plan be reviewed and revised?
9. As a materiel manager, how do you report to your supervisor and what is the frequency?
10. What kinds of information do you report?
11. In your opinion, who has the most influence over the importance and position of materiel management in your institution?
12. Who does the orientation of the materiel management concept to all new employees in your hospital and how often?

Chapter 3

The Making of the Materiel Manager

To buy or not to buy used to be the question, but today that interrogatory is much more complex. As Dr. Dean S. Ammer states in his recent book, *Hospital Materials Management: Neglect and Inefficiency Promote High Costs of Care:*

> In the ten years between 1962 and 1972—which hospital administrators remember as a period in which nurses and other hospital personnel first showed their bargaining muscle and began to win huge raises for themselves—hospital payroll costs increased by 236 per cent from the 1962 level of $13.12 per patient day to the 1972 level of $44.17 per patient day. Non-payroll costs increased during this same period by 349 per cent, from $6.41 per patient day to $29.72 per day. Thus, the rate of increase of non-payroll costs was almost half again greater than the rate of increase of payroll costs. The major villain, as far as hospital costs are concerned, is not the hospital employee but the various recipients of non-payroll costs. And, of course, hospital suppliers collectively are overwhelmingly the major beneficiaries of increases in non-payroll costs.[1]

In reference to hospital management, there are at least three distinct areas which cut horizontally across all departmental lines of authority and also have much impact vertically as well. These are often referred to as the three M's of

---

[1]Dean S. Ammer, *Hospital Materials Management: Neglect and Inefficiency Promote High Costs of Care,* (Boston, Mass.: Northeastern University, Bureau of Business and Economic Research, 1974), p. 1.

management. Namely, they are management of manpower, money, and materiel.

In the area of manpower management or personnel administration, hospitals for the most part have recruited and hired qualified and well trained personnel directors who have been instrumental in bringing about good personnel practices. As a result, hospitals have respected and well managed personnel departments. However, this has not always been the case. Not so many years ago, various hospital department heads advertised, screened, and hired their own employees. This decentralization of the personnel function in many cases resulted in unfair personnel practices, lack of uniformity and continuity in disciplinary action, and discrepancies in salary administration. One might ask what brought about the change. For sure, it was not just one single influence, but it is safe to assume among them were pressures from the outside.

What were some of those outside pressures? Changes in the wage and hour law policies and procedures certainly had their effects. The Equal Employment Opportunity Act brought about many changes, as did the retraction of the Taft-Hartley Act exemption for hospitals. Unions certainly made their presence felt. The Occupational Safety and Health Act changed many employee practices, as have the personnel surveys made by the Joint Commission on Accreditation of Hospitals. Exactly what caused the changes is not as important, though, as the fact that hospitals have made great strides in the area of personnel administration. Good personnel managers have been hired, uniform policies and procedures written, and effective wage and salary scales developed, resulting in an effective meeting of the objectives of both management and labor.

In the area of hospital financial management, most hospitals now have effective and credible financial systems. But, not too many years ago, many hospitals did not have approved budgets, did not prepare prospective budgets, and did not have annual independent financial audits. What happened to cause the dramatic changes? In many cases, it was pressure from third parties and government. For instance, Medicare and Medicaid regulations had a tremendous effect on the hospital financial systems. Audits are now mandatory. The computer has also had its impact, with cost analysis and cost accounting now household words. Blue Cross and other third party intermediaries were also influential. An article entitled "Naturally" from the February 24, 1977, issue of *The Wall Street Journal* included the following paragraph:

> The most telling detail in President Carter's budget revisions is his plan for dealing with steadily increasing hospital costs. He proposes to solve the problem by outlawing it. No longer will hospital costs

> increase by 15% a year; by edict of the Department of Health, Education and Welfare, they shall not increase more than 9% a year. After noticing what natural gas controls have done for energy, and what New York City rent controls have done for housing, the President naturally wants to do the same thing for medical care.

However, it is important to note that hospitals have responded to regulations, pressures, and controls and have developed effective financial management and systems in the process.

In the area of materiel management, not nearly enough has happened. It is time that hospitals turn their managerial efforts in this direction because materiel management will continue to grow in importance over the next five to ten years. Even today, governmental agencies, third party payers, and consumer groups are getting involved in the ever-increasing spiral of the costs of materiel and purchased services. In the words of Dr. Dean Ammer, "Competent purchasing and inventory control can reduce aggregate hospital charges by at least $1,000,000,000 per year but improvement is not likely without active encouragement of 'third party' payers."[2] However, in the area of materiel management, there is time for hospitals to respond individually and collectively. Hospitals can develop this area more effectively and efficiently without outside influence, but they must begin soon. The task can start with the development of good materiel managers and continue with hospital administrators providing leadership and support for them to carry out their responsibilities.

Who Is This Materiel Manager?

It may be simpler to state who he is not. Certainly he is not just a purchaser of goods and services, a shuffler of paper, or an interviewer of salesmen. He is much more. In fact, purchasing will become one of his minor tasks. Webster defines "manage" as "to handle and control." Today's materiel manager manages people, systems, money, publics, property, negotiations, and materiel. He is a thinker, planner, controller, organizer, director, and coordinator. His rightful place is not just in a line responsibility, but also in a staff or advisory relationship within the hospital organization. He should make decisions that cross interdepartmental lines of authority to permeate the entire institution.

The number of personnel in the materiel management sector may vary from 25 to 100, depending on the delineated and delegated areas of responsi-

---

[2] Ammer, *Hospital Materials Management,* p. 1.

bility. There may be as many as six or more departments or divisions reporting to and being supervised by this manager. The monetary budget may range into the millions of dollars. The decisions of this manager are so far-reaching that they can improve or impair the quality of patient care.

Interestingly enough, it is not rare to see this department directed by an assistant or associate administrator. But while the education and background of materiel managers may be varied, the position and its scope should be responsible and responsive. In fact, the quality and direction of a hospital's materiel program directly depends on the effectiveness of its manager, who should be flexible, innovative, and self-educated to the totality of the hospital.

The Managerial Profile of the Materiel Manager

Aside from the materiel and supply functions that are naturally associated with the materiel manager, the administrative perspective of this position makes the manager more responsible and responsive, and hence more effective, than his tasks alone might indicate. It is important to stress at this point that the total materiel management program must be an administrative concept and objective fully recognized and approved by top management. However, accountability must be placed on the materiel manager for developing and selling the concepts to top management. If materiel management is to be effective and promising, the entire hospital must be aware and committed to its precepts.

This author is often asked, "Where does one begin with the development of a total materiel management program?" It is a must that a functional snapshot be taken of the current handling of materiel management in one's own hospital. In order to plan for the future, present conditions should be surveyed and listed in a responsibility inventory. This is very similar to a supplies inventory, but is a tally of talents and tasks. This inventory should be written and dated. The following parameters should be taken into consideration in the process:

a. Number of personnel in the department;
b. Number of departments or units reporting to the materiel manager;
c. Square footage comprising the total department;
d. Annual budget in dollars;
e. Complete physical count of all "official" inventories by department;
f. Complete physical count of all "unofficial" inventories by department;
g. Average number of purchase orders processed annually;
h. Total number of vendors by category of supplies;
i. Dollar volume of service contracts listed individually by department;
j. Number of hospital patient days per year;

k. Average daily census of the hospital;
l. Average length of stay;
m. Total dollars purchased annually;
n. Number and dollar volume of the patient charges from this area;
o. The ratio of employees to occupied beds;
p. Man-hours per dollar purchased; and
q. Materiel costs per patient day.

After the responsibility inventory has been taken, the materiel manager is in an excellent position to plot direction for the future. The inventory should contain complete information about the present, and should be updated every six months to determine progress and future direction. It is further suggested that the materiel manager share this inventory and his progress with his administrator at frequent intervals.

Next, the materiel manager should develop a departmental management profile which will provide written standards of management in the areas of planning, organizing, directing, controlling, and evaluating. These standards should be developed and catalogued into a large manual according to subject for ready and frequent reference. It should be reviewed and revised as necessary, but no less often than twice a year. The departmental management profile consists of the following management criteria or standards.

a. An Organizational Chart With Current Staffing Pattern.

   The organizational chart is a graphic presentation of the authority relationships and chain of command in the department. It should be dated and approved by the appropriate administrative representative. Accompanying it should be a listing of the positions and persons staffing the department on each shift.

b. Departmental Objectives.

   Another managerial function of increasing importance to the materiel manager is that of developing and executing departmental objectives. Objectives should be drawn up and administratively approved at least a month before the beginning of the time period in which they should be achieved. They should be written in concise and clear terms, with a completion date stated in the body of the objective. To be most effective, the materiel manager should limit his objectives to a number that can be effectively achieved within the time period (for example, reduce both official and unofficial inventory from $300,000 to $100,000 by December 31).

   Objectives should be categorized as short, intermediate, and long term. They also should be tied directly into the budgetary process because there will be monetary expenditures associated with the accomplishment of most objectives even though they may be cost-saving in the long run. After the objectives have been approved, the materiel manager should review these again with his staff and assign responsibility for their accomplishment within certain specified time intervals. Management by objective is not new and there is nothing magical about the process, but it can be a source of motivation, enthusiasm, participation, and fulfillment for the employees of this vital department.

c. Policies and Procedures.

How effective can the managerial style of the materiel manager be without carefully thought out policies and procedures? Generally speaking, policy broadly states intent and procedure spells out the details for execution. It is very important that the departmental policies and procedures are in harmony with the administrative policies and procedures.

d. Job Descriptions.

The materiel manager must develop and contantly update employee job descriptions. They must be meaningful both to the supervisor and to the subordinate, indicating for and to whom the person is responsible. Then the major tasks of the position should be delineated. There is a crucial requirement for careful and thoughtful elaboration of the duties and responsibilities of all of the positions of the department. Remember, if it isn't written, it isn't done!

e. Performance Evaluation.

The materiel manager is responsible for the evaluation of the performance of key supervisory personnel. Proper evaluation of manpower is imperative to proper performance of the department. The appraisal should include the employee's tasks, the efficiency rating, justification of the rating, and a work improvement plan. Every employee should be evaluated objectively on his/her anniversary date. This is where the managerial training and education of the materiel manager can produce dividends in the development, motivation, and enhanced productivity of the employees of the department.

f. Minutes of Departmental Conferences.

Good communication is a must. Therefore, the materiel manager should meet with all departmental personnel at least monthly. Minutes should be kept of these meetings; one copy should be sent to administration and another filed in the departmental management profile.

g. Continuing Education Programs.

Continuing education programs for departmental personnel should be carefully planned and budgeted by the materiel manager. These programs should be documented and filed in the departmental management profile.

h. Orientation Programs.
   All new employees are to be oriented to the hospital and the materiel management department. The orientation outlines should be filed in the departmental management profile.
i. Preventive Maintenance Documentation.
   For all major equipment, especially patient care equipment, the materiel manager must keep a record of all repairs and preventive maintenance.
j. Contracts and Agreements.
   Any departmental commitment must be recorded and filed in the departmental management profile.
k. Annual Operational Budget.
   Each departmental director is responsible for submitting an annual operational budget for review and approval. After the budget has been approved, it must be followed. The budget process is to be written and referenced in the departmental management profile. However, the materiel manager must budget for the materiel management department, and also act in an advisory capacity to the other department managers. His expertise in this area of forecasting needs can make or break the entire budgetary process.
l. Licenses and Certifications of Registration.
   All licenses and certifications pertaining to the operation of the department are to be filed in the departmental management profile.
m. Departmental Reports and Statistics.
   The materiel manager submits many reports to administration, all of which should be filed by month in the departmental management profile.
n. Patient Care Audit Programs (If Applicable).
   If the materiel manager has input into the patient audit process, it should be documented.
o. Internal and External Disaster Plans.
   The hospital fire and disaster plans should be on reference file in the department. Additionally, the materiel manager should have a departmental fire and disaster plan posted on the bulletin board and filed in the departmental management profile.
p. Inspection Reports.
   If the department undergoes a city, state, regional, or national inspection, the report should be filed in the departmental management profile.

q. Standards: Joint Commission on Accreditation of Hospitals, (J.C.A.H.).
   The J.C.A.H. standards and departmental replies to each standard should be on file in each departmental management profile.
r. Safety Plan.
   The hospital and departmental safety plan should be filed in the departmental management profile.
s. Departmental Informational Brochures.
   Brochures to explain the department's services should be developed and a copy of each filed in the departmental management profile.
t. Statement of Services Offered.
   There should be a brief statement of services available to each of the consumer departments. This statement of services should be made available to all supply consumers.

A proposed schedule for the completion of some of these tasks is offered in Figure 3-1.

The departmental management profile is very helpful in making the materiel manager successful and effective. To receive the most benefit from this monumental work, the materiel manager should see that it reflects departmental organizational changes. For example, if there is a change in one of the employee's tasks or functions, the job description should be immediately updated. To be most effective, the profile should be reviewed and the necessary updates made at least twice per year.

The most important characteristic of the materiel manager is that he must be a manager. His or her success will lie in getting things done by, with, and through other people. To do so, the materiel manager must be able to motivate, evaluate, delegate, initiate, investigate, and activate. The materiel manager of tomorrow must take his position alongside the other capable and respected managers who are responsible for manpower, money, and materiel. To do so, the materiel manager must maintain a perspective that includes the entire organization, be responsive to ever-changing organizational needs, be able to promote change through the hospital political process, and be a representative of management to and for the employees.

Pertinent Points to Ponder

1. If managerial expertise is the primary characteristic of the materiel manager, what are some others and how would you rate their significance?
2. How does the materiel manager differ from the personnel director or the financial director? In what ways are they similar?

Figure 3-1 Schedule of Tasks of the Materiel Manager

A TIMELY ADMINISTRATIVE REVIEW OF THE MATERIEL MANAGEMENT DEPARTMENT
YEAR _____

DATE SCHEDULED	*PROJECT*	*DATE COMPLETED*
JANUARY	[a] Annual Objectives	☐
JANUARY	[b] Review and Update of Director's Job Description	☐
JANUARY	[c] Review and Update of Table of Organization	☐
JANUARY & JULY	[d] Review and Update of the Departmental Management Profile	☐
EACH MONTH	[e] Minutes of Departmental Meetings	☐
EACH MONTH	[f] Monthly Departmental Reports	☐
EACH MONTH	[g] Monthly Budget Review	☐
JUNE	[h] Review and update of Accreditation Standards for the Department	☐
ANNIVERSARY DATE	[i] Director's Performance Evaluation	☐
AT LEAST THREE MONTHS PRIOR TO NEXT BUDGET YEAR	[j] Budget Preparation	☐

3. What factors are involved in the ever-spiraling costs of hospital supplies and equipment?
4. Can these costs be reduced or contained? If so, in what ways can they be controlled?
5. Are third parties becoming involved in materiel management? How?

6. In what ways can you convince the third parties (government, insurance companies, the public, etc.) that you and the hospital are doing a good job in managing materiel?
7. What is the main criterion that the third parties will use in determining a hospital's materiel effectiveness?
8. How will good management practices help to reduce costs?
9. There are usually committees of the board of trustees which monitor the areas of personnel and finance. What influence does the board exercise in the area of materiel management?
10. If you were a hospital administrator in search of a materiel manager, where would you recruit?
11. What makes a materiel manager a "good" one?
12. Does the materiel manager have a role in patient care audits? If so, how and why?

Chapter 4

Job Descriptions for Key Departmental Positions

Good job descriptions are a must for the materiel manager. Employees have a right to know for what, to whom, and for whom they are responsible. Yet some managers and institutions seem to want to keep this information secret for fear that such knowledge will cause disgruntlement. In the initial departmental orientation, the individual employee should be given a copy of the pertinent job description and asked to review it in detail before returning to the supervisor with any questions. All employees should know that their job descriptions are subject to regular, periodic reviews and will be updated to reflect the changing milieu.

The purpose of this chapter is to delineate key position documents that can be easily adapted by a hospital regardless of its size, location, philosophy toward materiel management, or management expertise. The individual hospital management can choose to consider those aspects which are considered to be characteristic of its materiel management philosophy and objectives. The following key positions will be described in detail:

a. Director of materiel management
b. Assistant director of materiel management or purchasing director
c. Chief pharmacist
d. Supply, process, and distribution supervisor
e. Exchange cart coordinator
f. Cart attendant
g. Receiving clerk
h. Processing supervisor

Position Description for the Materiel Manager*

Unfortunately, most hospitals have not yet delineated a position description for the materiel manager. Many have simply taken the description of the duties of director of purchasing and changed the name to materiel manager. This is an anathema to effective materiel management!

Position Title

Materiel manager or director of materiel management.

Position Purpose

To manage and control supplies and equipment from acquisition to disposition.

Responsible To

The chief executive officer or a member of top management.

Responsible For

The direction, supervision, evaluation, and overall management of the following positions:

a. Assistant director of materiel management
b. Purchasing agent
c. Chief pharmacist
d. Central sterile supply supervisor or supply, process, and distribution manager
e. Supervisor of central stores

The effective position description should include a well defined organizational chart delineating both inter- and intradepartmental lines of authority.

Degree of Supervision

Supervision by top management will vary according to the degree of development and advancement of the concept of total materiel management in each hospital. In the early stages of development, administrative supervision should be direct, consistent, and frequent. This is to assure that the administrative philosophies, concepts, and objectives are being executed according to the plan devised by administration and materiel management.

In the advanced stages of development, administrative direction can be remote and would approximate that given to any other middle manager, such as director of laboratories, in the institution. Supervision at this stage

* Reprinted with the permission of DIMENSIONS in Health Service, Journal of the Canadian Hospital Association.

is usually through regularly scheduled conferences with top management and well-organized monthly reports.

Areas of Emphasis

a. Writing and adhering to product and equipment specifications;
b. Supervising the procurement of all supplies, services, and equipment through a centralized purchasing process;
c. Receiving and accounting for receipt of all supplies;
d. Stocking supplies for adequate periods of time only;
e. Studying and reviewing utilization of materiel within the institution;
f. Developing and adhering to effective policies and procedures for the management of supplies and materiel;
g. Standardizing and evaluating all products, equipment, and services;
h. Processing and reprocessing reusable supplies and equipment;
i. Distributing all goods and services;
j. Controlling "official" and "unofficial" inventories;
k. Accounting for equipment (more commonly called property or assets management);
l. Reviewing and servicing patient care equipment;
m. Controlling printing and all printed matter, including xerography;
n. Reviewing and evaluating patient charges; and
o. Disposing of waste products of the goods and services purchased efficiently and effectively.

Committee Representation

The materiel manager or his/her delegate should be a member of at least the following hospital committees:

a. Standardization
b. Pharmacy and Therapeutics
c. Patient Care Audit
d. Cost Containment
e. Patient Charge Review

Other optional committees are:

a. Group Purchasing if applicable
b. Shared Services
c. Budget
d. Infection

Experience

The candidate for the position of director of materiel management should have considerable familiarity (3 to 5 years) with the supply, process, and distribution phases of materiel management in the hospital or industrial setting. Furthermore, the candidate must be able to enumerate demonstrable results in his/her last position such as reduction of inventory, unification of supply, process, and distribution functions, and centralization of all purchasing.

Educational Requirements

The candidate should have an acceptable baccalaureate degree or an experiential equivalency.

A masters degree in hospital administration, business administration, industrial engineering, pharmacy, or any other appropriately related field is desirable.

Job Knowledge

The candidate should have a working knowledge of at least the following areas:

a. Logistics
b. Business management
c. Business ethics
d. Management principles
e. Business math
f. Basic personnel administration

Skills

The candidate must possess the following:

a. Fundamental management skills of planning, organizing, directing, controlling, and staffing.
b. The ability to get things performed through, with, and by people.
c. Good communication skills.
d. Effective negotiation skills.
e. Analytical ability.

Major Tasks and Scope of Responsibility

a. Supervises, assigns, and directs the activities of all personnel performing materiel functions.
b. Evaluates, at least annually, the performance of the key supervisory personnel of the Department of Materiel Management (i.e., purchasing agent, chief pharmacist, CSR supervisor, central stores supervisor, etc.).
c. Negotiates prime supplier contracts with major suppliers and distributors.

d. Sets the appropriate and necessary fiduciary, ethical, and professional tone of the materiel management effort both intra- and interdepartmentally.
e. Establishes and maintains a good professional rapport with the medical staff, administration, nurses, staff for patient care areas, and members of all other hospital departments.
f. Confers regularly on at least a monthly basis with all personnel of the department in a group session to discuss plans, objectives, problems, etc., and records minutes of such meetings.
g. Establishes departmental policies and procedures in accordance with hospital policies.
h. Reviews and makes appropriate recommendations in reference to all new supplies and equipment for the department and the entire hospital.
i. Updates on a regular basis all departmental managerial tools such as organizational charts, policies, procedures, job descriptions, and departmental orientation plans.
j. Assumes responsibility for the annual departmental budget preparation and assures adherence on a monthly basis.
k. Confers at least bimonthly on a regular basis with the administration to coordinate the hospital materiel management efforts with the objectives and plans of top management.
l. Establishes, in conjunction with administration, realistic, obtainable goals for the department on an annual basis.
m. Relates directly and through the proper committees with the medical staff concerning all aspects of supply, equipment, and property management.
n. Develops, schedules, conducts, and documents inservice and continuing education programs for personnel of the department.
o. Takes responsibility for controlling, counting, and reporting of all hospital supply inventories on a regular basis.
p. Establishes and maintains the proper and appropriate professional and ethical relationships with all sales representatives.
q. Conducts the business affairs of the department according to the principles and guidelines of the prudent buyer philosophy.
r. Meets or exceeds standards of compliance of all the accreditation and regulatory bodies and commissions, in relationship to supply management.
s. Supports and participates in group purchasing and shared services efforts with other hospitals and related health facilities.
t. Submits monthly reports to top management concerning the functional and administrative phases of the department.
u. Performs the appropriate committee functions as assigned.

v. Performs other related tasks as may be deemed necessary for the effective and efficient function of the Department of Materiel Management.

Evaluation

Every manager should be evaluated on a regularly scheduled basis. It is suggested that the new materiel manager be evaluated after 90 days on the job and then at least annually thereafter. The materiel manager should be evaluated by top management and reviewed on the basis of two criteria:

a. How well is he/she performing the major tasks?
b. Are the objectives of the position being met?

Authority Relationships

An up-to-date organizational chart should be attached to each job description to indicate authority and reporting relationships (Figure 4–1).

Salary

Commensurate with education, training, and assigned responsibilities.

Position Description for Assistant Director of Materiel Management or Director of Purchased Services

Position Title

Assistant director of materiel management.

Position Purpose

To provide managerial continuity to the Department of Materiel Management in certain specified areas and to act for the director in his absence.

Responsible To

The director of materiel management.

Responsible For

The direction, supervision, evaluation, and overall management of the following positions:

a. Supervisor of supply, process, and distribution
b. Receiving clerk

(See Figure 4-1 for lines of authority and reporting relationships.)

Figure 4-1 Key Supervisory Responsibilities of the Material Management Chain of Command

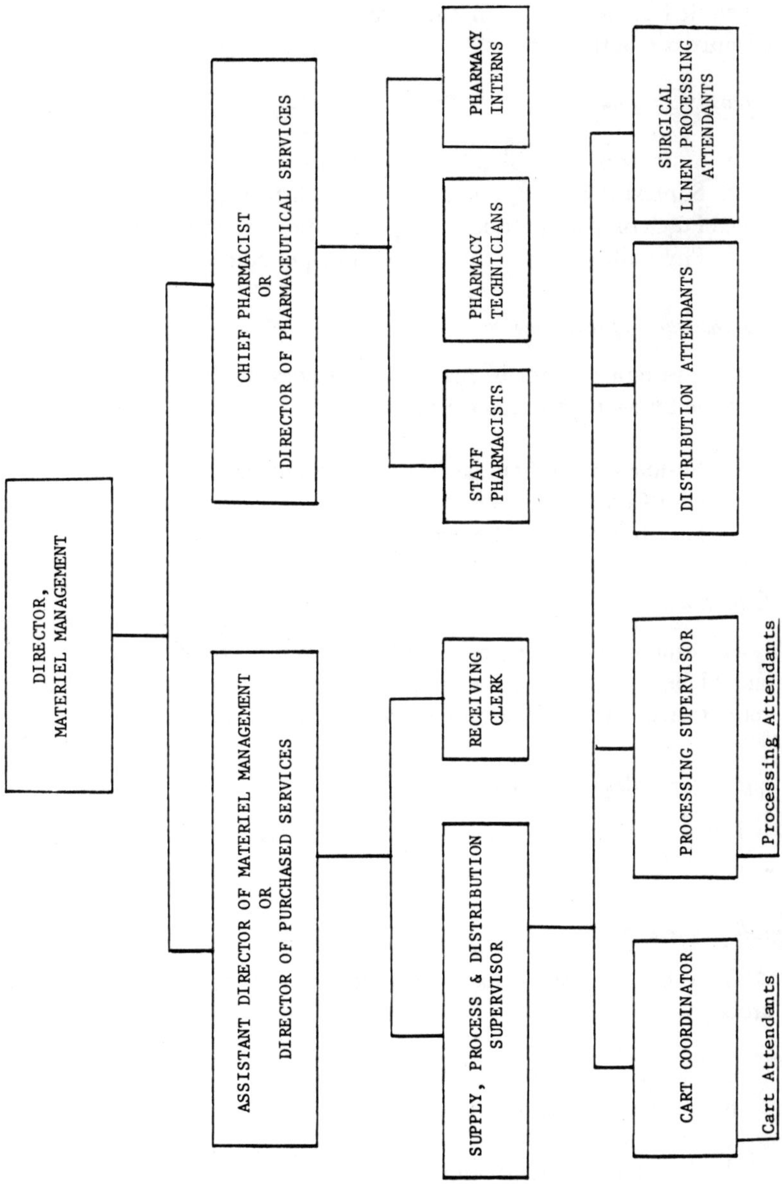

Degree of Supervision

Supervision will be rather remote and will occur through periodic, regularly scheduled conferences with the director of materiel management and well-organized monthly reports.

Areas of Emphasis

a. Writing of and adhering to product specifications;
b. Supervising all supply, process, and distribution areas;
c. Purchasing all products, drugs, equipment, and services;
d. Physically counting inventories on a periodic and regular basis.

Committee Representation

The assistant director of materiel management should be a member of at least the following hospital committees:

a. Evaluation and Standardization of Products
b. Cost Containment Review
c. Group Purchasing Committee

Experience

The candidate for the position of assistant director of materiel management should be familiar with the supply, process, and distribution phases of materiel management, either in a hospital or industrial setting.

Educational Requirements

The candidate should have a baccalaureate degree or an experiential equivalency.

Job Knowledge

The candidate should have a working knowledge of at least the following areas:

a. Purchasing administration and techniques
b. Business management
c. Business ethics
d. Fundamental management principles
e. Business math
f. Basic personnel administration

Skills:

The candidate must possess the following:

a. Fundamental management skills of planning, organizing, directing, controlling, and staffing;
b. Ability to get things performed through, with, and by people;
c. Good communication skills;
d. Effective negotiation skills; and
e. Analytical ability.

Major Tasks and Scope of Responsibility

a. Supervises the supply, process, and distribution functions;
b. Conducts daily purchasing rounds of the nursing units to check with head nurses regarding concerns involving the cart and supply systems;
c. Reviews daily special requisitions with appropriate management representative;
d. Prepares, researches, and coordinates all functions involving the Evaluation and Standardization of Products Committee;
e. Performs all purchasing for the hospital;
f. Assumes responsibility for the quarterly physical inventories of all official and unofficial supply areas;
g. Interviews sales representatives and keeps current on supply publications and price changes;
h. Evaluates annually the supply, process, and distribution supervisor and the receiving clerk;
i. Negotiates prime supplier contracts with major suppliers and distributors;
j. Establishes and maintains a good professional rapport with the medical staff, administration, nurses, employees of patient care areas, and staff of all other hospital departments;
k. Establishes departmental policies and procedures in accordance with hospital policies;
l. Assists the director in the annual departmental budget preparation and assures adherence on a monthly basis;
m. Establishes in conjunction with the director realistic and obtainable goals for the division on an annual basis;
n. Establishes and maintains the proper and appropriate professional and ethical relationships with all sales representatives;
o. Conducts the business affairs of the division according to the principles and guidelines of the prudent buyer philosophy;

p. Supports and participates in group purchasing and shared services efforts with other hospitals and related health facilities;
q. Submits monthly reports to the director of materiel management concerning the functional, budgetary, and administrative phases of the department;
r. Performs the appropriate committee functions as assigned;
s. Develops and distributes information on supplies, drugs, and equipment to all members of the medical staff and all other related hospital personnel;
t. Evaluates the effectiveness of services available to the various supply consumers from materiel management.
u. Performs other related tasks as may be deemed necessary for the effective and efficient function of the department.

Evaluation

The assistant director of materiel management will be evaluated after 90 days on the job and then at least annually thereafter by the materiel manager on the basis of two criteria:

a. How well is he/she performing the major tasks?
b. Are the objectives of the position being met?

Authority Relationships

An up-to-date organizational chart should be attached to each job description to indicate authority and reporting relationships (Figure 4-1).

Salary

Commensurate with education, training, and assigned responsibilities.

Position Description for the Chief Pharmacist

Position title

Chief pharmacist or director of pharmaceutical services.

Position Purpose

To provide professional and managerial supervision and direction to the division of pharmaceutical services.

Responsible To

The director of materiel management.

Responsible For

The direction, supervision, evaluation, and overall management of the following positions:

a. Staff pharmacists
b. Pharmacy technicians
c. Pharmacy interns

Degree of Supervision

Supervision will be somewhat remote and will occur through periodic regularly scheduled conferences with the director of materiel management and monthly reports.

Areas of Emphasis

a. Unit dose systems
b. Intravenous admixture programs
c. Radio-pharmaceuticals
d. Narcotics and controlled substances
e. Outpatient pharmacy
f. Pharmacy management
g. Clinical pharmacy
h. Patient drug profiles
i. Drug informational systems

Committee Representation

The chief pharmacist should be a member of at least the following committees:

a. Pharmacy and Therapeutics
b. Evaluation and Standardization of Products
c. Cost Containment
d. Patient Care Audit
e. Infection
f. Accreditation Review

Experience

The candidate for the position of chief pharmacist should have considerable familiarity (3 to 5 years) with pharmaceutical services in the hospital or retail setting. Furthermore, the candidate should have at least two years of supervisory or management experience.

Educational Requirements

The candidate should have at least a B.S. in pharmacy. A masters degree in pharmacy with a hospital residency is desirable.

Job Knowledge

The candidate should have a working knowledge in at least the following areas:

a. Hospital pharmacy administration
b. Basic personnel administration
c. Business ethics
d. Fundamental management principles

Skills

The candidate should possess the following:

a. Fundamental management skills of planning, organizing, directing, controlling, and staffing;
b. The ability to get things performed through, with, and by people; and
c. Good communication skills.

Major Tasks and Scope of Responsibility

a. Sets the ethical and professional tone of the pharmacy;
b. Supervises, assigns, and directs the activities of personnel performing pharmaceutical services;
c. Evaluates the performance, at least annually, of the key personnel reporting directly to him or her;
d. Develops specifications to be used by the purchasing agent in negotiating the purchase of drugs;
e. Establishes and maintains a good professional rapport with the medical staff, nurses, and staff of all other patient care departments;
f. Confers regularly on at least a monthly basis with all personnel in the division of pharmacy to discuss plans, objectives, problems, etc., and records minutes of such meetings;
g. Updates on a regular basis all managerial tools such as organizational charts, policies, procedures, job descriptions, and orientation plans;
h. Prepares the annual pharmaceutical services budget and assures adherence to it on a monthly basis;
i. Confers at least bimonthly on a regular basis with the administration and other key members of materiel management to coordinate hospital

materiel management efforts with the objectives and plans of top management;

j. Establishes realistic, obtainable goals for the department on an annual basis;
k. Relates directly and through the proper committees with the medical staff concerning all aspects of the delivery of pharmaceutical services;
l. Develops, schedules, conducts, and documents inservice and continuing education programs for the personnel in the pharmacy;
m. Establishes and maintains the proper and appropriate professional and ethical relationships with all pharmaceutical representatives;
n. Cooperates and complies with the policies of centralized purchasing for all pharmaceutical purchases;
o. Meets or exceeds standards of compliance of all the accreditation and regulatory bodies and commissions in relationship to the pharmacy;
p. Submits monthly reports to the director of materiel management concerning the functional, budgetary, and administrative phases of the pharmacy;
q. Performs the appropriate committee functions as assigned;
r. Makes pharmaceutical rounds of all nursing units at least three times per week;
s. Serves as a source of drug information to the medical staff, nursing staff, and all others, including the various student disciplines;
t. Serves as a preceptor for programs with pharmacy internships and residencies; and
u. Performs other related tasks as deemed necessary for the effective and efficient functioning of the Department of Materiel Management.

Evaluation

It is suggested that the new chief pharmacist be evaluated after 90 days in the position and then at least annually thereafter by the materiel manager on the basis of two criteria:

a. How well is he/she performing the major tasks?
b. Are the objectives of the position being met?

Authority Relationships

An up-to-date organizational chart should be attached to each job description to indicate authority and reporting relationships. In this case, the chief pharmacist reports directly to the materiel manager (Figure 4-1).

Salary

Commensurate with education, training, and assigned responsibilities.

Position Description for the Supply, Process, and Distribution Supervisor

Position Title

Supply, process, and distribution (S.P.D.) supervisor.

Position Purpose

To provide supervision and direction to the supply, process, and distribution functions.

Responsible To

The assistant director of materiel management.

Responsible For

The direction, evaluation, and overall supervision of the following positions:

a. Cart coordinator
b. Process supervisor
c. Stock clerks
d. Surgical linen attendants
e. Printer

Degree of Supervision

Supervision should be rather frequent and direct on a regular basis. Several key reports will be generated from this position.

Areas of Emphasis

a. Supply, process, and distribution
b. Exchange cart replenishment
c. Cart and supply distribution
d. Supply processing
e. Linen processing
f. Copy center

Committee Representation

The supply, process, and distribution supervisor should be a member of at least the following hospital committees:

a. Evaluation and Standardization of Products
b. Other appropriate committees as deemed necessary

Experience

The candidate for this position should be familiar with the supply, process, and distribution functions of hospital materiel management.

Educational Requirements

The candidate should possess at least a high school education.

Job Knowledge

The candidate should have a working knowledge of at least the following areas:

a. Supply management
b. Inventory techniques
c. Basic math
d. Distribution patterns
e. Distribution equipment and systems
f. Nursing unit supply needs

Skills

The candidate must possess the following:

a. Fundamental management skills of planning, organizing, directing, controlling, and staffing;
b. Ability to get things performed through, with, and by people;
c. Good communication skills; and
d. Basics of supervision.

Major Tasks and Scope of Responsibility

a. Supervises the S.P.D. center, exchange cart replenishment, exchange cart distribution, supply and linen processing, supply distribution, printing and copy center;
b. Reviews and evaluates the:

    - Cart coordinator
    - Process supervisor
    - Stock clerks
    - Surgical linen attendants
    - Printer;

c. Reviews and updates cart quotas with the appropriate nursing personnel on each unit at least quarterly;
d. Establishes maximum and minimum volumes for all central stores supplies;
e. Assumes responsibility for the esthetics and cleanliness of the central stores (S.P.D. center);
f. Conducts tours of the S.P.D. center for visitors and staff;
g. Provides emergency backup for all positions in the S.P.D. area;
h. Assigns supply costs to the applicable departments and units as the supplies are issued;
i. Develops a credible perpetual inventory system in conjunction with data processing and accounting;
j. Verifies annual inventory volumes;
k. Prepares an annual budget and adheres to it on a monthly basis;
l. Assumes responsibility for all patient charges on a daily basis; and
m. Performs other duties as may be assigned by the assistant director of materiel management.

Evaluation

The S.P.D. supervisor should be evaluated by the assistant director of materiel management (or purchasing director) after 90 days in the position and then at least annually thereafter on the basis of two criteria:

a. How well is he/she performing the major tasks?
b. Are the objectives of the position being met?

Authority Relationships

An up-to-date organizational chart should be attached to each job description to indicate authority and reporting relationships (Figure 4-1).

Salary

Commensurate with education, training, and assigned responsibilities. Salary should be somewhere midrange of other hospital first line supervisory levels.

Position Description for the Exchange Cart Coordinator

Position Title

Exchange cart coordinator.

Position Purpose

To assure that all supply exchange carts measure up to the established quotas both qualitatively and quantitatively. Also, to see that all patient supply charges are accounted for in the shortest time period possible.

Responsible To

The S.P.D. supervisor.

Responsible For

The direction, evaluation, and general overall supervision of the cart attendants.

Degree of Supervision

Supervision is frequent and direct on a regular basis. This person will be responsible for providing the lost charge report on a monthly basis.

Areas of Emphasis

a. Cart supply quotas
b. Patient supply charges
c. Cart distribution
d. Quality and quantity checks of the carts
e. Lost charges

Committee Representation

This position has no specific committee involvement; however, the person could serve on various hospital committees as deemed appropriate.

Experience

Central supply or central stores experience would be helpful.

Educational Requirements

Entry level education is sufficient.

Job Knowledge

The candidate should have a working knowledge of at least the following areas:

a. Central stores
b. Patient charge processing
c. Basic math
d. Distribution patterns

Skills

The candidate should possess good communication skills and the fundamentals of supervision.

Major Tasks and Scope of Responsibility

a. Supervises supply cart attendants;
b. Evaluates all supply cart attendants on their anniversary dates;
c. Assists in taking annual physical inventories;
d. Tracks down all lost supply charges;
e. Completes the monthly lost charge report;
f. Supervises replenishment of the supply carts in the following manner:
    1. Separates and arranges tab card charge cards from the previous day's charge tray by appropriate category for each item.
    2. Receives cart paperwork from the cart attendant for the current day.
    3. Computes shortage from each unit by comparing the difference column and number of charge slips received from each individual unit and enters this figure in the "S" column (Figures 4-2, 4-3, 4-4).
    4. Attempts immediately to track down any shortage by phone or by a visit to the unit.
    5. Completes summary report for both charge and noncharge items using all the paper flow from the replenished carts. Takes completed daily summary reports to the S.P.D. supervisor.
    6. Completes daily total on the monthly shortage report. At end of month, computes the grand total for each floor and sends one copy of the report to the materiel manager and the other to administration.
    7. Takes daily accumulation of tab cards to data processing as soon as possible.
    8. Performs a final check of all carts for completeness and quality and sees that necessary changes are made.
    9. Keeps all forms current, making necessary changes when needed.
    10. Orients the ward clerks and unit personnel as needed to facilitate the charging function and supply flow.
g. Performs other duties as may be assigned from time to time by the S.P.D. supervisor.

Evaluation

The Exchange Cart Coordinator should be evaluated by the S.P.D. supervisor after 90 days in the position and then at least annually thereafter.

Figure 4-2 Sample Cart Quota Profile for the Orthopedic Unit

COLUMN LEGEND:
Q—Quota
I—Inventory
Is—Issued
R—Requisitions
S—Shortage

St. Anthony Hospital **MOBILE CART EXCH. - CART QUOTA PROFILE**

NORTH 5 - 635.31

ITEM	UNIT	CAT. NO.	Q	I	Is	R	S
BASINS-EMESIS-DISP.	EA/1	00126482	6				
BASIN-WASH-PLASTIC	EA/1	00130609	6				
URINAL DISP.	EA/1	00976480	6				
BED PAN W/COVER	EA/1	00141440	3				
PADS-SANITARY-NON-STERILE	PK/12	11530102	3				
BELT-SANITARY	EA/1	00168641	3				
URIMETER	EA/1	00966960	1				
UNDERPADS 23 x 36	EA/1	00964684	6				
KIDNEY STONE FILTERS	EA/1	00487017	2				
TRAY-IRRIGATION	EA/1	17426099	3				
TRAY BLADDER CARE-W/O CATH	EA/1	17186404	1				
TRAY CATH-15 FR. RED-RUB	EA/1	17186628	2				
TRAY CATH-16 FR. FOLEY	EA/1	17186529	3				
COLLECTOR URINE MID-STREAM	EA/1	00295980	1				
ENEMA ADMIN. SET	EA/1	00414805	6				
SPECI-CONTAINER (TOILET TYPE)	EA/1	00312256	3				
BAG DRAINAGE CLOSED SYSTEM	EA/1	00046144	3				
TRAY-PREP SET	EA/1	17599853	4				
TRAY-TRACHE-OSTOMY CARE	EA/1	17866450	1				
INTRACATH 8"	EA/1	10133809	1				
INTRACATH 12"	EA/1	10133908	1				
INTRACATH 24"	EA/1	10134104	1				
TRAY IRRIGATING VAG	EA/1	17520883					
TRAY LUMBAR PUNCTURE	EA/1	17559865	1				
AIRWAY-CHILD	EA/1	00005447					
AIRWAY-MED. ADULT	EA/1	00006809					
AIRWAY-LGE. ADULT	EA/1	00008169					
STOCKINGS ANTI-EMB. SM. NYLON	PR/1	11874203					
STOCKINGS ANTI-EMB. MED. NYLON	PR/1	11877305	1				
STOCKINGS ANTI-EMB. LGE. NYLON	PR/1	11880408	1				
BALLS COTTON MED.	CS/4000	11018603					
APPL. COTTON TIP 6 STERILE	CS/1000	00021873					
BINDER SURGICAL	EA/1	00173849					
COLOPLAST BAG #2	PK/10	00304632	1				
COLOPLAST BAG #3	PK/10	00306001	1				
SLIPPERS-PILLOW PAWS MED.	PR/1	00758888	3				
SLIPPERS-PILLOW PAWS LGE.	PR/1	00760249	3				
LOTION-DER-MASSAGE 8 OZ.	BOT/1	00648725	6				
POWDER 4 OZ.	CAN	00716720	6				
CEPACOL 5 OZ.	BOT/1	00269282	6				
BLADES-KNIFE #10	BX/50	00190405					
BLADES-KNIFE #11	BX/50	00191767					
BLADES-KNIFE #12	BX/50	00191783					
BLADES-KNIFE #15	BX/50	00193128					
BLADES-KNIFE #20	BX/50	00194480					
TUBE SALEM SUMP 16 FR.	EA/1	18616961	2				
TUBE SALEM SUMP 18 FR.	EA/1	18617019					
BANDS-I.D. ADULT	BX/250	00114249					
BANDAGES-ELASTIC 2"	ROLL/1	11282100					
BANDAGES-ELASTIC 3"	ROLL/1	11285202	2				
BANDAGES-ELASTIC 4"	ROLL/1	11288305	2				
BANDAGES-ELASTIC 6"	ROLL/1	11294501	2				
DRAPE-BANDAID 24 x 30	BX/10	11381308					
DRESSING 3 x 3 STERILE ADAPTIC	BX/50	11421609					
DRESSING 3 x 8 STERILE ADAPTIC	BX/36	11424702					
EYE PADS-OVAL	BX/50	11440203					
GAUZE 1/4" IODOFORM PACKING	BOT/1	11458809					
GAUZE 1/2" IODOFORM PACKING	BOT/1	11461902					
GAUZE 1" IODOFORM PACKING	BOT/1	11465002					
GAUZE 2" IODOFORM PACKING	BOT/1	11468105					

ITEM	UNIT	CAT. NO.	Q	I	Is	R	S
GAUZE 1/4" PLAIN PACKING	BOT/1	11471208					
GAUZE 1/2" PLAIN PACKING	BOT/1	11474301					
GAUZE 1" PLAIN PACKING	BOT/1	11477403					
GAUZE 2" PLAIN PACKING	BOT/1	11480506					
TRAY SUTURE REMOVAL-DISP.	EA/1	17826462					
THERMOMETER-KIT ORAL	EA/1	00921262					
THERMOMETER-KIT RECTAL	EA/1	00930883					
FULLER-SHIELDS	EA/1	00504563	3				
MASK FILTER BARD.	BX/50	00652800					
ASEPTEX SURG. MASK 1800	BX/50	00663682					
MASK SURG. FILTRON DISP.	BX/50	00666602					
TISSUE KLEENEX	BX/150	00939769	3				
BANDAGE 2" SELF-ADHERING	PK/12	11310000					
BANDAGE 3" SELF-ADHERING	EA/1	11313103	2				
BANDAGE 4" SELF-ADHERING	PK/12	11316205					
BANDAGE 6" SELF-ADHERING	EA/1	11319308	2				
GAUZE VASELINE 3 x 9	EA/1	11499308	2				
GAUZE VASELINE 3 x 18	BX/12	11499126					
GAUZE VASELINE 3 x 36	BX/12	11502200					
BRUSH-SURG. PREP SPONGE-HEX.	BX/36	00224402					
BRUSH-SURGEON	BX/30	00229864					
CAP SURGEON DISP.	BX/100	00253104					
STRAP MONTGOMERY 8½ x 11	EA/1	11892809	1				
PADS-COMBINE DR. 5 x 9 STERILE	BX/25	11520806					
SPONGES-COTTON FILLED 4 x 3 STER.	TR/25	11725405					
SUSPENSORY, MED.	EA/1	00874487					
SUSPENSORY, LGE.	EA/1	00876219					
SUSPENSORY, X-LGE.	EA/1	00877209					
DEODORANT ASEPTICARE 12 OZ.	CAN/1	31104698	1				
CATH MED. 14-16 FR.	EA/1	10874162					
ROUTINE SUCTION KIT	EA/1	17199985	3				
FOLEY-CATH 14FR. 2 WAY 5cc	EA/1	10374882					
FOLEY-CATH 16 FR. 2 WAY 5cc	EA/1	10374932					
FOLEY-CATH 18 FR. 2 WAY 5cc	EA/1	10374981	2				
FOLEY-CATH 20 FR. 2 WAY 5cc	EA/1	10375046					
FOLEY-CATH 22 FR. 2 WAY 5cc	EA/1	10375095					
FOLEY-CATH 24 FR. 2 WAY 5cc	EA/1	10375137					
FOLEY-CATH 20 FR. 2 WAY 30cc	EA/1	10420255					
FOLEY-CATH 22 FR. 2 WAY 30cc	EA/1	10420313					
FOLEY-CATH 24 FR. 2 WAY 30cc	EA/1	10420370					
FOLEY-CATH 24 FR. 3 WAY 30cc	EA/1	10446003					
FOLEY-CATH 26 FR. 3 WAY 30cc	EA/1	10450468					
NEEDLE-CATH. 1963T	EA/1	10080281	1				
NEEDLE-CATH. 1964T	EA/1	10084747	5				
CATH-AROUND THE NEEDLE 1972T	EA/1	10088649	3				
TUBING-PENROSE STERILE 5/8" x 12"	EA/1	18258863					
TUBING-PENROSE STERILE 1/4" x 12"	EA/1	18264887					
TUBING-PENROSE STERILE 1"	EA/1	18307108					
TUBING-PENROSE STERILE 3/8" x 12"	EA/1	18331108					
TUBING-PENROSE STERILE 1/2" x 12"	EA/1	18361204					
CONNECTORS 5 in 1	EA/1	00311449					
INTER INFUSION SET 19-GA.	EA/1	14122451	2				
INTER INFUSION SET-21 GA.	EA/1	14175004	2				
D 5 W 150 cc	EA/1	14251300	2				
D 5 W 250 cc	EA/1	14251359					
D 5 W 500 cc	EA/1	14251409	2				
D 5 W 1000 cc	EA/1	14251458	4				
10% DEX INJ 1000ML.	EA/1	14252456					
5% DEX + 0.9% SOD. CHL 250 ML.	EA/1	14256051	2				
5% DEX + 0.9% SOD.CHL 500 ML.	EA/1	14256101	2				

ITEM	UNIT	CAT. NO.	Q	I	Is	R	S
5% DEX + 0.9% SOD. CHL 1000 ML.	EA/1	14256150	4				
5% DEX + 0.45% SOD. CHL 1000 ML.	EA/1	14257604	4				
5% DEX + 0.2% SOD. CHL 1000 ML.	EA/1	14260350	4				
0.45% SOD. CHL IN WATER 1000 ML.	EA/1	14262174					
0.9% SOD. CHLO INJECT 50 ML.	EA/1	14262208					
SOD. CHL INJECTION 0.9% 150 ML.	EA/1	14263800	2				
SOD. CHL INJECTION 0.9% 250 ML.	EA/1	14263859					
SOC. CHL INJECTION 0.9% 500 ML.	EA/1	14263909	2				
SOD. CHL INJECTION 0.9% 1000 ML.	EA/1	14263958	2				
SOD. LACTATE INJ 500 ML. 1/6 MOLAR	EA/1	14264121					
5% DEX + LAC. RINGERS 500 ML.	EA/1	14265201					
5% DEX + LAC. RINGERS 1000 ML.	EA/1	14265250	6				
LAC. RINGERS INJ 500 ML.	EA/1	14292700					
LAC. RINGERS INJ. 1000 ML.	EA/1	14292759	2				
5% AMIGEN 1000 cc INJECTION	EA/1	14300040					
5% AMIGEN, 5% DEX 1000 cc	EA/1	14300875					
5% DEX ADMIXTURE 50 ML.	EA/1	14301857					
GENT.6%-75+0.9% SOD. CHL. 500 ML.	EA/1	14302202					
STERILE WATER FOR INJ. 1000 ML.	EA/1	14303556					
5% DEX. IN WATER 5% ALCOH. 1000 ML.	EA/1	14304091					
5% SOD. BICARB. IN WATER 500 ML.	EA/1	14309983					
PLASMA-LYTE 148 IN WATER 1000 ML.	EA/1	14311179					
PLASMA-LYTE 56 IN 5% DEX. 1000 ML.	EA/1	14313159	4				
ELECTROLYTE NO.1 1000 ML.	EA/1	14319404					
ELECTROLYTE NO. 2 1000 ML.	EA/1	14319636					
GENTRAN 10%-40 IN 0.9% SOD-C 500 ML.	EA/1	14320857					
GENTRAN 10%-40 IN 5% DEX. 500 ML.	EA/1	14320964					
DIANEAL WITH 1.5% DEX 1000 ML.	EA/1	14321145					
DIANEAL WITH 1.5% DEX 2000 ML.	EA/1	14321236					
STERILE WATER FOR IRRIG. 500 ML.	EA/1	14326185					
0.9% SOD. CHL. IRRIG 1000 ML.	EA/1	14329353	3				
0.9% SOD. CHL. IRRIG 1500 ML.	EA/1	14329957					
EVACUATED 500 ML. CONTAINER	EA/1	14334007					
EVACUATED 1000 ML. CONTAINER	EA/1	14334148					
0.9% SOD. CHL. IRRIG 3000 ML.	EA/1	14400428					
VENOUS PRESSURE SET	EA/1	14463335					
Y-Type Blood-Sol. ADM SET & PRES-PUMP	EA/1	14465280	2				
CYSTO INTERMITTENT IRRIGATION SET	EA/1	14489306					
Y-Type Cont. BLADDER IRRIG. c̄ DRIP CHAMB.	EA/1	14489355					
ADMIN. SET c̄ AIRWAY CONNECTOR	EA/1	14489405					
ADMIN. SET TWO MEDICATION SITES	EA/1	14500029	8				
MINI-DRIP ADM. SET Y MEDICATION SITE	EA/1	14500037	3				
EXTENSION SET TWO MEDICATION SITES	EA/1	14500045	4				
HYPODERMOCLYSIS SET	EA/1	14500052	1				
CONTINU-FLO ADMIN. SET	EA/1	14500060	4				
ADD-A-LINE MEDICATION SET	EA/1	14500078	4				
BLOOD COLLECTION SET	EA/1	14500086					
FILTER CONNECTOR	EA/1	14500094					
HYPERELIMENTATION KIT	EA/1	14570113					
SMALL VEIN SET 19 x ¾	EA/1	14605455	6				
SMALL VEIN SET 21 x ¾	EA/1	14605521					
SMALL VEIN SET 21 x 1	EA/1	14605711	6				
SMALL VEIN SET 23 x ¾	EA/1	14605828					
FEMALE CATH. KIT	EA/1	17001009					
ANGIOCATH 20 x 1¼	EA/1	10116051	3				
HEMO-VAC #1500	EA/1	00533125					
HEMO-VAC #1530	EA/1	00533653					
FILLED BY:		DATE:					

Figure 4-3 Sample Cart Quota Profile for the Medical Unit

COLUMN LEGEND:
Q—Quota
I—Inventory
Is—Issued
R—Requisitions
S—Shortage

St. Anthony Hospital **MOBILE CART EXCH. - CART QUOTA PROFILE**

WEST 3 - 645.31

ITEM	UNIT	CAT. NO.	Q	I	Is	R	S
BASINS-EMESIS-DISP.	EA/1	00126482	5				
BASIN-WASH-PLASTIC	EA/1	00130609	5				
URINAL DISP.	EA/1	00976480	5				
BED PAN W/COVER	EA/1	00141440	5				
PADS-SANITARY-NON-STERILE	PK/12	11530102	2				
BELT-SANITARY	EA/1	00168641	2				
URIMETER	EA/1	00966960					
UNDERPADS 23 x 36	EA/1	00964684	2				
KIDNEY STONE FILTERS	EA/1	00487017	2				
TRAY-IRRIGATION	EA/1	17426099	3				
TRAY BLADDER CARE-W/O CATH	EA/1	17186404	1				
TRAY CATH-15 FR RED-RUB	EA/1	17186628	2				
TRAY CATH-16 FR FOLEY	EA/1	17186529	2				
COLLECTOR URINE MID-STREAM	EA/1	00295980	2				
ENEMA ADMIN. SET	EA/1	00414805	3				
SPECI-CONTAINER (TOILET TYPE)	EA/1	00312256	3				
BAG DRAINAGE CLOSED SYSTEM	EA/1	00046144					
TRAY-PREP SET	EA/1	17599853					
TRAY-TRACHE-OSTOMY CARE	EA/1	17866450	1				
INTRACATH 8"	EA/1	10133809					
INTRACATH 12"	EA/1	10133908					
INTRACATH 24"	EA/1	10134104					
TRAY IRRIGATING VAG	EA/1	17520883					
TRAY LUMBAR PUNCTURE	EA/1	17559865					
AIRWAY-CHILD	EA/1	00005447					
AIRWAY-MED. ADULT	EA/1	00006809					
AIRWAY-LGE. ADULT	EA/1	00008169					
STOCKINGS ANTI-EMB. SM. NYLON	PR/1	11874203					
STOCKINGS ANTI-EMB. MED. NYLON	PR/1	11877305					
STOCKINGS ANTI-EMB. LGE. NYLON	PR/1	11880408					
BALLS COTTON MED.	CS/4000	11018603					
APPL. COTTON TIP 6 STERILE	CS/1000	00021873					
BINDER SURGICAL	EA/1	00173849					
COLOPLAST BAG #2	PK/10	00304632					
COLOPLAST BAG #3	PK/10	00306001					
SLIPPERS-PILLOW PAWS MED.	PR/1	00758888	6				
SLIPPERS-PILLOW PAWS LGE.	PR/1	00760249	6				
LOTION-DER-MASSAGE 8 OZ.	BOT/1	00648725	10				
POWDER 4 OZ.	CAN	00716720	10				
CEPACOL 5 OZ.	BOT/1	00269282					
BLADES-KNIFE #10	BX/50	00190405					
BLADES-KNIFE #11	BX/50	00191767					
BLADES-KNIFE #12	BX/50	00191783					
BLADES-KNIFE #15	BX/50	00193128					
BLADES-KNIFE #20	BX/50	00194480					
TUBE SALEM SUMP 16 FR.	EA/1	18616961					
TUBE SALEM SUMP 18 FR.	EA/1	18617019					
BANDS-I.D. ADULT	BX/250	00114249					
BANDAGES-ELASTIC 2"	ROLL/1	11282100					
BANDAGES-ELASTIC 3"	ROLL/1	11285202					
BANDAGES-ELASTIC 4"	ROLL/1	11288305					
BANDAGES-ELASTIC 6"	ROLL/1	11294501					
DRAPE-BANDAID 24 x 30	BX/10	11381308					
DRESSING 3 x 3 STERILE ADAPTIC	BX/50	11421609					
DRESSING 3 x 8 STERILE ADAPTIC	BX/36	11424702					
EYE PADS-OVAL	BX/50	11440203					
GAUZE 1/4" IODOFORM PACKING	BOT/1	11458809					
GAUZE 1/2" IODOFORM PACKING	BOT/1	11461902					
GAUZE 1" IODOFORM PACKING	BOT/1	11465002					
GAUZE 2" IODOFORM PACKING	BOT/1	11468105					

ITEM	UNIT	CAT. NO.	Q	I	Is	R	S
GAUZE 1/4" PLAIN PACKING	BOT/1	11471208					
GAUZE 1/2" PLAIN PACKING	BOT/1	11474301					
GAUZE 1" PLAIN PACKING	BOT/1	11477403					
GAUZE 2" PLAIN PACKING	BOT/1	11480506					
TRAY SUTURE REMOVAL-DISP.	EA/1	17826462	3				
THERMOMETER-KIT ORAL	EA/1	00921262	7				
THERMOMETER-KIT RECTAL	EA/1	00930883	7				
FULLER-SHIELDS	EA/1	00504563					
MASK FILTER BARD.	BX/50	00652800					
ASEPTEX SURG. MASK 1800	BX/50	00663682					
MASK SURG. FILTRON DISP.	BX/50	00666602					
TISSUE KLEENEX	BX/150	00939769	10				
BANDAGE 2" SELF-ADHERING	PK/12	11310000					
BANDAGE 3" SELF-ADHERING	EA/1	11313103					
BANDAGE 4" SELF-ADHERING	PK/12	11316205					
BANDAGE 6" SELF-ADHERING	EA/1	11319308					
GAUZE VASELINE 3 x 9	EA/1	11499308	2				
GAUZE VASELINE 3 x 18	BX/12	11499126					
GAUZE VASELINE 3 x 36	BX/12	11502200					
BRUSH-SURG. PREP SPONGE-HEX.	BX/36	00224402					
BRUSH-SURGEON	BX/30	00229864					
CAP SURGEON DISP.	BX/100	00253104					
STRAP MONTGOMERY 8½ x 11	EA/1	11892809	1				
PADS-COMBINE DR. 5 x 9 STERILE	BX/25	11520806					
SPONGES-COTTON FILLED 4 x 3 STER.	TR/25	11725405					
SUSPENSORY, MED.	EA/1	00874487					
SUSPENSORY, LGE.	EA/1	00876219					
SUSPENSORY, X-LGE.	EA/1	00877209					
DEODORANT ASEPTICARE 12 OZ.	CAN/1	31104698	1				
CATH MED. 14-16 FR.	EA/1	10874162					
ROUTINE SUCTION KIT	EA/1	17199985					
FOLEY-CATH 14FR. 2 WAY 5cc	EA/1	10374882					
FOLEY-CATH 16 FR. 2 WAY 5cc	EA/1	10374932					
FOLEY-CATH 18 FR. 2 WAY 5cc	EA/1	10374981					
FOLEY-CATH 20 FR. 2 WAY 5cc	EA/1	10375046					
FOLEY-CATH 22 FR. 2 WAY 5cc	EA/1	10375095					
FOLEY-CATH 24 FR. 2 WAY 5cc	EA/1	10375137					
FOLEY-CATH 20 FR. 2 WAY 30cc	EA/1	10420255					
FOLEY-CATH 22 FR. 2 WAY 30cc	EA/1	10420313					
FOLEY-CATH 24 FR. 2 WAY 30cc	EA/1	10420370					
FOLEY-CATH 24 FR. 3 WAY 30cc	EA/1	10446003					
FOLEY-CATH 26 FR. 3 WAY 30cc	EA/1	10450468					
NEEDLE-CATH. 1963T	EA/1	10080281	1				
NEEDLE-CATH. 1968T	EA/1	10084747	5				
CATH-AROUND THE NEEDLE 1972T	EA/1	10088649	3				
TUBING-PENROSE STERILE 5/8" x 12"	EA/1	18258863					
TUBING-PENROSE STERILE 1/4" x 12"	EA/1	18264887					
TUBING-PENROSE STERILE 1"	EA/1	18307108					
TUBING-PENROSE STERILE 3/8" x 12"	EA/1	18331108					
TUBING-PENROSE STERILE 1/2" x 12"	EA/1	18361204					
CONNECTORS 5 in 1	EA/1	00311449					
INTER INFUSION SET 19-GA.	EA/1	14122451	2				
INTER INFUSION SET-21 GA.	EA/1	14175004	2				
D 5 W 150 cc	EA/1	14251300	3				
D 5 W 250 cc	EA/1	14251359					
D 5 W 500 cc	EA/1	14251409	3				
D 5 W 1000 cc	EA/1	14251458	3				
10% DEX INJ 1000ML.	EA/1	14252456					
5% DEX + 0.9% SOD. CHL 250 ML.	EA/1	14256051	3				
5% DEX + 0.9% SOD CHL 500 ML.	EA/1	14256101	3				

ITEM	UNIT	CAT. NO.	Q	I	Is	R	S
5% DEX + 0.9% SOD. CHL 1000 ML.	EA/1	14256150	3				
5% DEX + 0.45% SOD. CHL 1000 ML.	EA/1	14257604	3				
5% DEX + 0.2% SOD. CHL 1000 ML.	EA/1	14260350	3				
0.45% SOD. CHL IN WATER 1000 ML.	EA/1	14262174					
0.9% SOD. CHLO INJECT 50 ML.	EA/1	14262208					
SOD. CHL INJECTION 0.9% 150 ML.	EA/1	14263800	3				
SOD. CHL INJECTION 0.9% 250 ML.	EA/1	14263859					
SOC. CHL INJECTION 0.9% 500 ML.	EA/1	14263909	3				
SOD. CHL INJECTION 0.9% 1000 ML.	EA/1	14263958	3				
SOD. LACTATE INJ 500 ML. 1/6 MOLAR	EA/1	14264121					
5% DEX + LAC. RINGERS 500 ML.	EA/1	14265201					
5% DEX + LAC. RINGERS 1000 ML.	EA/1	14265250	3				
LAC. RINGERS INJ 500 ML.	EA/1	14292700					
LAC. RINGERS INJ. 1000 ML.	EA/1	14292759	3				
5% AMIGEN 1000 cc INJECTION	EA/1	14300040					
5% AMIGEN, 5% DEX 1000 cc	EA/1	14300875					
5% DEX ADMIXTURE 50 ML.	EA/1	14301857					
GENT.6%-75+0.9% SOD. CHL. 500 ML.	EA/1	14302202					
STERILE WATER FOR INJ. 1000 ML.	EA/1	14303556					
5% DEX. IN WATER 5% ALCOH. 1000 ML.	EA/1	14304091					
5% SOD. BICARB. IN WATER 500 ML.	EA/1	14309983					
PLASMA-LYTE 148 IN WATER 1000 ML.	EA/1	14311179					
PLASMA-LYTE 56 IN 5% DEX. 1000 ML.	EA/1	14313159					
ELECTROLYTE NO.1 1000 ML.	EA/1	14319404	3				
ELECTROLYTE NO. 2 1000 ML.	EA/1	14319636					
GENTRAN 10%-40 IN 0.9% SOD-C 500 ML.	EA/1	14320857					
GENTRAN 10%-40 IN 5% DEX. 500 ML.	EA/1	14320964					
DIANEAL WITH 1.5% DEX 1000 ML.	EA/1	14321145					
DIANEAL WITH 1.5% DEX 2000 ML.	EA/1	14321236					
STERILE WATER FOR IRRIG. 500 ML.	EA/1	14326185					
0.9% SOD. CHL. IRRIG 1000 ML.	EA/1	14329353	3				
0.9% SOD. CHL. IRRIG 1500 ML.	EA/1	14329957					
EVACUATED 500 ML. CONTAINER	EA/1	14334007					
EVACUATED 1000 ML. CONTAINER	EA/1	14334148					
0.9% SOD. CHL. IRRIG 3000 ML.	EA/1	14400428					
VENOUS PRESSURE SET	EA/1	14463335					
Y-Type Blood-Sol. ADM SET & PRES-PUMP	EA/1	14465280	2				
CYSTO INTERMITTENT IRRIGATION SET	EA/1	14489306					
Y-Type Cont. BLADDER IRRIG. c̄ DRIP CHAMB.	EA/1	14489355					
ADMIN. SET c̄ AIRWAY CONNECTOR	EA/1	14489405					
ADMIN. SET TWO MEDICATION SITES	EA/1	14500029	8				
MINI-DRIP ADM. SET Y MEDICATION SITE	EA/1	14500037	1				
EXTENSION SET TWO MEDICATION SITES	EA/1	14500045	3				
HYPODERMOCLYSIS SET	EA/1	14500052	1				
CONTINU-FLO ADMIN. SET	EA/1	14500060	4				
ADD-A-LINE MEDICATION SET	EA/1	14500078	4				
BLOOD COLLECTION SET	EA/1	14500086					
FILTER CONNECTOR	EA/1	14500094					
HYPERELIMENTATION KIT	EA/1	14570113					
SMALL VEIN SET 19 x ¾	EA/1	14605455	6				
SMALL VEIN SET 21 x ¾	EA/1	14605521					
SMALL VEIN SET 21 x 1	EA/1	14605711	6				
SMALL VEIN SET 23 x ¾	EA/1	14605828					
FEMALE CATH. KIT	EA/1	17001009					
ANGIOCATH 20 x 1¼	EA/1	10116051	3				
HEMO-VAC #1500	EA/1	00533125					
HEMO-VAC #1530	EA/1	00533653					
FILLED BY:		DATE:					

Figure 4-4 Sample Cart Quota Profile for the Surgical Unit

ST. ANTHONY HOSPITAL

LINEN CART QUOTA PROFILE

LOCATION: SURGERY

FORM NO. 142

ITEM	Q	INV	ISS	Q	INV	ISS	Q	INV	ISS	Q	INV	ISS	Q	INV	ISS	Q	INV	ISS	Q	INV	ISS	Q	INV	ISS	Q	INV	ISS	Q	INV	ISS	Q	INV	ISS	Q	INV	ISS	Q	INV	ISS	Q	INV	ISS	Q	INV	ISS
1 SCRUB DRESSES:																																													
2 SIZE 30-32	24			24			24			24			24			24			24			24			24			24			24			24			24			24			24		
3 SIZE 34-36	24			24			24			24			24			24			24			24			24			24			24			24			24			24			24		
4 SIZE 38-40	24			24			24			24			24			24			24			24			24			24			24			24			24			24			24		
5 SIZE 44-48	6			6			6			6			6			6			6			6			6			6			6			6			6			6			6		
6 SIZE 48	2			2			2			2			2			2			2			2			2			2			2			2			2			2			2		
7 LINEN HAMPER BAGS	10			10			10			10			10			10			10			10			10			10			10			10			10			10			10		
8 SCRUB PANTS:																																													
9 SMALL	24			24			24			24			24			24			24			24			24			24			24			24			24			24			24		
10 MEDIUM	24			24			24			24			24			24			24			24			24			24			24			24			24			24			24		
11 LARGE	12			12			12			12			12			12			12			12			12			12			12			12			12			12			12		
12 BATH TOWELS	6			6			6			6			6			6			6			6			6			6			6			6			6			6			6		
13 WASH CLOTHS	6			6			6			6			6			6			6			6			6			6			6			6			6			6			6		
14 SCRUB BLOUSES:																																													
15 SMALL	24			24			24			24			24			24			24			24			24			24			24			24			24			24			24		
MEDIUM	24			24			24			24			24			24			24			24			24			24			24			24			24			24			24		
LARGE	12			12			12			12			12			12			12			12			12			12			12			12			12			12			12		

DATE FILLED																
WEIGHT																
DATE RETURNED																
WEIGHT RETURNED																TOTAL
NO. OF LBS. IN USE																
COMPLETED BY																

Authority Relationships

An up-to-date organizational chart should be attached to each job description to indicate authority and reporting relationships (Figure 4–1).

Salary

Commensurate with education, training, and assigned responsibilities. Salary should be at the supervisory entry level rate.

Position Description for the Cart Attendant

Position Title

Cart attendant.

Position Purpose

To replenish the supply and linen exchange carts according to a preprinted cart quota profile (Figures 4-2, 4-3, 4-4).

Responsible To

The exchange cart coordinator.

Responsible For

The daily output of supply and linen carts that are replenished on a quality and quantity basis.

Degree of Supervision

The supervision for this position is direct and frequent to assure a quality product.

Areas of Emphasis

a. Cart supply quotas
b. Distribution patterns
c. Storeroom logistics
d. S.P.D. cleanliness standards
e. Assembly line processing of carts
f. Quality checks

Committee Representation

Not applicable as such, but could be a member of a hospital committee at large such as the Safety Committee.

Experience

Entry level experience.

Educational Requirements

The candidate should have a high school education or an acceptable experiential equivalency.

Job Knowledge

a. Basic math
b. Good telephone manners

Skills

The Candidate must possess the following:

a. Ability to plan and organize the workflow in a constantly changing environment
b. Basic communication skills
c. Good hand-eye coordination

Major Tasks and Scope of Responsibility

a. Folds the cart cover neatly onto the top of the cart;
b. Takes the patient charge tray from the cart and gives it to the cart exchange coordinator;
c. Takes a complete inventory of all cart supplies by using the preprinted cart quota profile;
d. Computes the difference between the quota and the actual inventory and puts this amount in the appropriate column "D";
e. Replenishes the cart by using the difference column and putting this amount in the issue column;
f. Fills both charge and noncharge items at the same time;
g. Returns completed cart paperwork to the exchange cart coordinator immediately after replenishing items on the cart;
h. Places the replenished cart in the appropriate storage area, leaving cover up so that the exchange cart coordinator can make a quality check of the cart;
i. Repeats same procedure for all carts (Figure 4-5); and
j. Assists in exchanging the carts on the units if necessary after all carts have been replenished.

NOTE: It is imperative that the duties of this position be spelled out in detail for proper and quality supply replenishment.

Figure 4-5 Daily Cart Replenishment Schedule

8:00 a.m.	—	BEGIN PROCESSING THE MEDICAL-SURGICAL CARTS *ONLY.*
8.45 a.m.	—	THREE MEDICAL-SURGICAL CARTS COMPLETED (Assuming there are three cart attendants on duty).
9:30 a.m.	—	THREE ADDITIONAL MEDICAL-SURGICAL CARTS COMPLETED.
10:15 a.m.	—	THREE ADDITIONAL MEDICAL-SURGICAL CARTS COMPLETED.
10:15 a.m. to 10:30 a.m.	—	BREAK
11:15 a.m.	—	THREE ADDITIONAL MEDICAL-SURGICAL CARTS COMPLETED.
11:15 a.m. to 12:00 a.m.	—	a] PERFORM THE MISSING CHARGE REVIEW b] PUT THE FINISHING TOUCHES ON THE MEDICAL-SURGICAL CARTS (QUALITY AND QUANTITY CONTROL)
12:00 noon to 12:30 p.m.	—	LUNCH
12:30 p.m.	—	BEGIN PROCESSING THE LINEN CARTS *ONLY.*
1:00 p.m.	—	THREE LINEN CARTS COMPLETED.
1:30 p.m.	—	THREE ADDITIONAL LINEN CARTS COMPLETED.
2:00 p.m.	—	THREE ADDITIONAL LINEN CARTS COMPLETED.
2:30 p.m.	—	THREE ADDITIONAL LINEN CARTS COMPLETED.
3:00 p.m.	—	THREE ADDITIONAL LINEN CARTS COMPLETED.
3:00 p.m. to 3:15 p.m.	—	PUT THE FINISHING TOUCHES ON THE LINEN CARTS.
3:15 p.m. to 3:30 p.m.	—	BREAK
3:30 p.m. to 4:30 p.m.	—	PROCESS ALL NECESSARY PAPERWORK INCLUDING CHARGE VOUCHERS AND GET AREA READY FOR NEXT DAY.

Evaluation

The cart attendants are evaluated 90 days after hiring and at least annually on the anniversary date thereafter.

Authority Relationships

An up-to-date organizational chart should be attached to each job description to indicate authority and reporting relationships (Figure 4-1).

Salary

Entry level salary.

Position Description for the Receiving Clerk

Position Title

Receiving clerk.

Position Purpose

To assure that all supplies, drugs, and equipment are received in accordance with proper and prudent practices.

Responsible To

The assistant director of materiel management or the director of purchased services.

Responsible For

a. Centralized receiving of all goods and services
b. Proper and approved receiving policies
c. Appropriate recordkeeping
d. "Stockless" receiving
e. Returned goods procedure

Degree of Supervision

Supervision should be direct and at frequent intervals.

Areas of Emphasis

a. Strict adherence to receiving policies and procedures
b. "Aged" receiving reports
c. Supervision of the entire centralized receiving process
d. "Stockless" receiving
e. Tagging and recording of capital equipment
f. Internal control measures

Committee Representation

The position has no specific committee responsibilities; however, the employee may be requested to serve on hospital committees such as Safety and Risk Management.

Experience

No specific experience is required, but previous hospital or industrial shipping and receiving experience is desirable.

Educational Requirements

The candidate should have at least a high school education.

Job Knowledge

a. Basic math
b. Hospital logistics
c. Distribution patterns
d. Proper lifting and heavy handling techniques
e. Ethical business principles

Skills

The candidate should possess the following:

a. Ability to organize sizeable workload
b. Good communication skills
c. Good hand-eye coordination

Major Tasks and Scope of Responsibility

a. Supervises the entire centralized receiving process;
b. Processes and receives all supplies and equipment and distributes them into the respective areas;
c. Reviews the purchase order file weekly for overdue shipments and back orders and reports this information to the director of purchased services;
d. Transports furniture and equipment inter- and intradepartmentally as the need arises;
e. Assumes responsibility for internal control in the receiving process;
f. Keeps the staging and dock areas clean and orderly at all times by sweeping the area at least once per day and removing all cartons and boxes from the staging area by at least 4:00 p.m. daily;

g. Tags all capital equipment as it is received, initiating the property management system of accountability;
h. Follows the returned goods policy to the letter;
i. Takes responsibility for paper flow from the receiving process to data processing and accounting;
j. Delivers supplies or works in the S.P.D. areas occasionally; and
k. Performs other related duties as may be assigned by the immediate supervisor.

Evaluation

The receiving clerk should be evaluated after 90 days on the job and then at least annually thereafter.

Authority Relationships

An up-to-date organizational chart should be attached to each job description to indicate the authority and reporting relationships (Figure 4-1).

Salary

Commensurate with education, training, and assigned responsibilities. The compensation should be at the entry supervisory level.

Position Description for the Processing Supervisor

Position Title

Processing supervisor.

Position Purpose

To maintain a maximum level of quality control in the supply, processing, reprocessing, and sterilization functions.

Responsible To

S.P.D. supervisor.

Responsible For

The direction, evaluation, and overall supervision of the following:

a. Processing attendants
b. Sterilization and processing quality control programs

Degree of Supervision

Supervision is fairly remote but rather frequent with periodic quality control checks by the S.P.D. supervisor.

Areas of Emphasis

a. Quality control programs in the areas of processing and sterilization
b. Supervision of attendants
c. Inservice and quality continuing education programs
d. Effective policies and procedures for the clean and soiled divisions
e. Equipment rounds
f. Preventive maintenance programs for patient care equipment
g. Accreditation standards

Committee Representation

The processing supervisor should be a member of the following hospital and/or medical staff committees:

a. Infection Control
b. Evaluation and Standardization of Products
c. Cost Containment
d. Patient Charge Review
e. Others, as deemed appropriate by immediate supervisor

Experience

The candidate should have considerable familiarity (3 to 5 years) with the hospital supply processing function.

Educational Requirements

The candidate should have at least a high school education with considerable central supply experience. A baccalaureate degree in biology, bacteriology, zoology, or industrial engineering is highly desirable.

Job Knowledge

a. Sterilization and quality control techniques and programs
b. Appropriate accreditation standards
c. Emergency items
d. Code blue procedures
e. Infection control standards
f. The various instrument and linen pack requirements

g. Basic personnel policies and procedures
h. Pack dating and numbering systems

Skills

The candidate must possess:

a. Ability to organize workload
b. Ability to cope well under emergency and stressful conditions
c. Good hand-eye coordination
d. Good supervisory skills
e. Ability to converse with various health care professionals
f. Communication skills

Major Tasks and Scope of Responsibility

a. Supervises, assigns, and directs the activities of all personnel performing processing functions;
b. Evaluates the performance at least annually of the personnel in the unit on all appropriate shifts;
c. Establishes and maintains a good professional rapport with the medical staff, nurses, and staff of patient care areas and all other applicable departments and units;
d. Establishes and enforces unit policies and procedures in accordance with departmental policies;
e. Reviews and makes the appropriate recommendations in reference to all new supplies and equipment for the unit;
f. Develops, schedules, conducts, and documents inservice and continuing education programs for the personnel of the unit;
g. Meets or exceeds standards of compliance of all the accreditation and regulatory bodies and commissions in relationship to supply processing and sterilization;
h. Submits periodic reports to the S.P.D. supervisor concerning the functional phases of the unit;
i. Performs the appropriate committee functions as assigned;
j. Conducts equipment rounds to all nursing units at 10:00 a.m. and 2:00 p.m. daily, initiating patient charge vouchers accordingly and returning any applicable equipment to S.P.D. for reprocessing;
k. Operates the gas and steam sterilizers according to specified policies and procedures;
l. Develops and requires strict adherence to maximum quality control processing standards;

m. Develops and accomplishes unit objectives on a regular basis; and
n. Performs other related duties as may be assigned by the S.P.D. supervisor.

Evaluation

The processing supervisor should be evaluated after 90 days on the job and then at least annually thereafter.

Authority Relationships

An up-to-date organizational chart should be attached to each job description to indicate the authority and reporting relationships (Figure 4-1).

Salary

Commensurate with education, training and assigned responsibilities. Compensation is at the upper levels of the hospital supervisory salary scale.

Good job descriptions are indicative of good management. In the materiel management department, where the positions range from professional to entry level, it is imperative to have well delineated, well written job descriptions. Furthermore, it is equally important to keep these descriptions current to reflect changing times, attitudes, goals, personnel, and technologies.

Pertinent Points to Ponder

1. How many different positions are there in the area of materiel management?
2. Who should be involved in the writing and updating of job descriptions?
3. Could it be that certain positions such as purchasing agent and C.S.R. supervisor have become outdated and should be renamed and restructured? Name other such job titles that could be given new life by the same process.
4. Would you consider the position of director of materiel management to be line or staff? Why?
5. How are new position descriptions developed and approved in your hospital?
6. Do any of your employees report to two bosses? Is this good practice and why?
7. As a supervisor in the department of materiel management, if you should quiz your employees regarding for and to whom are they responsible, what would be their most likely responses?

8. How often should job descriptions be reviewed and updated? How long has it been since you have reviewed the job descriptions of the employees that report to you?
9. What aspect of the job description do you consider to be the most important? The least important?
10. What method do you think is best for making an employee completely knowledgeable and aware of his or her position description?
11. Under what circumstances do you consider good job descriptions to be of the most importance?
12. How do job descriptions for the same position differ from hospital to hospital?

Chapter 5

Pertinent Policies and Procedures Set the Pace for Progress

In the past, hospital purchasing has received much attention and discussion. Unfortunately, purchasing has been associated with getting the best initial price from the vendor, even though there is much more to the process than just negotiating a low price from various dealers. In fact, the lowest price may turn out to be the highest one. In actuality, purchasing is only one of a myriad of essential elements that comprise the total function of hospital materiel management. How, how much, when, why, and what happens to the supply once it is purchased are far more important than from whom and at what price the hospital purchases.

The materiel management thrust of a hospital must be developed and sold to the administration by the materiel manager or purchasing director, who must convince top management to fully recognize and approve the plan. If the total materiel program is to be effective, furthermore, the entire hospital must be aware and committed to its precepts. Materiel managers and purchasing directors often complain that they do not get the proper administrative and departmental support to effectively perform their duties. This symptom is most likely the result of policies and procedures which have been inadequately communicated. The managerial effectiveness of the materiel manager can be greatly limited without thoughtful, written, and administratively approved policies and procedures for the entire program. Quite simply, policies and procedures are the building blocks upon which the materiel program is built, and careful attention must be given to their construction.

AN ORGANIZATIONAL FORMAT FOR POLICY AND PROCEDURE DETERMINATION

The main objective of policy and procedural determination is to have them written in a common sense and meaningful manner that can be used for managerial direction and guidance. A policy is a statement of intent and a procedure spells out that intent in detail. The essentials of a results-oriented policy and procedure format are as follows:

Subject

This subject is often difficult to state in explicit words. The question that must be answered is, "To whom are the policy and procedure directed?" Once this has been determined, the subject can be expressed in language understandable to the appropriate person. Most often, subjects have many synonymous terms to describe them, and all commonly recognized ones should be listed. For example, if the subject is "contract purchasing," it should also be listed as "prime supplier approach," "prime vendor concept," and "solo purchasing."

Objective

It is imperative that a reason be given for the requested protocol. It should be concisely stated and represent a reasonable approach to a problem or situation. In many cases, it is important to state the present situation and proceed to give the intended goal. For example, in reference to the reduction of supply inventories it would be appropriate to state the objective as, "to reduce the inventory in central stores from $300,000 to $100,000 by end of the fiscal year."

Policy Statement

After delineating the purpose or goal, the policy of the hospital regarding this subject must be indicated. In other words, what will be the mission of the institution in relationship to the topic. For example, it may be the policy of the hospital not to accept back orders. At this point, it is important to note that there may be many policy statements in reference to only one objective. If this is so, they should be enumerated in order of priority.

Correlation of Departmental Policy to Hospital Policy

It is important that each department establish policies and procedures that are in coordination with the overall administrative or hospital policies. The materiel manager should refer to the hospital policy number or title that is addressed by this particular departmental policy.

Procedural Documentation

In order to meet or exceed an objective, the involved parties are to perform in a certain prescribed manner. The manager should enumerate the important steps which must be taken so that everyone will be familiar with the procedure and execute action accordingly.

Exceptions

If certain departments, units, or employees do not have to follow this enumerated policy and procedure, they should be listed. In keeping with fair and uniform standards, it is imperative also to state why each exception is made. For example, if a policy allowed only a two-week maximum of a certain supply, but the lead time between procurement and receipt was three weeks, this would be a justifiable exception. Of course, all exceptions must be rational and realistic or the entire process will be meaningless.

Dates of Approval and Reviews

To be meaningful, all policies and procedures should be reviewed and updated accordingly at least twice per year. It is important that the initial approval date remain on the document and that all review dates be listed in sequence.

Attachments

If there are pertinent accompanying documents, they should become an integral part of the policy and procedural documentation. For example, if the subject is ordering of supplies, then an appended copy of the purchase order would be appropriate.

Authorized Signatures

For policy and procedure to be effective, they must be based on and supported by an accepted authority. In other words, recognized authority is the essence of delegation. It is suggested that all materiel management policies and procedures be signed by the administrator, the materiel manager, and others as may be appropriate.

Using these criteria, the materiel manager can more than meet the requirements for quality policy and procedural documentation. For the average hospital, there are between 100 and 150 subjects that should be addressed and carefully documented in this manner. Following is a representative cross-section of 25 of these subjects.

Materiel Management Policy and Procedure Number 1

Subject

Cost containment philosophy.

Objective

To reduce or contain the ever-spiraling costs of supplies, labor, and equipment in the most effective manner.

Policy Statements

- To obtain quality health care supplies at the lowest possible cost.
- To maintain wages and salaries of supply personnel at a comparable industry level.
- To enter into shared service endeavors whenever feasible.
- To participate in group purchasing whenever the conditions indicate.
- To continually monitor the cost of supplies and equipment within the hospital.
- To provide for a standardization process which will allow for a total review of all products before purchase.

Correlation of Departmental Policy to Hospital Policy

The above materiel management policy statements refer directly to hospital cost containment policy #10 (example only).

Procedural Documentation

- The director of materiel management should negotiate prime supplier contracts on all major categories of supplies based on largest volume discount regardless of the quantities to be purchased.
- Supply, process, and distribution functions will be coordinated and amalgamated in order to reduce the number of personnel needed to staff the entire materiel management department.
- All unofficial departmental inventories will be kept to a two-week maximum. These inventories will be monitored by taking quarterly physical inventories.
- All official inventories are to be kept to a $300 per bed maximum.
- All new supplies and equipment must be reviewed and approved by the hospital standardization committee before being purchased.
- The materiel manager and purchasing director are to investigate and participate in group purchasing and shared services endeavors that will be cost beneficial to the hospital.

- The materiel manager and purchasing director will participate in legitimate supply price comparisons on local, regional, and statewide levels. These indicators will in turn be used to negotiate more prudently.

Exceptions

There will be no exceptions to the cost containment philosophy.

Attachments

None

Dates of Approval and Reviews

Approval: January 3, 1976
Review: July 1, 1976
Review: January 1, 1977
Review: July 1, 1977
Review: January 2, 1978
Review: July 1, 1978

Authorized Signatures

Administration
Materiel manager

Materiel Management Policy and Procedure Number 2

Subject

Returned goods.

Objective

To develop an effective process for returning unwanted or defective supplies and equipment to the vendor or manufacturer.

Policy Statement

It shall be the responsibility of the Department of Materiel Management to return all supplies and equipment that are either ordered by mistake, erroneously shipped, obsolete, or defective as soon as possible.

Correlation of Departmental Policy to Hospital Policy

The above delineated policy is in compliance with hospital policy #25 (example only).

Procedural Documentation

- After the decision has been made to return a supply or piece of equipment to the vendor or manufacturer, the receiving clerk is contacted to begin shipment preparation.
- The director of materiel management shall notify the company or its representative that the goods are being returned and by what means. He also requests the approval to return the goods.
- The returned items should be appropriately and securely packaged.
- The most appropriate vehicle or means of transportation must be selected in accordance with the nature of the goods.
- A letter explaining the reasons for and conditions of returns must accompany all returned goods.
- The replacement value of the returned products or equipment must be determined and the shipment insured at its total replacement value.
- If the reason for returning the goods is because of an erroneous shipment on the part of the company, then the shipment will be made at no cost to the hospital (F.O.B. hospital.—*see glossary*).
- The transportation is arranged and returned goods are shipped accordingly.
- A returned goods ledger is completed with the following information:

  1. Name and description of item
  2. Date returned
  3. Transportation source
  4. How shipped
  5. Insured amount
  6. Cost of shipment
  7. Initials of person responsible for the shipment.

- This ledger will remain active until full credit has been received or restitution has been made.

Exceptions

This procedure will be followed unless the company or its representative stipulates otherwise.

Attachments

None

Dates of Approval and Reviews

Approval: January 1, 1976
Review: July 1, 1976
Review: January 1, 1977
Review: July 1, 1977
Review: January 1, 1978
Review: July 1, 1978

Authorized Signatures

Administration
Materiel Manager

Materiel Management Policy and Procedure Number 3

Subject

Statement of services offered.

Objective

To delineate to all concerned parties those services that are provided by the Department of Materiel Management.

Policy Statement

The scope of services of this department shall encompass the management and control of goods and services from acquisition to disposition.

Correlation of Departmental Policy to Hospital Policy

This departmental policy is supportive of hospital policy #3 (example only).

Procedural Documentation

- Required patient care supplies shall be provided to all nursing units and pertinent departments by means of a total supply cart exchange program. This program will provide 95 to 99 percent of all the supply needs of that unit for a 24-hour period.
- Needed supply items not found on the exchange cart will be provided via a 24-hour, seven day a week hotline delivery service.
- Patient care equipment, such as suction machines, is to be controlled and inspected twice daily by means of equipment rounds conducted by the processing supervisor. Charges for all such equipment also will be noted during these rounds.

- Miscellaneous equipment rounds will be conducted weekly to each nursing unit to ensure that equipment such as stethoscopes, otoscopes, scales, flashlights, etc., are in proper working order.
- All supplies and services for the hospital will be procured by means of centralized purchasing through the materiel management department.
- All capital equipment will be requested on a special requisition form.
- All supplies and equipment entering the hospital, even those for evaluation purposes, will be received through the centralized receiving process and be delivered directly to the appropriate areas.
- The standardization and evaluation of all supplies and equipment will be conducted by the materiel management department with the assistance of a multidisciplined committee.
- All reusable patient care supplies and equipment are to be processed or reprocessed by trained competent S.P.D. personnel in a quality controlled manner.
- Materiel management will conduct quarterly physical reviews of all official and unofficial inventories within the hospital.
- Proper accountability of all capital equipment shall be the responsibility of materiel management.
- Periodic review of patient care supplies shall be conducted jointly by nursing service and materiel management.
- Activities of sales representatives within the hospital will be monitored and controlled.
- All transport and transfer of supplies and equipment within the hospital shall be performed by this department.
- This statement is to be posted in all departments and nursing units.

Exceptions

None

Attachments

None

Dates of Approval and Reviews

Approval: January 1, 1977
Review: July 3, 1977
Review: January 4. 1978
Review: July 5, 1978
Review: January 2, 1979

Authorized Signatures

Administration
Materiel manager

Materiel Management Policy and Procedure Number 4

Subject

Departmental administrative reports.

Objective

To keep administration informed and knowledgeable of supply activity within the hospital.

Policy Statement

The Department of Materiel Management shall submit timely and meaningful reports to administration concerning the operational, budgetary, professional, and planning aspects of the department.

Correlation of Departmental Policy to Hospital Policy

The above delineated policy is in compliance with hospital policy #15 (example only).

Procedural Documentation

- The materiel manager will submit the following reports at periodic intervals:
  - a. **Prime Supplier Report.** This is a monthly report delineating the amounts purchased from prime suppliers on a monthly and year-to-date basis.
  - b. **Pharmacy Supplier Report.** This report provides the total dollar volume purchased from pharmaceutical vendors on a monthly and year-to-date basis.
  - c. **S.P.D. Usage Report.** This report delineates the total dollar volume of S.P.D. issues and each department's supply cost on a monthly basis.
  - d. **Linen Usage Report.** This report gives the linen usage in the various patient care areas on a monthly and year-to-date basis.
  - e. **Pharmacy Summary.** This report summarizes the activity in pharmacy and the adjustments to the purchase and inventory cycles.

f. **Cart Shortage Report.** This report, published daily and monthly, indicates shortages of any of the patient charge items incurred by the nursing unit and the corresponding patient charge associated with the loss.
g. **Inventory Turnover Report.** This is a helpful indicator which provides total dollar volume of supplies which move in and out of central stores on a monthly and yearly basis.
h. **Monthly Budget Report.** This report provides any exceptions to the forecasted budget projections and indicates personnel costs, supply costs, overtime costs, and number of full-time equivalent positions utilized for the month.
i. **Physical Inventory Report.** This quarterly report indicates the amount of supplies in stock in the various official and nonofficial areas at the time of reporting.

- Administration shall receive a copy of all departmental reports in an expeditious manner.
- Any variances from the normal operating range are to be justified in writing.

Exceptions

In some cases, administration will ask for a special report on a certain supply or cost activity.

Attachments

Not applicable

Dates of Approval and Reviews

Approval: July 1, 1977
Review: January 1, 1978
Review: July 1, 1978
Review: January 1, 1979

Authorized Signatures

Administration
Materiel manager

Materiel Management Policy and Procedure Number 5

Subject

Contracts and agreements.

Objective

To assure the proper development, approval, and documentation of all contracts and commitments of the hospital in reference to supplies, equipment, and equipment services.

Policy Statement

The Department of Materiel Management will develop guidelines and format for the entering into all contracts and agreements in reference to purchase commitments for supplies, equipment, and equipment services.

Correlation of Departmental Policy to Hospital Policy

The above delineated policy is in compliance with hospital policy #3 (example only).

Procedural Documentation

- The materiel manager or director of purchasing shall initiate all negotiations for all such contracts for the hospital.
- The following items should be considered in the development of such contracts:

  1. Length of contract
  2. Enumeration of services purchased
  3. Payment terms
  4. Insurance and indemnity notification clause
  5. Assignment and governing law reference
  6. Transportation charges
  7. Terms of cancellation

- All contracts and commitments for services are to be initiated through the normal hospital purchasing procedure. Therefore, a purchase order number is assigned to each contract.
- All contracts and long-term agreements must be approved by administration.
- All contracts and service commitments in excess of $15,000 must receive the approval of the board of trustees.
- The costs of providing the services must be a budgeted item.

Exceptions

None

Attachments

Not applicable

Dates of Approval and Reviews

Approval: January 1, 1978
Review: July 2, 1978
Review: January 5, 1979

Authorized Signatures

Administration
Materiel manager

Materiel Management Policy and Procedure Number 6

Subject

Departmental visitation by sales representatives.

Objective

To monitor and to provide guidelines for the activities of sales representatives within the hospital.

Policy Statement

All sales representatives seeking contact with hospital personnel are required to register with the materiel management department.

Correlation of Departmental Policy to Hospital Policy

The above delineated policy is in compliance with hospital policy #19 (example only).

Procedural Documentation

- It is considered desirable that sales representatives notify the materiel management secretary by letter or phone at least a week in advance of their visit.
- Sales representatives should also observe the departmental hours for appointments.
- All sales representatives, regardless of their supply specialty, must register with the materiel management secretary.
- If a sales representative desires to confer with a department head or other departmental personnel, the materiel management secretary will call to arrange the conference.

- The secretary will issue a visitor's identification badge which is to be worn while in the hospital and will properly route these individuals to their desired destinations.
- Sales representatives are not to attempt to contact personnel during working hours without prior arrangement through the Department of Materiel Management.
- All hospital personnel contacted shall inquire as to whether proper hospital procedure has been followed. If the answer is negative, the sales representative shall be instructed as to the proper procedure.
- Likewise, hospital personnel seeking contact with sales representatives should do so through the Department of Materiel Management.
- Sales representatives are not permitted in the processing areas of S.P.D. or pharmacy, nor are they invited to participate in the standardization process.
- Any supplies or samples that are to be evaluated are to be given to the director of purchasing for presentation to the Standardization Committee.
- Any equipment requested by hospital personnel to be brought in for evaluation purposes only must also undergo the entire purchase order process.
- No piece of equipment or new product will be put into service without the prior and proper notification of the Department of Materiel Management.
- Only designated materiel management personnel will be permitted to make purchase commitments on behalf of the hospital.
- A copy of this procedure and other procedures of interest to sales representatives are to be made available through the materiel management secretary.

Exceptions

None

Attachments

Not applicable

Dates of Approval and Reviews

Approval: January 1, 1978
Review: July 1, 1978
Review: January 1, 1979
Review: July 1, 1979

Authorized Signatures

Administration
Materiel manager

Materiel Management Policy and Procedure Number 7

Subject

Movement and transfer of hospital equipment and furnishings.

Objective

To assure that all hospital equipment and furnishings are transferred in a documented and uniform manner.

Policy Statement

All equipment and hospital furnishings shall be transferred or delivered by trained materiel management attendants.

Correlation of Departmental Policy to Hospital Policy

The above delineated policy is in compliance with hospital policy #15 (example only).

Procedural Documentation

- All departments and nursing units desiring the transport or transfer of equipment must request it from the Department of Materiel Management.
- The requests shall be in writing on the proper form and must indicate what items are to be moved and/or stored and desired destination.
- At least a 24-hour notice is required for all requests.
- Upon the receipt of the transfer request, the Department of Materiel Management will dispatch personnel to the requested department and transport the equipment to the designated area.
- After the transfer is completed, the necessary changes are made in the appropriate property management ledger.

Exceptions

Setting up of rooms or areas for meetings and special events is to be handled by the Department of Housekeeping.

Attachments

Not applicable

Dates of Approval and Reviews

Approval: January 1, 1976
Review: July 1, 1976
Review: January 1, 1977
Review: July 1, 1977
Review: January 1, 1978

Authorized Signatures

Administration
Materiel manager

Materiel Management Policy and Procedure Number 8

Subject

Processing of back orders.

Objective

To ensure an effective and standardized process for handling supply back orders.

Policy Statement

Back orders are to be discouraged and kept to a minimum. However, when they do occur, they should be handled in a prescribed, uniform manner which should be made known to receiving, accounting, data processing, and the requesting department.

Correlation of Departmental Policy to Hospital Policy

The above delineated policy is in compliance with hospital policy #7 (example only).

Procedural Documentation

- When a purchase order is placed to a vendor, the vendor is instructed to call and notify the hospital of a back order situation immediately.
- The item or items are eliminated from the initial purchase order and placed on a separate purchase order with indication of the estimated time of delivery.
- All such orders are kept in a back order file in the receiving department and are reviewed at least weekly.
- Any back order over 14 days shall be reevaluated to determine if reordering from another vendor is probable or necessary.

- Any back order over 30 days, unless otherwise stipulated, shall be cancelled automatically.
- Back order statistics are kept on all prime suppliers, and this information is summarized and put into the vendor performance appraisal which is sent to the appropriate company representative on an annual basis.
- Back orders are to be kept to an absolute minimum and any unnecessary expenses involved will be paid by the suppliers.

Exceptions

None

Attachments

Not applicable

Dates of Approval and Reviews

Approval: July 1, 1977
Review: January 1, 1978
Review: July 1, 1978

Authorized Signatures

Administration
Materiel manager

Materiel Management Policy and Procedure Number 9

Subject

Linen processing.

Objective

To set forth guidelines for the proper laundering, sanitation, and transportation of patient care linen.

Policy Statement

All linen shall be processed in an approved, inspected, sanitary manner.

Correlation of Departmental Policy to Hospital Policy

The above delineated policy is in compliance with hospital policy #12 (example only).

Procedural Documentation

- All linen shall be collected by housekeeping and nursing service in a predescribed sanitary manner and deposited in the appropriate linen chutes (see nursing and housekeeping procedures).
- Soiled linen is placed in linen hampers and covered appropriately.
- All linen is centrally collected in the soiled linen room by housekeeping personnel.
- Linen is transported in a separate elevator to the laundry.
- Contaminated linen which has been placed in water soluble bags shall be deposited directly into the washer without being opened.
- All other linen not placed in water soluble bags shall be placed directly into the washer.
- The linen shall be placed into 180° water with soap and concentrated chlorine bleach.
- The linen shall then be treated with a fabric softener and a bacteriostat in the final rinse.
- All linen either will be ironed at 325° or tumble dried at 350° for further sanitation.
- The processed linen is transported to S.P.D. for delivery to the nursing units.
- Finally, the processed linen stored in the S.P.D. area is spot-cultured periodically.

Exceptions

None

Attachments

Not applicable

Dates of Approval and Reviews

Approval: January 1, 1978
Review: July 1, 1978
Review: January 1, 1979
Review: July 1, 1979

Authorized Signatures

Administration
Materiel manager

Materiel Management Policy and Procedure Number 10

Subject

Charging of patient supply items.

Objective

To ensure an effective, standardized method of individually charging for patient supply items.

Policy Statement

It should be the policy of the Department of Materiel Management that all individual patient charge items will be processed in a standardized manner in order to minimize loss of revenue through lost charges.

Correlation of Departmental Policy to Hospital Policy

The above delineated policy is in compliance with hospital policy #30 (example only).

Procedural Documentation

- Appropriate preprinted charge vouchers are to be placed upon all patient charge supply items in the S.P.D. processing area.
- Patient charge items are to be transferred to the patient care units with the appropriate charge voucher attached.
- Nurses in charge of patient treatment shall process the charge voucher when an item is used by affixing the necessary patient information via the addressograph machine.
- Processed charge tickets will be placed in the appropriate charge container located on the supply cart.
- Processed charge tickets are to be returned to S.P.D. daily for verification against the supplies issued. If shortages exist, the supply cart coordinator will make every attempt possible to obtain the appropriate charge. If he or she is unable to do so, the cost of that item will be charged to the responsible nursing unit.
- All processed charge vouchers are to be taken daily to data processing for transferring to the patient's account.
- On special delivery items by S.P.D. attendant, the attendant shall obtain the necessary information, process the charge voucher and return it to S.P.D.
- The loss of patient charges must be kept at an absolute minimum through total cooperation of materiel management and nursing service.

Exceptions

None

Attachments

Not applicable

Dates of Approval and Reviews

Approval: January 1, 1978
Review: July 1, 1978
Review: January 1, 1979
Review: July 1, 1979
Review: January 1, 1980

Authorized Signatures

Administration
Materiel manager

Materiel Management Policy and Procedure Number 11

Subject

Receiving of radioisotopes.

Objective

To ensure that radioactive materials are received and handled in a safe and expeditious manner.

Policy Statements

- The Department of Materiel Management will coordinate the delivery of radioactive material to coincide with the normal receiving hours of the department if at all possible.
- The hospital will order, receive, and handle all radioactive material in accordance with the accreditation standards of the National Regulatory Commission (NRC).

Correlation of Departmental Policy to Hospital Policy

The above delineated policies are in compliance with hospital policy #22 (example only).

Procedural Documentation

- All radioactive materials will be purchased in accordance with the standardized purchase procedure of the Department of Materiel Management.
- The receiving copy of the purchase order is to be routed to the receiving clerk for delivery processing.
- Every attempt is to be made to coordinate the delivery of the radioactive material with the standard receiving hours of Monday through Friday, 7:30 a.m. to 4:30 p.m.; Saturday, 7:30 a.m. to 12:00 noon.
- If the delivery coincides with these hours then the procedure is as follows:

    1. The receiving clerk keeps a reference file on all vendors of radioactive material and is knowledgeable of these deliveries.
    2. He immediately calls the nuclear technician on duty and informs him or her of the delivery.
    3. The technician immediately responds and processes the delivery in accordance with NRC regulations.
    4. The technician takes the package to the hot lab and monitors it before opening. He also monitors the packing material for spillage after opening.
    5. The technician verifies the number and items in the package with the receiving clerk.
    6. The receiving clerk processes the paperwork according to standard policy.
    7. This procedure is applicable for all deliveries made during standard receiving hours.

- If the delivery of the radioactive material is made after the standard receiving hours then the following procedure is followed:

    1. The transportation courier uses the telephone at the receiving dock to notify the hospital operator of the delivery.
    2. The telephone operator immediately notifies the radiology technician on duty of the delivery.
    3. The technician processes the delivery and takes the radioactive material to the hot lab for monitoring.

- Sometimes, irregular deliveries made at night or on holidays can be misdirected and delivered to undesignated receiving areas of the hospital such as the laboratory or the emergency room. If this happens, then the following procedure is followed:

1. Packages containing radioactive material are always clearly marked and labeled as "Radioactive."
2. All possible areas of undesignated delivery are notified and periodically instructed not to receive such deliveries or sign the receiving slip.
3. The transportation courier should be instructed to take such material directly to the Radiology Department, where standard procedure then will be followed.

Exceptions

None

Attachments

Not applicable

Dates of Approval and Reviews

Approval: January 15, 1978
Review: July 1, 1978
Review: January 2, 1979

Authorized Signatures

Administration
Materiel manager

Materiel Management Policy and Procedure Number 12

Subject

Use of a drug formulary and therapeutic guide.

Objective

To bring about standardization of pharmaceuticals and develop a drug informational source for members of the medical and nursing staffs.

Policy Statements

- All drugs shall be reviewed under the standardization process on a regular basis.
- The Pharmacy and Therapeutics Committee, a multidisciplined committee composed of medical staff members and those from other patient care areas, shall meet at least monthly and provide the functions of drug standardization and updating of the therapeutic guide.

- The pharmacy shall be responsible for the distribution of all of this information to the applicable areas on a regular basis.
- The chief pharmacist will be a member of the Pharmacy and Therapeutics Committee.

Correlation of Departmental Policy to Hospital Policy

The above delineated policies are in compliance with hospital policy #50 (example only).

Procedural Documentation

- All requests for new stock drugs must be submitted on a new drug request form to the chief pharmacist. This request will be researched and all pertinent information submitted to the Pharmacy and Therapeutics Committee for review, action, and recommendation to the Executive Committee of the medical staff for its review and approval.
- The pharmacist shall continually review generic categories of drugs and make appropriate recommendations as to the brand name to be standardized and published in the formulary.
- The therapeutic guide, developed from the formulary, shall include the form and use of selected therapeutics agents. This informational guide is to be updated as new information is made available.
- Investigational drugs shall not be used in the hospital unless they are approved by the Pharmacy and Therapeutics Committee.
- If a drug that is not listed in the formulary and for which substitutions are not available is ordered by a physician in an emergency situation, it is obtained in limited quantities from the most local source as soon as possible.
- If it is unlikely that a certain drug needed in an emergency situation will be used again for some time, every attempt is made to borrow or purchase it from another hospital.
- The chiefs of all medical and surgical departments are notified in advance if deletion of a listed formulary drug is being considered. They will notify the members of their appropriate departments and report the responses back to the Pharmacy and Therapeutics Committee.

Exceptions

Intravenous solutions and sets are not under the purview of the Pharmacy and Therapeutics Committee.

Attachments

Not applicable

Dates of Approval and Reviews

Approval: January 15, 1978
Review: June 30, 1978
Review: January 2, 1979

Authorized Signatures

Administration
Materiel manager
Chief pharmacist

Materiel Management Policy and Procedure Number 13

Subject

Outdated sterile supplies.

Objective

To ensure that no outdated sterile supplies are utilized for patient care purposes.

Policy Statement

No outdated sterile supplies shall be maintained in stock or on the units at any time, and appropriate measures shall be taken to ensure that these supplies do not exist.

Correlation of Departmental Policy to Hospital Policy

The above delineated policy is in compliance with hospital policy #44 (example only).

Procedural Documentation

- All supply items of a sterile nature are listed by name and departments or units using them in a sterile supply ledger. A safe sterile shelf life for each item is determined and recorded in the ledger.
- All supplies that are sterilized in the S.P.D. area are affixed with a load control number to indicate a safe expiration date.
- Congruent with each load control number, the following information shall be recorded and maintained in S.P.D.:

    1. Number of items sterilized in the load
    2. Identity of items sterilized

3. The initials of the attendant who was responsible for the sterilization
4. Date the load was sterilized
5. Time and temperature exposure.

- All sterile supplies are rotated in a First In, First Out (FIFO) manner to ensure usage of the oldest stock first.
- Supply cart items are rotated in a similar manner, and sterile supplies are checked each day before being delivered to the nursing units.
- Daily routine checks of S.P.D. stock are conducted by the S.P.D. supervisor to ensure that no outdated supply exists or is used.
- If supplies from a vendor become outdated, they are returned for credit or exchanged for like items.
- Outdated supplies which have been processed by S.P.D. personnel are opened, examined, and if found to be in order, resterilized.
- If for some reason resterilization is not possible, the items are disposed of by the S.P.D. supervisor and adjustments made to the proper account.

Exceptions

None

Attachments

Not applicable

Dates of Approval and Reviews

Approval: December 5, 1978
Review: June 30, 1979
Review: December 30, 1979
Review: June 15, 1980

Authorized Signatures

Administration
Materiel manager
S.P.D. supervisor

Materiel Management Policy and Procedure Number 14

Subject

Evaluation of personnel.

Objective

To provide for the objective, constructive evaluation of the performance of all personnel in the Department of Materiel Management.

Policy Statements

- All employees within the department will receive an annual performance appraisal by their respective supervisors.
- The evaluation is to be in writing and a copy filed in the personnel department.

Correlation of Departmental Policy to Hospital Policy

The above delineated policies are in compliance with hospital policy #11 (example only).

Procedural Documentation

- Both in the hospital and departmental orientation, the new employee is informed of the performance evaluation.
- After 90 days on the job, the employee is given an initial evaluation by the appropriate supervisor. Here, the employee's performance is thoroughly discussed with him/her, with the strong and weak points noted and a plan of action for improved performance delineated.
- Each employee is reevaluated on his/her anniversary date by the respective supervisor.
- The evaluation will consist of at least the following criteria:

    1. A review of the employee's major tasks
    2. A numerical rating of each task
    3. Comments and justification of the rating
    4. A written work improvement program

- After the evaluation has been completed by the supervisor, the employee is notified and scheduled for an evaluation conference.
- At least an hour or two should be given to each employee for a thorough appraisal.
- The employee should also be given a copy of the evaluation to follow as the supervisor reviews it with him or her.
- The evaluation should be performed objectively and the employee given ample time to respond if he or she desires.

- After the evaluation interview is finished, the employee is requested to sign the evaluation as to whether he agrees or disagrees with the appraisal and the work improvement plan.
- The employee is given one copy of the evaluation and another is made a part of his permanent file in the Department of Personnel.
- The main thrust of the evaluation is to assist the employee in his progress and growth with the department as well as with the hospital.
- Salary increases are not discussed in conjunction with the performance evaluation, but are handled separately.
- An evaluation may be performed at any time if deemed necessary by the supervisor.

Exceptions

None

Attachments

Not applicable

Dates of Approval and Reviews

Approved: January 5, 1978
Review: June 1, 1978
Review: January 10, 1979

Authorized Signatures

Administration
Materiel manager

Materiel Management Policy and Procedure Number 15

Subject

Lending of supplies and equipment.

Objective

To provide a control system for any supplies or equipment that is borrowed by other health care institutions.

Policy Statements

- The hospital shall lend needed supplies and equipment to other health care institutions if there is not anticipated need for them, but only for short, specified periods of time.

- The director of materiel management must be consulted before permission for the loan is granted.

Correlation of Departmental Policy to Hospital Policy

The above delineated policies are in compliance with hospital policy #36 (example only).

Procedural Documentation

- All requests to borrow supplies or equipment are to be approved by the director of materiel management.
- He or she should confer with the other department heads if there is some question as to whether the hospital may need the supplies or equipment before the loaned items are returned.
- If the decision is made to loan the requested item or items, then the requesting hospital must:

    1. Furnish roundtrip transportation for the loaned items
    2. Sign a release of responsibility of the lending hospital for any harm to a patient or employee by the requesting hospital because of misuse, malfunction, or use of the supply or equipment
    3. Agree to repair or replace the supplies or equipment in case of damage or loss
    4. Sign an equipment lending form which states the date, the supply description, the date of return, and the signature of the person obtaining the item

- No equipment will be loaned to patients or employees of the hospital.

Exceptions

Physicians who have knowledge of the use of the supplies or equipment may be granted permission to borrow equipment under the same above conditions.

Attachments

Not applicable

Dates of Approval and Reviews

Approval: December 5, 1977
Review: June 30, 1978

Authorized Signatures

Administration
Materiel manager

Materiel Management Policy and Procedure Number 16

Subject

Use of supply and drug locator lists.

Objective

To facilitate the location of needed supplies and drugs.

Policy Statements

- A supply and drug locator list shall be supplied to all departments and nursing units and kept current by the materiel management department.
- Drug and supply continuity will be provided in case of emergencies.

Correlation of Departmental Policy to Hospital Policy

The above delineated policies are in compliance with hospital policy numbers 41 and 51 (example only).

Procedural Documentation

- A format for the supply and drug locator list must be developed and should include the following information:
    1. A list of all supplies and drugs that are kept in stock.
    2. The location of each should be indicated using supply area, aisle, and shelf.
    3. All departments and units which use the items should be indicated.
    4. Suppliers and their telephone numbers should be furnished in case of an emergency in which the hospital has exhausted its total supply of an item.
- The supply and drug locator list should be kept in all departments and nursing units.
- This locator list should include a cross reference of all brand, generic, and common names for all supplies and drugs.
- Since the S.P.D. area should be staffed around the clock, the locator list can still be of invaluable use in personnel orientation, absence of key supervisory persons, and in smaller hospitals where the central stores is not staffed around the clock.

Exceptions

None

Attachments

Not applicable

Dates of Approval and Reviews

Approval: January 5, 1978
Review: June 30, 1978
Review: January 2, 1979
Review: June 29, 1979
Review: January 5, 1980

Authorized Signatures

Administration
Materiel manager

Materiel Management Policy and Procedure Number 17

Subject

Centralized purchasing of supplies, equipment, and service.

Objective

To ensure a standardized and controlled purchasing process.

Policy Statement

All supplies, equipment, and service shall be procured according to a centralized purchasing procedure through the Department of Materiel Management.

Correlation of Departmental Policy to Hospital Policy

The above delineated policy is in compliance with hospital policy #52 (example only).

Procedural Documentation

- All purchasing is to be performed through the Department of Materiel Management.
- All stock items are ordered routinely and automatically upon the reaching of the supply minimum.

- The director of purchasing uses the economic order quantity (E.O.Q.) factor to reorder stock supplies. In other words, when the volume reaches the minimum level, the volume representing the difference between the maximum and minimum supply on hand is ordered.
- For nonstock items, the consuming departments and units use a special requisition form. The departments provide the appropriate specifications on this form and send it to the director of purchasing.
- Upon the receipt of the special requisition form, the purchasing director checks the provided information to see if it is correct and complete. The purchasing director then negotiates price, terms, and delivery dates.
- The special requisition form also provides information as to whether the supply and dollar volume were included in the current budget.
- The purchasing director then forwards the completed requisition to administration for review, comment, and approval.
- All requisitions are then immediately returned to materiel management for appropriate action.
- The purchasing director will assign the requisition a purchase order reference number, have the purchase order processed, attach a copy to the appropriate copy of the requisition, and forward to the requesting department for their files.
- The purchasing director shall transmit the purchase order either by telecopier, sales representative, or mail to the supplier. Also, the designated copies are sent to receiving, data processing, and accounting.
- No purchase order shall be considered valid unless it bears the authorized signature of either the purchasing director or the materiel manager.
- A purchase order must be issued for all contractual arrangements in which some form of financial liability for the hospital exists.
- Equipment or supplies for evaluation must also be ordered through the centralized process.
- Requisitions for capital equipment are to be submitted to the director of maintenance and biomedical engineer for review and comments before being processed.
- Requisitions in the amount of $15,000 or more must be approved by the board of trustees.

Exceptions

None

Attachments

Special requisition form (Figure 5-1)

Figure 5-1 Sample Requisition Form

NAME OF HOSPITAL

REQUISITION
FOR SUPPLIES AND/OR EQUIPMENT
– NOT STOCK ITEMS –

DATE________

SUGGESTED VENDOR

THIS SPACE FOR PURCHASING DEPARTMENT ONLY

VENDOR________ REQUISITION NO.________

ADDRESS________ PURCHASE ORDER NO.________

CITY AND STATE________ TERMS:________

CONFIRMING TO:________ DELIVERY BY________ DELIVERY DATE:________

QUANTITY	ITEM AND DESCRIPTION	UNIT	PRICE

DEPARTMENT DATE REQUIRED REQUESTED BY

COMPLETE THE FOLLOWING IF COST EXCEEDS $50.00 OR IF FOR EQUIPMENT

WAS THIS AMOUNT INCLUDED IN BUDGET? ☐ YES ☐ NO ESTIMATED COST $

WILL ADDITIONAL OR CHANGE OF PERSONNEL BE REQUIRED? ☐ YES ☐ NO IF "YES" STATE ADDED COST $

WILL ADDITIONAL SUPPLIES BE REQUIRED? ☐ YES ☐ NO IF "YES" STATE ADDED COST $

WILL STRUCTURAL CHANGE BE REQUIRED? ☐ YES ☐ NO INSTALLATION COST $

TOTAL ESTIMATED COST________ $________

STATE REASON FOR THIS REQUEST:________

APPROVED BY:

SUPERVISOR________

PURCHASING________

ADMINISTRATIVE APPROVAL:

ADMINISTRATOR________

TREASURER________

PRESIDENT, BOARD OF TRUSTEES________

MATERIEL MANAGER________

ESTIMATED REVENUE $________ SOURCE OF THIS REVENUE________

DO NOT SEPARATE - - - FORWARD COMPLETE FORM TO PURCHASING DEPARTMENT

PR-1/66

Dates of Approval and Reviews

Approval: January 30, 1978
Review: June 15, 1978
Review: January 15, 1979

Authorized Signatures

Administration
Materiel manager

Materiel Management Policy and Procedure Number 18

Subject

Distribution of supply and linen carts.

Objective

To ensure a standardized and systematic method of supply cart delivery.

Policy Statements

- The supply distribution system shall be via a manual total supply cart exchange program.
- All supply carts will be exchanged in a designated manner and according to a predetermined schedule.

Correlation of Departmental Policy to Hospital Policy

The above delineated policies are in compliance with hospital policy #55 (example only).

Procedural Documentation

- All supply carts are to be processed and ready for delivery by 5:00 a.m.
- Manual exchange of all carts will be performed between 5:00 a.m. and 7:00 a.m. daily.
- Supply and linen carts will be delivered according to a designated schedule which was determined by individual hospital time and motion studies.
- Linen carts will be delivered twice daily, in the morning in conjunction with the supply carts and in the afternoon around 2:00 p.m.
- Depleted supply and linen carts are to be returned to S.P.D. for reprocessing upon delivery of a replenished cart.

Exceptions

Exchange isolation technique carts are delivered as needed.

Attachments

Not applicable

Dates of Approval and Reviews

Approval: January 2, 1977
Review: June 30, 1977
Review: January 15, 1978
Review: July 1, 1978
Review: January 3, 1979

Authorized Signatures

Administration
Materiel manager

Materiel Management Policy and Procedure Number 19

Subject

Delivery of supplies and equipment.

Objective

To ensure a standardized and systematic process of delivering supplies and equipment not available via the cart system.

Policy Statement

There shall be a continuous delivery service of supplies and equipment to all departments and nursing units on an "as needed" basis.

Correlation of Departmental Policy to Hospital Policy

The above delineated policy is in compliance with hospital policy #55 (example only).

Procedural Documentation

- S.P.D. will remain open at all times in order to process and deliver needed supplies and equipment.
- All supply requests are to be telephoned via the hotline service to S.P.D., and S.P.D. personnel are to make all deliveries. No departmental or unit personnel are to come to S.P.D. for supplies.
- S.P.D. personnel will be dispatched to the receiving unit within 15 minutes of the request if the item is in stock.
- S.P.D. personnel will complete the necessary requisition and charge information for all telephone orders.

- If telephone request is not in stock, it will be obtained as quickly as possible.
- For items requested and not in stock, S.P.D. personnel shall inform the requesting party of the situation and indicate the action to be taken. For example, if the item is to be borrowed, S.P.D. will take the action to obtain it in the most expeditious manner.

Exceptions

None

Attachments

Not applicable

Dates of Approval and Reviews

Approval: January 1, 1978
Review: June 30, 1978
Review: January 5, 1979

Authorized Signatures

Administration
Materiel manager

Materiel Management Policy and Procedure Number 20

Subject

General sanitation of the S.P.D. area.

Objective

To provide a safe and sanitary area in which to work and store patient care supplies.

Policy Statement

All S.P.D. personnel are to be involved in maintaining the sanitation of the S.P.D. area at a desired high level of cleanliness on a scheduled basis.

Correlation of Departmental Policy to Hospital Policy

The above delineated policy is in compliance with hospital policy #2 (example only).

Procedural Documentation

- In order to ensure a desired level of cleanliness, all work surfaces, tables,

and countertops shall be cleaned thoroughly each day with an approved germicidal solution.
- All floors in the area are to be wet mopped daily by the Housekeeping Department and given a thorough cleaning and buffing each month.
- S.P.D. attendants shall maintain the supply area by daily wiping shelves, removing empty containers, and sweeping floors.
- All work equipment (carts, etc.) shall be sanitized on a daily basis to ensure proper cleanliness.
- The entire S.P.D. area, including vents, lights, etc., is to be vacuumed twice weekly.
- The exchange supply carts are to be cleaned daily and wet washed under pressure at least quarterly.
- Cultures from the general S.P.D. area will be taken periodically to monitor the effectiveness of the above procedures.

Exceptions

None

Attachments

Not applicable

Dates of Approval and Reviews

Approval: June 30, 1978
Review: January 1, 1979

Authorized Signatures

Administration
Materiel manager

Materiel Management Policy and Procedure Number 21

Subject

Processing of isolation carts.

Objective

To provide nursing service with all of the sterile supplies and equipment needed to properly care for the isolated patient.

Policy Statement

Hospital isolation technique is to be assisted and supported by the use of an isolation supply cart exchange program developed in accordance with guidelines approved by the Infection Control Committee.

Correlation of Departmental Policy to Hospital Policy

The above delineated policy is in compliance with hospital policy #33 (example only).

Procedural Documentation

- Supply quotas are established for the patient isolation procedure through the coordinated efforts of materiel management, nursing services, and the Infection Control Committee.
- These supplies are properly packaged and put into a specially designed isolation cart.
- Effort is made to use disposable supplies and equipment whenever possible.
- When the isolation technique is initiated on a nursing unit, an isolation supply cart is ordered from S.P.D. via the telephone hotline service.
- S.P.D. personnel immediately dispatch the isolation cart to the designated space outside the patient's room.
- Supplies are used from the cart by the medical and nursing staffs as needed. When the supplies have been depleted, nursing requests an isolation cart exchange and the procedure is repeated.
- Upon return to the S.P.D. area, the isolation cart is properly cleaned and disinfected by the approved procedure set forth by the Infection Control Committee.
- The isolation cart is completely replenished according to the designated cart quota.
- After being replenished, isolation carts are properly sealed to ensure proper quotas upon arrival to the patient care area.
- A completed charge voucher is attached to the cart for proper charging.
- The isolation cart is stored in the designated clean area for delivery to the units as needed.

Exceptions

None

Attachments

Not applicable

Dates of Approval and Reviews

Approval: June 30, 1978
Review: January 15, 1979

Authorized Signatures

Administration
Materiel manager
Infection control officer

Materiel Management Policy and Procedure Number 22

Subject

Product substitution.

Objective

To assure that the desired quality of supplies is attained in the purchasing process.

Policy Statements

- No product substitutions on behalf of the supplier will be allowed without the prior approval of the materiel manager.
- No product substitutions for standard items will be permitted without the prior approval of the Product Standardization Committee.

Correlation of Departmental Policy to Hospital Policy

The above delineated policies are in compliance with hospital policy #45 (example only).

Procedural Documentation

- Product substitutions are not unacceptable per se, but must be reviewed on an individual basis by the Product Standardization Committee.
- Products may not be substituted in any manner by the supplier without prior approval of the materiel manager.
- Any unauthorized substitutions will be returned to the supplier at the supplier's expense.
- After approval of the committee, the materiel manager or director of purchasing can purchase a substitute if a standard item is unavailable from suppliers and stocks are sufficiently low to warrant substitution.

- Product substitutions will be encouraged under the right conditions because many substitutions are as good as or better and less expensive than the standard item.
- The Product Standardization Committee is always on call for reviewing substitute items.

Exceptions

Emergency items

Attachments

Not applicable

Dates of Approval and Reviews

Approval: June 30, 1977
Review: January 5, 1978
Review: June 15, 1978

Authorized Signatures

Administration
Materiel manager

Materiel Management Policy and Procedure Number 23

Subject

Stockless purchasing.

Objective

To maintain only limited and controlled quantities of unofficial inventory in all departments and nursing units.

Policy Statements

- Unofficial inventory is that which has been dispensed and expensed to the using areas.
- No departments or unit shall have more than a 14-day inventory of supplies at any time.
- Quarterly physical inventories shall be made to assure compliance with this policy.

Correlation of Departmental Policy to Hospital Policy

The above delineated policies are in compliance with hospital policy #55 (example only).

Procedural Documentation

- Items that are used by only one or two departments are prime items for stockless purchasing.
- Stockless purchasing is extremely suited to such departments as laboratory, radiology, respiratory therapy, surgery, and other specialties.
- The materiel manager and the director of each applicable department develops a total list of supplies with corresponding quotas for a certain period of time.
- After the quota list has been established, it is preprinted and used by that department for ordering purposes.
- Any changes in the quota list must be approved by the materiel manager and the respective department director.
- Exact lead times for the acquisition of the items must be carefully determined by the materiel manager for effective results.
- When the stockless supplies are received, they are checked in and forwarded directly to the appropriate department.
- This procedure is repeated over and again with excellent cost containment results both for the respective departments and the hospital in general.
- Quarterly inventories will be taken by the department of materiel management in order to monitor the volume and dollar amounts of this unofficial inventory.
- In order to determine what is exactly a two-week supply, the materiel manager can easily obtain this figure by dividing the respective department's annual supply budget by 26.

Exceptions

None

Attachments

Not applicable

Dates of Approval and Reviews

Approval: January 1, 1978
Review: June 30, 1978
Review: January 2, 1979

Authorized Signatures

Administration
Materiel manager

Materiel Management Policy and Procedure Number 24

Subject

Product standardization.

Objective

To monitor and control the usage of supplies within the hospital with emphasis on the quality of care and the containment of costs.

Policy Statement

Any product which is used within the hospital must undergo evaluation and approval by the Standardization Committee.

Correlation of Departmental Policy to Hospital Policy

The above procedure is in compliance with hospital policy #7 (example only).

Procedural Documentation

- All potential products are to be submitted to the purchasing director either by sales representatives, physicians, hospital personnel, or patients.
- The purchasing director shall perform an initial screening of all items prior to submitting them to the Standardization Committee.
- The purchasing director may contact the concerned departments for their recommendations and comments.
- The samples are requested and evaluation reports are prepared for each item to be reviewed.
- Possible committee actions include:

    1. Acceptance of product
    2. Rejection of product
    3. Request for extensive review with periods of evaluation being 30, 60, or 90 days.

- Products to be evaluated are to be provided at the expense of the supplier if at all possible.
- Once an item has been reviewed, the product will not be reconsidered by the committee for at least a period of one year, unless there is a favorable price or product change.
- The concerned department is responsible for submitting a product orientation and utilization procedure to the Standardization Committee for review before the newly accepted product is purchased.
- The Standardization Committee shall submit a list of all newly accepted

standard items to the Patient Charge Review Board for their review and determination of patient charge before the item is purchased.
- The minutes of each Standardization Committee meeting are sent to the administration for review and approval. His/her approval constitutes authority to purchase the new item as a standard in its category.

Exceptions

Supplies needed in an emergency situation. However, at the next meeting of the Standardization Committee, this situation will be reviewed in detail and necessary action delineated.

Attachments

None

Dates of Approval and Reviews

Approval: June 3, 1978
Review: January 1, 1979

Authorized Signatures

Administration
Materiel manager

Materiel Management Policy and Procedure Number 25

Subject

Hospital compliance with the prudent buyer principle.

Objective

To ensure that the hospital is obtaining supplies and equipment at prices which are within or below the comparable range of prices paid for similar products by hospitals in the surrounding area.

Policy Statements

- The hospital and Department of Materiel Management will closely adhere to the concept of obtaining quality supplies and equipment at the lowest possible costs if all other factors remain equal.
- The department also recognizes that there is much more to materiel management than the price of purchased goods, so it works toward cost containment and excellent service in all functions of materiel management from acquisition to disposition.

Correlation of Departmental Policy to Hospital Policy

The above delineated policies are in compliance with hospital policy #49 (example only).

Procedural Documentation

- The department will encourage and will participate in any and all legitimate programs of supply cost comparisons.
- All purchasing of supplies, equipment, and services will be performed through centralized purchasing and a uniform procurement procedure.
- Purchase orders are to be issued for all purchase obligations of the hospital, even for supplies and equipment brought in for evaluation.
- Purchase orders always show terms and total price paid. If rebates or discounts are given by the supplier, they are to be reflected in the stated price on the purchase order and not taken off the face of the invoice or the final monthly statement. If the hospital will get a discount for paying the total amount of the invoice by a certain date, then this discount is also reflected in the stated purchase order price and the hospital will always pay the invoice by that date.
- Purchases are made only on the basis of hospital requisitions that have been approved by authorized personnel.
- Competitive bids are obtained on all purchases of materials, supplies, and services over the amount of $1,000.
- Competitive bids from at least three sources are always obtained on construction contracts.
- All bid information that was requested and received is filed with the hospital copy of the purchase order to the selected vendor.
- In all cases where the hospital selects other than the lowest bidder, the materiel manager provides a thorough written explanation which is filed with the hospital copy of the purchase order to the selected vendor.
- The Department of Materiel Management maintains an up-to-date list of all approved vendors, supplies, and contractors.
- The hospital also provides a written policy and procedure for the selection of vendors and contractors.
- The Department of Materiel Management maintains effective up-to-date maximums and minimums on all approved supplies and equipment.
- The department, in conjunction with the Product Standardization Committee, establishes workable specifications on all standard supplies and equipment.
- The Department of Materiel Management in cooperation with financial management has established a written procedure of internal control for the comparison of invoiced prices, quantities ordered, and terms on the

original purchase order with the receiving copy and the final invoice. There are at least three independent parties involved in the process.

- Where there are alternatives to providing a certain commodity, such as contracting laundry services versus hospital operation of these services, the materiel manager will enumerate the alternatives and provide in writing the criteria for considering all alternatives and making the final selection.
- The entire materiel management function is appropriately involved in the hospital annual independent audit.
- This prudent purchasing policy and procedure will be communicated and posted in all departments.
- Any and all potential conflicts of interest are to be delineated and avoided in the area of purchasing and management of materiel.
- Supply cost comparisons of similar hospitals in similar localities with similar supplies will be conducted at regular intervals and used as a purchasing and negotiation tool.
- Group purchasing contracts will be entered into whenever there is a cost, quality, or service advantage for the hospital.
- The director of purchasing will not purchase supplies or equipment that has not first been approved by the Hospital Product Standardization Committee.
- Distribution and handling of supplies and equipment will be kept to an absolute minimum.

Exceptions

None

Attachments

Not applicable

Dates of Approval and Reviews

Approval: June 30, 1977
Review: January 5, 1978
Review: June 29, 1978
Review: January 10, 1979

Authorized Signatures

Administration
Materiel manager

These delineated examples give a good view of the thoroughness, quality, and exactness that should go into the development of materiel management policies and procedures. However, there are many more topics that must be addressed in the same manner. The following subject list can be used as a guide to develop pertinent policies and procedures for your own hospital.

In the area of pharmaceutical services

- Administration of medication
- Adverse drug reaction
- Alcohol control
- Antidote stocks and information
- Approved services
- Control of cocaine
- Disaster contingency plan
- Drug recalls
- Drug sample policy
- Drug transaction control and accountability
- Employee purchase of pharmaceuticals
- Filling of medication orders
- Heparin flush
- Hyperalimentation solution preparation
- Medication checks
- Medications brought to the hospital by the patient
- Narcotics control
- Emergency cabinet stocking utilization
- Outpatient prescriptions
- Periodic pharmacy inspection of nursing units
- Pharmacy departmental meetings
- Physician medication orders
- Pricing policy for pharmacy
- Procurement of approved drugs, chemicals, and biologicals
- Purchase of all drugs, except schedule II
- Purchase of schedule II drugs
- Receiving of drugs, except schedule II
- Receiving of schedule II drugs
- Reconstitution of chemotherapy agents
- Reporting of medication errors
- Requisition of non-stock drugs
- Self-administration of medication
- Usage of abbreviations and chemical symbols
- Use of investigational drugs

In the areas of S.P.D. and purchased services

- Aeration of gas sterilized supplies
- Authorization to purchase
- Back-door purchasing
- Blanket purchase orders
- Biological monitoring of sterilization system
- Care of the staging and dock area
- Centralized purchasing philosophy
- Competitive bidding
- Conflict of interest in purchasing
- Contributions from suppliers
- Delineation of purchasing organization
- Delineation of S.P.D. organizational function
- Desirable inventory
- Desired inventory levels
- Displays by sales representatives
- Distribution of mail
- Economic order quantities
- Emergency delivery of supplies and equipment
- Employee acceptance of gifts and gratuities
- Exploration of purchasing alternatives
- Gas sterilization of surgery supplies
- General usage requisitions
- Group purchasing
- Leasing policy
- Limited access to S.P.D.
- Linen collection
- Linen transportation
- Load control numbers
- Preventive maintenance records and reports
- Prime supplier philosophy
- Processing and sterilization of reusable patient care supplies
- Processing of isolation carts

- Product obsolescence
- Product recalls
- Product specifications
- Purchase of capital equipment
- Purchasing for and/or selling to employees
- Receiving of supplies and equipment
- Reproduction of inhouse forms
- Service and supply of copier machines
- Spot culturing of the S.P.D. area
- S.P.D. departmental meetings
- S.P.D. internal disaster contingency plan
- S.P.D. inventory process
- Storage of supplies and equipment
- Supply cart processing
- Tours of the S.P.D. area
- Training of new personnel
- Unification of all S.P.D. functions
- Use of elevators by S.P.D. personnel
- Vendors list

Policy and procedure writing represents a lot of work, but the feeling is one of accomplishment after the task has been completed. Policy and procedures in essence set standards of expected performance that have been reduced to writing. They represent what is to be done.

For policies and procedures to be really effective, they must be simply stated, clearly defined, understandable, known to all appropriate parties, updated on a timely basis, reviewed, revised, approved and enforced by top management.

Pertinent Points to Ponder

1. Why are policies and procedures important to the materiel management philosophy?
2. What should be the connection between a policy and a procedure?
3. Who should be responsible for the development of materiel management policies and procedures?
4. What are the reasons that most hospitals do not have good materiel management policies and procedures?
5. Can the Department of Materiel Management have policies and procedures without the hospital having administrative policies and procedures? Why?
6. On the average, how many policies should the Department of Materiel Management have?
7. Will policies and procedures differ with the size of the institution?
8. What factors will cause a variance in materiel management policies and procedures from one hospital to another?
9. Why is it important to correlate the materiel management policies with those of the hospital?

10. Can a hospital department such as materiel management have policies without having procedures? Which are the most important?
11. In your opinion, what should be the basis of all departmental policies and procedures?
12. What happens if a hospital or departmental policy is ignored or administered improperly?

Chapter 6

The Act of Purchasing Should Be Simple and Results Oriented*

A Simple System Must Be Planned and Initiated

The purchase order has long been the umbilical cord of the purchasing process. This document represents a maze of red tape that is both duplicative and expensive. Presently, the average hospital system requires that five to ten copies of this form be made, and the average cost of this process is five to fifteen cents per copy. If the purchase order has become a costly artifact that is not really essential to the procurement cycle, what can replace it?

Some hospitals have experimented with several methods of data transmission that would be virtually paperless, and a device that offers promise is the Xerox Telecopier. The dilemma, which is characteristic of most hospitals, is that the requesting departments want to know that an item has been issued, ordered, and/or received. For instance, receiving must know that an order has been placed in order that it be received properly. Likewise, data processing needs certain information to update the computerized inventory readout if applicable. Last, accounting must be able to validate receipt of an order to be able to issue payment. Consideration of all these factors resulted in the creation of a Purchasing-Accounting-Receiving-Data Processing (P.A.R.D.) system of purchase data transmission (Figure 6-1).

The Telecopier is both a transmitter and a receiver. With this method, one piece of paper is generated by the hospital and another one by the supplier. A single preprinted form is the input document. To be effective, the document should be a listing of the frequently used supply items referenced only by a supplier number and a space to enter the quantity. The input document

*Reprinted with the permission of DIMENSIONS in Health Service, Journal of the Canadian Hospital Association.

Figure 6-1 P.A.R.D. System of Purchase Ordering

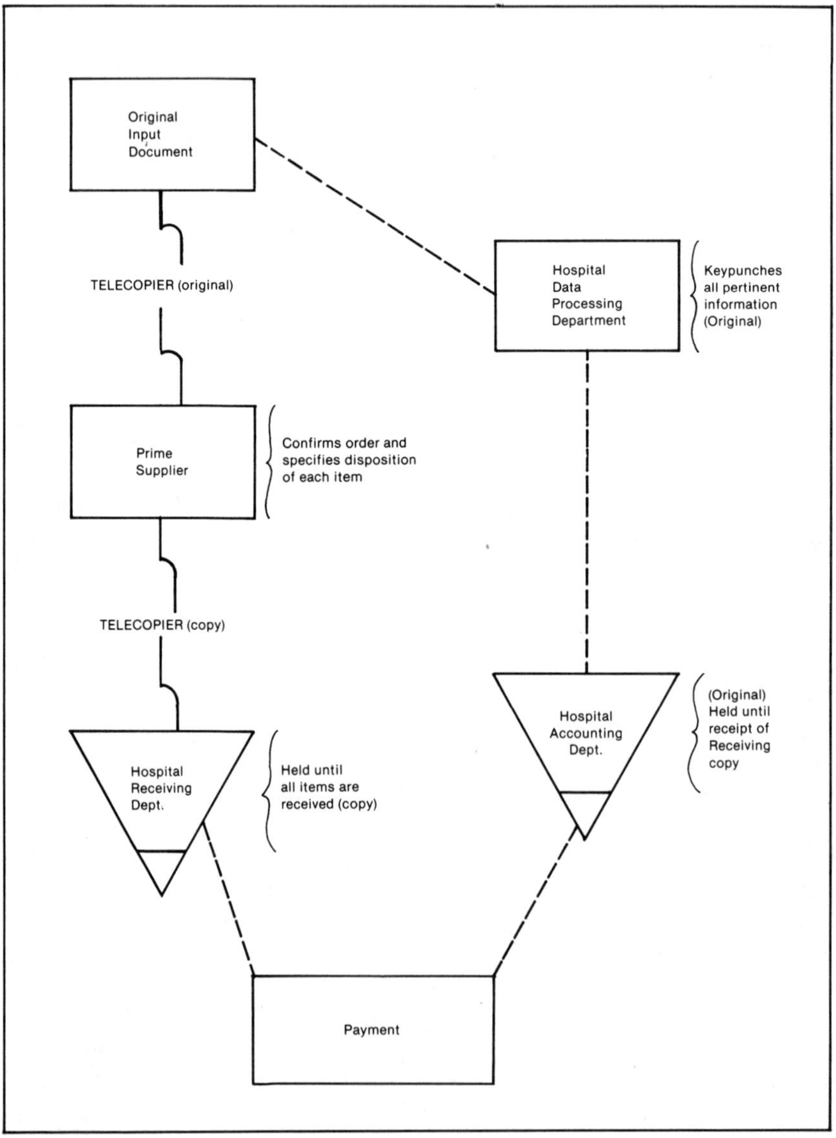

also has space to write the names of seldom used items. After the input document is completed, the purchasing agent or secretary transmits it over the Telecopier to the supplier. The original is then forwarded to data process-

Exhibit 6-1 The purchasing agent uses the Telecopier to transmit purchase orders to the supplier.

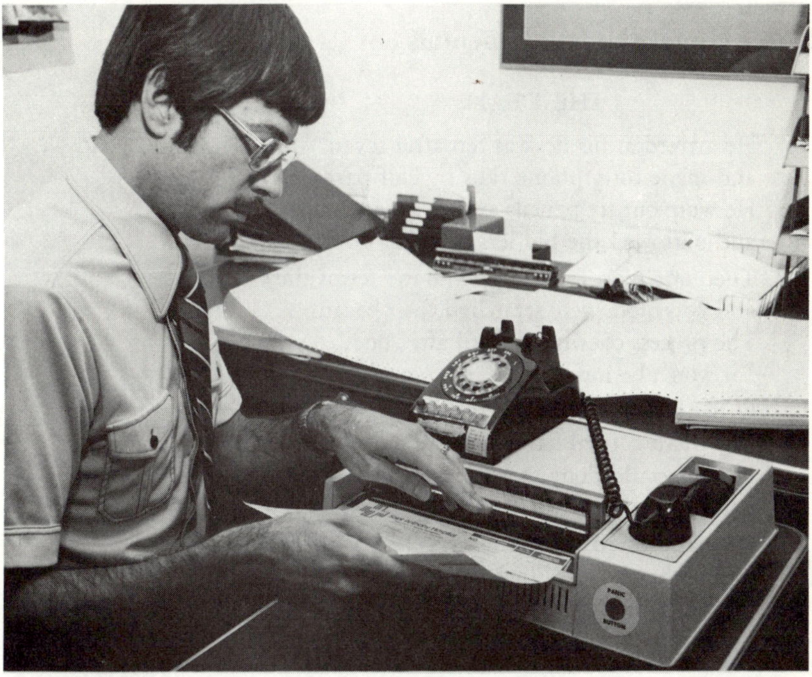

ing, which then sends it on to the Accounting Department where it is held until the supplies are received and payment is made.

After the supplier receives the order, the disposition of each item is determined and the pertinent information is transmitted back to the hospital within minutes. This copy is then kept by receiving until the supplies have arrived, at which time it is sent along with the supplier's invoice to accounting to be checked against the original. As can be seen, the entire process involves the hospital in handling only two pieces of paper. Furthermore, a very simple numbering system allows purchase order numbers to be used for control. Simply indicate on the original document the numbers representing the day, month, year, and the number of that transaction for the day. For example, the fourth purchasing transaction of July 12, 1979, would be indicated as 71279-4. In addition, under this P.A.R.D. system all back orders are identified and transferred to a separate purchase order.

Reduction of paperwork should be one of the goals of every materiel manager, an objective which this procedure achieves. The act of purchasing should become a repetitive, simple task, which ultimately should not be in the job description of the true materiel manager. In the long run, after automating or mechanizing its function for maximum utilization of time and talent, the manager should have only to supervise it.

Don't Forget the Fundamentals

THE DEAL

He arrived at his desk at ten after seven,
and made forty phone calls by half past eleven.
He wore out six pencils and emptied his pen
and narrowed the bidders list clear down to ten.

Then one more was dropped—the terms they were net,
and two more were scratched, just because. . . I forget.
The process continued until after one,
"it won't be long now. . . the work's about done."

Other bids were cast out for this reason or that,
and the two final names carefully dropped in the hat.
No one could deny that the process was fair,
and the name of the winner was pulled out with much flair.

He was pleased with himself as he paced on the floor,
and dashed out to lunch and returned about four.
He was quite satisfied, his pleasure immense
on the three dollar purchase—he saved 13¢.

Anonymous

In this day of computers and advanced technology, it is easy to lose sight of the basic principles of materiel management. It seems that a system has to be complex to be worth considering. It must be computerized, centralized, pressurized, automated, integrated, or amalgamated to get our attention. However, it is sobering to consider that all of those systems and concepts must be built around very simple, fundamental principles. In all my consultations with hospitals that are having problems in managing materiel, I frequently find that the simple fundamentals have most often been violated. For example, a hospital that was having problems with its perpetual inventory system is having more problems than ever now that the inventory has been computerized. This is because computers will not correct human mistakes.

Underlying all the sophisticated and innovative materiel management concepts, such as automated cart systems, electronic ordering systems, and computerized moving averages for inventory pricing, are some basic functions that must be operating well or all of the technology goes for naught. The seven fundamentals that must be practiced religiously for materiel management concepts to be implemented effectively are as follows:

1. Effective management and supervision
2. Sound purchasing methods
3. An efficient purchase system
4. A simple inventory control program
5. Results-oriented requisition and distribution system
6. Written policies and procedures
7. A practical receiving program

Fundamental one, effective management and supervision, cannot be emphasized enough. The entire materiel management thrust must be built on the managerial functions of planning, organizing, directing, controlling, and staffing. These functions, if effectively applied, can cover a multitude of technical blunders. Effective supervision can seek out the simple mistakes and correct them before they become major problems. Good management practices and results-oriented supervision must permeate the entire materiel management effort from the basics to the complexities.

Fundamental two, sound purchasing methods, accentuates the art and skill of ethical, hard-nosed negotiation. "Negotiation" is a word that is not heard often today in hospital purchasing circles. Words like "buy," "purchase," "procure," and "acquire" are in vogue. The word "negotiation," however, suggests that some effort is expended to bring about a mutual agreement, so that negotiation involves both the hospital and the supplier. Some rules of negotiation for hospitals to follow are:

- Never purchase at list price.
- Ask for the quantity price, and then try to get that price for any amount purchased.
- Always ask for a discount regardless of how little you buy.
- Always ask for price protection on negotiated prices. Begin with two years and work downward. Remember, price protection for even 30 days is better than no price protection at all.
- Assume you will get at least 2 percent if you pay the total invoice by the tenth of the next month.
- Never feel sorry for the supplier or the sales representative.
- Try quoting prices at which the supplier will sell, rather than having the supplier quote prices at which the hospital must buy.
- Always keep in mind that regardless of how good a price you are getting, most likely somebody is getting a better one.

The purchasing act is one of the fundamental functions in the supply cycle (Exhibit 6-2). In calculating how the act is executed, hospitals generally can obtain better prices than they are presently getting by either requesting or negotiating them. In reference to good prices, studies have shown that it is not the size of the hospital which counts, but rather the quality and determination of the person who does the purchasing.

Fundamental three, an efficient purchase system, again stresses simplicity. If the purchase system adds substantially to the price of the commodity being bought, then it is highly inappropriate. For instance, some authorities have stated that it costs between $35 and $40 to initiate an uncomplicated purchase order (one with no back orders). If, for instance, the entire order is under $100, the purchasing system has increased cost by some forty percent. In order to start simplifying the system, the materiel manager can try to have the requisition double as the purchase order, not type purchase data, limit the purchase document to only one copy, and have the companies supply the purchase orders.

Exhibit 6-2 The act of purchasing is a fundamental function in the supply cycle.

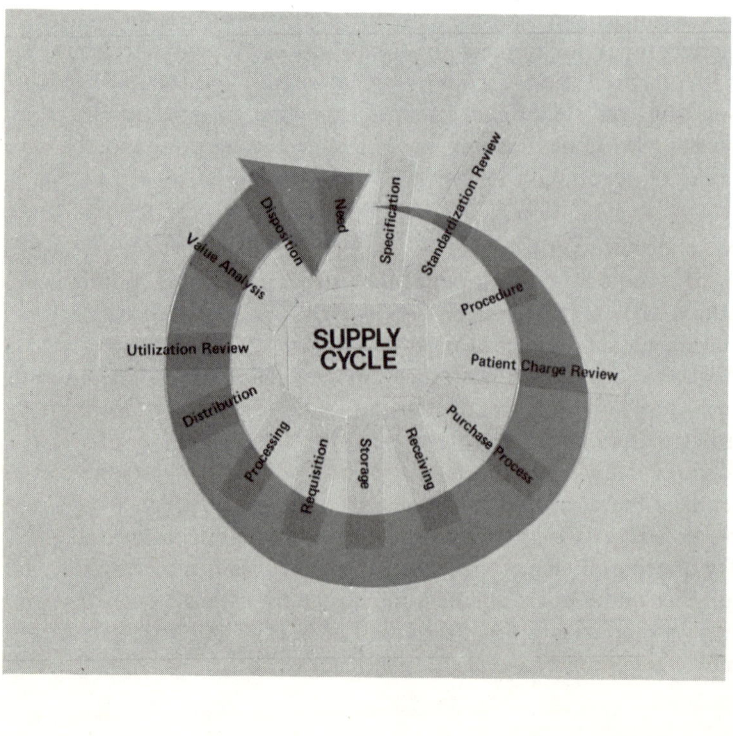

Fundamental four, a simple inventory control program, is very meaningful. If you have more than 500 items in central stores, you probably have too many! Computerization of inventories is an outward expression that your inventory got so big you had to have a computer to control it. The inventory should be small enough to keep it replenished without relying on computerization to supply the information. The secret to an inventory is to control it, not count it.

Fundamental five, a results-oriented requisition and distribution system, is imperative to the materiel management function. The materiel manager must develop a sound and credible requisition and distribution procedure which results in having the right supply, at the right place and time, in the right quantities.

Fundamental six, written policies and procedures, provides the foundation for the building of the materiel management structure. In the efficient materiel management setting, there is a need for some 100 to 150 policies and procedures.

Fundamental seven, a practical receiving program, denotes the need for accountability and responsibility. A good receiving program will have internal control built directly into it. For the best results, the purchasing, receiving, and paying of invoices should be done by separate persons. Receiving of supplies and equipment is one of the most important functions in the materiel management continuum and should be executed in a professional and ethical manner.

If your materiel management program is giving you troubles that were not anticipated, chances are you have violated some or all of the fundamentals. Remember, when all else fails, return to the basics.

The Necessity for Centralized Purchasing

The concept of centralized purchasing has been around for decades, but while hospital managers vow that it is right and proper, they continue to allow decentralized purchasing to exist and prosper. Decentralization of purchasing is as direct a violation of good materiel management practices as centralized purchasing is an essential element of it.

Generally speaking, there are five major violators of the principle of centralized purchasing in most hospitals—the pharmacy, dietary, radiology, laboratory, and plant maintenance departments. When queried as to why they should perform their own purchasing, the answer most likely will be that their needs and products are different and special and only they have the expertise to buy them. This is a very poor argument at best! No product or supply is so special that it cannot be purchased by a capable materiel manager or purchasing agent if he or she is given the proper specifications. In reality, many departmental directors do not know what they want well enough to instruct the purchasing agent on what to buy. For the sake of efficiency and cost effectiveness, they should be required to figure out and specify what they really need so that all goods and services may be purchased by the designated purchasing department. This policy should be made explicitly clear to any prospective directors of pharmacy, laboratory, radiology, dietary, and maintenance to avoid any future misunderstanding.

Why is the precept of centralized purchasing so important? For one, it sets the tone for the entire materiel management program of the hospital. It emphasizes that purchasing is important and that persons with certain training, competency, and authority should perform this function. In addition, it is safe to predict that an effective and efficient materiel management effort cannot be made upon decentralized purchasing.

Centralized purchasing promotes uniformity of the purchasing and receiving process, which includes specification clearance, price negotiation, hospital policy adherence, time determinations, product receiving, invoice payment, and proper file documentation. Furthermore, it assures that all of these tasks are executed in an efficient and uniform manner. These days, with the function of purchasing more complex than ever, and pressure and attention placed on this area by management, government, and third party payers, purchasing and supply negotiations must be done by a competent full-time professional who knows the appropriate legalities and the various related regulations.

Centralized purchasing also encourages adherence to product specifications. All department heads should be responsible for determining the quality and specifications of the products they use. However, there are very few good product specifications provided to the supplier by the hospitals, and value analysis and product service standards are rarely found. The necessary impetus for hospitals to put more emphasis in this area should be provided by centralized purchasing.

Centralized purchasing also greatly assists the product standardization process. When several departments are utilizing similar but different products, the centralized purchasing department can readily spot this common phenomenon and take the necessary steps to standardize these items. Saving to the hospital will result because the purchasing agent will be able to negotiate a better price based on combined volumes. This aspect would have gone unnoticed under decentralized purchasing.

Suppliers are often criticized for their "back door selling" techniques. In other words, they will market, sell, and ship to anyone in the hospital that shows an interest in their product. However, hospitals are just as guilty for their "back door buying" practices. As long as decentralized purchasing is tolerated and overlooked, it will be done. Centralized purchasing, of course, does away with both back-door selling and buying.

Finally, centralized purchasing relieves the various departments of the tasks of interviewing and negotiating with sales representatives. Certainly, departmental directors have enough to do without getting into the purchasing act. If the concept of total centralized purchasing is presented and implemented in the right manner, it will sell itself, and the hospital will be the ultimate benefactor. Unfortunately, in a recent survey of 500 U.S. hospitals, only six percent indicated that they practiced true centralized purchasing.

Hospitals Should Share Prices

With every purchasing agent, buyer, and materiel manager, there is reluctance to share openly supply prices with their colleagues. Everyone is looking for the elusive best price for hospital commodities, and almost everyone thinks he or she has obtained it. But how can you tell if your hospital is getting even a good price? Even if there is information sharing, conditions such as "This is just a tentative price," or "I also get a certain discount off that price," or "This is the last price I received, however, the next price will be lower" go along with it. Unfortunately, in acting in this manner, purchasing agents are playing right into the suppliers' hands. Surveys have shown that the lowest price is not necessarily characteristic of any certain type of hospital, and even group purchasing associations do not always get the best price. What then determines who will get the best price? The truth is that no one knows because there is no knowledge of who is getting the best price.

The one known constant is that prices for the same product vary from hospital to hospital, region to region, and dealer to dealer. Why do prices for identical supplies differ? The major reasons are as follows:

a. In some cases, volume is a factor of price. The greater the volume, the lower the price.
b. Location can make a difference. The greater distance the supply must be transported, the higher the price.
c. The negotiation skill of the purchasing agent is a factor.
d. The type of supply sometimes makes a difference.
e. The prestige of the institution can have a distinct effect on prices. Large teaching hospitals oftentimes get their products at cost because there is the likelihood that these products will become standards of practice for future physicians.
f. The supplier's need to make a quota or promotional sale is a factor.

All this indicates that hospital purchasing personnel should share supply prices on a frequent and scheduled basis. Hospital associations, hospital councils, and purchasing groups, in the same vein, should develop, implement, and participate in a supply price comparison survey to serve as a purchasing index for individual hospital purchasing agents. In the art of negotiation, the more knowledgeable agent can better achieve the objective of purchasing at an advantageous price. However, there seems to be a certain security in not knowing the pertinent information. It must be stressed that the important issue is not that one is paying the highest prices, but that one is taking the necessary steps to prevent this from happening over and over. Supply price comparisons should be looked upon only as an organizational tool to assist the purchasing department to do a more intelligent job of negotiation. After all, there may well be legitimate reasons for paying more.

Who should take the initiative and implement a supply price comparison index? It can be performed by almost anyone at any level; however, the more support it has the more credibility it will receive. A hospital council or association representing several hospitals is an ideal vehicle. It is imperative that the concept behind the comparison index be communicated to the administrators as well as to the purchasing agents and materiel managers. Top management support is a must in such a sensitive endeavor.

The survey can be divided into three components: the construction of an effective survey form, information retrieval, and information dissemination. To begin, it might be advisable to select ten of the highest dollar volume supplies in ten supply categories used by a majority of the hospitals participating in the survey. Also, it is advisable, wherever possible, to specify brand names instead of generic equivalents. However, in categories such as linen and dietary items, it is difficult to compare brand names, so a space should be provided to indicate the manufacturer or supplier. After the initial list of 100 frequently used items has been compiled, it should be decided what other general information, such as size and location of hospital, type of purchasing practice, and group purchasing affiliation, should be included. This information can have a great bearing on the survey. For instance, if the sample is large enough, one might find that prices are lower in hospitals that practice centralized purchasing or are higher in a rural setting.

After the survey form has been devised, it should be sent to all participating hospitals with a concise set of instructions for its completion and a specified return date. Don't be too concerned to find that the initial return rate is disappointing. My experience indicates that an effort is successful if it produces a 25 percent return rate.

After the prices have been correlated to the informational hospital statistics, summarize the data and distribute it only to those hospitals which participated in the survey. To be effective, the report should not refer to any of the hospitals, but to all hospitals in general. Price data for each supply should be referenced as to the lowest, highest, and average price paid. This format can be very helpful to the purchasing agent or the materiel manager. The entire survey should be repeated quarterly or semiannually to determine any changes in the price index.

Pertinent Points to Ponder

1. Why should the purchasing process be simplified?
2. What is the difference between purchasing and negotiation?
3. Can the hospital alter the purchase process without involving the supplier? Why or why not?
4. Who should pay for the purchase orders, the hospital or the supplier? Why?
5. Why do computerized systems appeal to hospital purchasing agents and materiel managers?
6. Why hasn't centralized purchasing been practiced by more hospitals?
7. What departments do their own purchasing in your hospital? Why?
8. Why is it important for hospitals to centralize the purchasing function?
9. Is getting the best price always the most important objective of purchasing? Why or why not?
10. In your opinion, why don't hospitals openly share their supply prices?
11. How do the prudent buyer auditors obtain their prices for determining maximum allowable costs?
12. If you find you are paying exorbitant prices for supplies and equipment, what alternatives are available to you?

Chapter 7

All About The Product Standardization Process

The prudent purchasing principle outlines several requirements for hospitals to meet in order to carry out responsible purchasing from the standpoint of governmental regulations. However, it is more concerned with price than anything else. For instance, a hospital can buy a ten-year supply of an item if the price is right. This does not, however, take into account the total cost of having the right supply in the right quantities at the right place and time. If third parties really wanted to bring about cost containment and cost avoidance in hospitals on a large-scale basis, nothing could do it better than mandatory product standardization.

Under federal mandate and regulation, hospitals were forced to develop and maintain utilization committees to review appropriateness of care and to determine that it was provided at the proper level. As a result, hospital stays were shortened and inpatient occupancy decreased. As a corollary to this, a product standardization committee is nothing more than a utilization committee for supplies, and a hard-nosed hospital standardization program would surely decrease the number of products and the cost of supplies per diem. Should product standardization committees become mandatory for all hospitals? The answer is an unqualified "yes," with hospital management mandating their development and use before government and third parties beat us to the punch.

Planning for Effectiveness

There always have been standardization programs in hospitals. The important question is if they have been effective. Since the expenses of hospital supplies are increasing at a never-ending rate, emphasis must be placed on the containment and reduction of costs. It has been demonstrated that the best way to achieve the money-saving benefits of product standardization and evaluation is through a well organized and results-motivated committee. Despite this, a recent U.S. survey indicated that only half of the hospitals use standardization committees in making purchasing decisions, even though hospital supply costs rank second only to labor costs. Why, then, don't all hospitals initiate and operate such committees? The answer most likely is that most standardization efforts in the past have just not been effective. The two main reasons for this ineffectiveness have been the lack of total commitment and involvement in the process by the various hospital disciplines and the lack of standards by which to measure success.

Administrative Support Through Policy Delineation

Support from top management is the key element in any successful standardization endeavor. An administrative policy and procedure should be drawn up at the earliest possible date setting forth the objectives, duties, and responsibilities of everyone involved in the standardization efforts. Then this policy statement or directive should be delineated in writing and distributed to all concerned parties. A guideline is as follows:

Subject

Administrative policy for product and equipment evaluation and standardization.

Objective

To monitor and control the use of supplies and equipment within the hospital with emphasis on the quality of care and the containment of costs.

Policy Statement

It shall be the policy of this hospital that any product or piece of equipment which is proposed for use within the hospital must first undergo evaluation and approval by the Evaluation and Standardization of Products Committee.

Procedural Documentation

- All potential products (either for use or evaluation) must be submitted to the Department of Materiel Management by physicians, hospital personnel, sales representatives, patients, etc.
- The department will initially screen all items before submitting them to the Standardization Committee.

- The materiel manager will contact the concerned departments for their recommendations and comments before the item is brought to the committee for review.
- A product standardization profile (Figure 7–1) is prepared for each item to be reviewed. The profile of each item is distributed to each committee member at the meeting.
- An agenda is prepared and distributed at least one week prior to the next committee meeting.
- The committee shall meet at least monthly and also on an ''as needed'' basis.
- If the requesting department is not represented on the committee, then it may send a representative to present the item. This representative may vote in this one case.
- Possible committee actions are:

    a. Acceptance of the product
    b. Nonacceptance of the product
    c. A 30-day evaluation
    d. A 60-day evaluation
    e. A 90-day evaluation.

- The products to be evaluated are to be paid for by the supplier if at all possible.
- Once an item has been reviewed and rejected, the product will not be reconsidered by the committee for at least a year unless there is a favorable price or product change.
- If an item is approved, the respective department is responsible for submitting a product orientation and utilization procedure to the Standardization Committee for review before the newly accepted product is actually purchased.
- The Committee also shall submit a list of all newly proposed items to the Patient Charge Committee for their review and determination of patient charge (if applicable) before the item is reviewed by the Standardization Committee.
- The minutes of all committee meetings must be sent to the administrator or his delegate before any action is taken. If the administration does not approve of the stated action or actions, this is communicated back to the committee and the item or items are not purchased.

Exceptions

All items must undergo the above procedure with one exception. If the product is requested on an emergency basis by a physician, it can be

Figure 7-1 Product Standardization Profile

DATE:______________ HOSPITAL PRODUCT NUMBER______________

REQUESTED PRODUCT:______________

MANUFACTURER:______________

SUPPLIED BY:______________

REQUESTED BY:______________

REQUESTED ITEM WILL:

- ☐ BE AN ADDITIONAL ITEM
- ☐ REPLACES:______________
- ☐ REDUCES USE OF ANOTHER ITEM:______________
- ☐ OTHER:______________

PRODUCT COMPARISONS:

CHARACTERISTICS	PRESENT ITEM	REQUESTED ITEM
MANUFACTURER		
SUPPLIER		
ANNUAL USE		
USE AND/OR EVALUATION RESULTS		
AVAILABILITY		
PATIENT CHARGE		
PACKAGING DATA		
HOSPITAL STOCK ITEM		
MINIMUM ORDER QUANTITY		
ADVANTAGES		
DISADVANTAGES		
QUANTITY ON HAND		
COST PER UNIT		
NET SAVINGS (OR LOSS)		
OTHER		

Figure 7-1 continued

STANDARDIZATION COMMITTEE ACTION:

☐ ACCEPTED

☐ NOT APPROVED

☐ APPROVED FOR 30 DAYS EVALUATION

☐ APPROVED FOR 60 DAYS EVALUATION

☐ APPROVED FOR 90 DAYS EVALUATION

☐ TABLED PENDING FURTHER INFORMATION

☐ OTHER:______________________________

ADDITIONAL COMMENTS:______________________________

____

____

____

DATE:____

SIGNATURE OF CHAIRMAN:______________________________

____

purchased. However, this item and action will be reviewed at the next committee meeting.

Review and Comment

At least annually.

Authorized Signature

Administrator.

This policy and procedure format can serve as the organizational structure for the entire standardization process. With this key document and proclamation, it now is up to the other members of the Standardization Committee to cooperate in the team effort required to accomplish the goals.

Committee Representation

After administration has expressed the necessary concern and interest, it is imperative to involve key members of the medical staff in the process. There must be a genuine attempt to interest members of the medical staff in the process because the physician is the ultimate consumer of most products and equipment. Therefore, it only stands to reason that the physicians should be included and properly oriented to the purpose and function of product standardization. Furthermore, every possible attempt should be made to elevate this committee to the position it deserves, and representation by the medical staff is an important element in this effort. Committee leadership, however, should come from a hospital rather than medical department.

Physicians should be appointed by the chief of the medical staff, and service on the Standardization Committee should help fulfill the physician's committee membership responsibilities. In other words, to the physician the product standardization effort becomes a medical staff duty. Why haven't physicians been involved in standardization efforts in the past? Some indicate that they do not have the time to participate in such a menial task. Others have stated that the physicians will dominate and intimidate the other members of the standardization committee. These are just excuses! After all, like the other members, each physician has only one vote. Experience has shown that physicians will participate vigorously and unselfishly in such programs. They feel they receive an excellent product orientation and education for a minimum expenditure of time and effort. In fact, if presented properly, the Standardization Committee can become the best attended and most active committee in the organizational structure. Furthermore, it is beneficial to rotate medical staff membership at least annually because physicians who have served on this committee are more knowledgeable and hence more appreciative of the entire materiel management philosophy.

Since a large number of the products that come before the review process are patient care oriented in some way, nursing service also must be well represented on the standardization team. Nursing representation should almost parallel that of the medical staff, with nursing administration and each of the major nursing divisions providing at least one member. Additionally, experience has demonstrated that "nursing inservice" can create havoc with the standardization process. Through the use of samples of new products on the nursing units without prior knowledge of materiel management or purchasing. Invariably, when the samples are used up, the nurses request more of these nonstocked items. The resulting conflict between nursing and materiel management can be eliminated by including appropriate nursing personnel in the standardization review, thereby involving them in the effort to follow all the procedures. Finally, the traditional concern over nursing representatives sticking together to exercise a bloc vote has been shown in practice to be unfounded.

Since standardization represents a team approach, other participants should be recruited (Table 7-1, Exhibit 7-1). The hospital financial director is an excellent draft choice, because often cost analysis of one product versus another must be performed before a decision can be made. Since the purchasing agent or materiel manager is ultimately involved with the supply scene, he or she also must be an active participant in the standardization process.

However, a bit of caution should be exercised against having too many members from materiel management. Laboratory and radiology should be involved because they represent the major stockless purchasing areas, as should

Table 7-1: Membership of product evaluation committees, according to a U.S. national survey.

Hospital Position	Membership on Committee
Purchasing Agent	81%
Central Supply Supervisor	77
Nursing Service Representative	74
Director of Nursing	57
In-Service Education Coordinator	57
Operating Room Supervisor	57
Physician	50
Materiel Manager	41
Infection Control Nurse	37
Administrator	32
Pharmacist	30
Engineer	24
Administrative Coordinator	14
Assistant Administrator	10
Director of Finance/Comptroller	8

Source: Reprinted, with permission, from Robert B. Rock, Jr., and Cecelia Meshelany, "Studying the Statistics on Standardization Committees," *Hospitals, Journal of the American Hospital Association, 50,* Dec. 16, 1976, pp. 81–88.

Exhibit 7-1 Product standardization for hospitals can best be performed by a well structured multi-disciplinary committee.

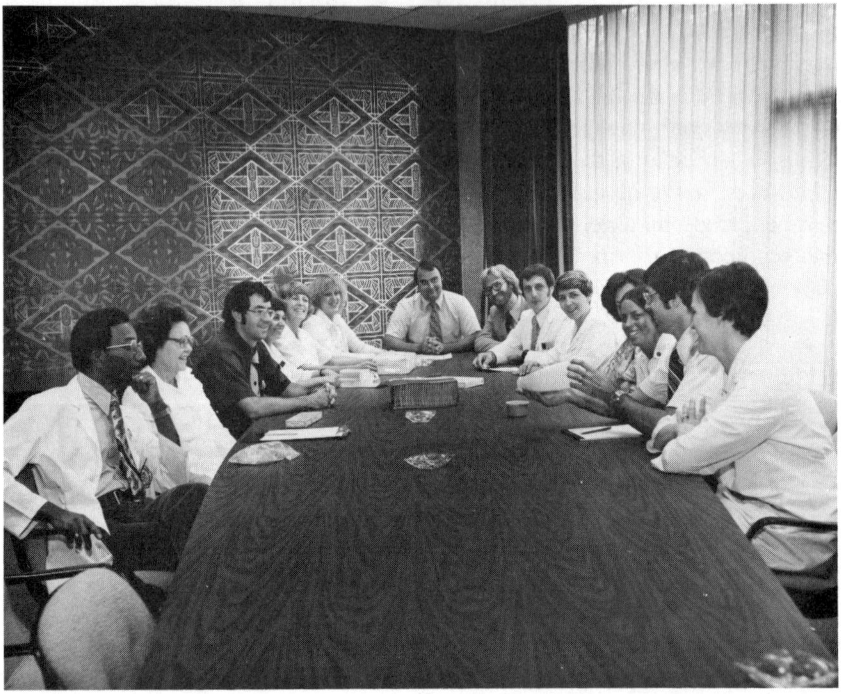

maintenance and housekeeping, the major service departments. Finally, any department or area not represented on the Standardization Committee can send a representative to present items and provide needed consultation whenever appropriate.

It is strongly recommended that sales representatives not be allowed to attend committee meetings. The committee must be objective at all times and not swayed by sales presentations or promotions. After all, the goals of the sales representative are hardly those of the committee.

Many hospitals have tried to get the standardization review performed by as few members as possible because of the time involved and the difficulty of obtaining a concensus from a large number of people. However, the Standardization Committee seems to be an exception to the normal committee stereotype. It is recommended that it have no fewer than 15 members, and is seen as effectively functioning with as many as 25 interested members. In other words, there is a direct correlation between the number of representatives on the standardization team and the objectivity achieved.

Objectives, Scope, and Mission of the Standardization Committee

For a standardization committee to be worthwhile, there must be a concise delineation of its purpose and objectives before it is even formed. It is suggested that these objectives be set forth by administration with the input of all concerned disciplines. The following are examples of the objectives of standardization:

- To provide the mechanism to ensure an improved level of patient care through product evaluation with emphasis on the quality of care and the containment of costs;
- To evaluate the voluminous and continuous flow of new and improved products;
- To reduce the expense of educating and training personnel to many and varied products and techniques through standardization;
- To keep administration and department heads informed and abreast of changes in equipment and products;
- To assist department heads in understanding mutual problems in reference to supplies and equipment; and
- To minimize the quantities of inventory by reducing the variety of products.

The following description concerns the scope and mission of the committee:

> The next consideration will be the scope and mission of the Standardization Committee. Here there are five areas to look at. First, representatives from hospitals around the country think this Committee should provide a system for the introduction, review, and analysis of products and equipment used within the hospital. Second, they think the Committee should be responsible for reviewing the use of established standards. Third, the Committee should have the responsibility for evaluating and choosing the product best for patient care. This assumes consideration of such elements as patient benefit, service, availability, and price. For the purpose of consistency and clarity, we define a patient-care related product as any item used in providing care to the patient. (While the criteria should apply equally to equipment, this chapter will emphasize products rather than equipment.) Fourth, the Committee should bring only those products and equipment to the hospital that can produce the desired result. This means developing procedures to obtain the best use of the product or equipment. And, fifth, the Committee should strive

to promote discipline in the selection of products aimed at the upgrading of patient care. [1]

Fundamental Policies and Guidelines for the Standardization Committee

The very definition of the word "standardize" means to compare with or to bring into conformity with a standard. So a major task of a Standardization Committee is to set standards of product acceptability. This takes time and expertise and should not be done haphazardly or subjectively.

The Standardization Committee must have a set, published time to meet, and it is recommended that this occur no less than monthly. In addition, it should be prepared to convene on an as-needed basis. An agenda should be printed and distributed to all members at least a week in advance of the next meeting. Also, the minutes of the last meeting should be distributed as soon as possible to allow each committee member ample time for preparation.

The nonphysician members should be appointed by the administrator; the chairman should either be a member of the administration or the materiel manager. Again, this is an attempt to provide the committee with the necessary clout, dignity, and continuity to perform its important task.

Furthermore, nonmembers should be invited to attend meetings for advisory purposes whenever the occasion arises.

The product entry-review process is the most important phase of standardization. This step must be well structured, but at the same time flexible so that the employees will feel free to use the process. Anyone from sales representatives to physicians and hospital personnel to patients may request that items be put on the standardization agenda for consideration, and one person—perhaps the purchasing agent—should be designated to receive all potential standard items (Figure 7-2). This person then would perform an initial screening of all items, including contacting the manufacturer or supplier to obtain all requisite information. He then completes a product standardization profile, solicits comments and recommendations from the department that will be using the item, and requests samples of the item from the manufacturer or supplier. A copy of the product standardization profile is sent to each committee member and the item then added to the monthly agenda. This process is repeated for each product to be considered.

The item may be presented to the committee by the person who suggested it or by the purchasing agent. The committee hears the presentations, solicits

---

[1]Johnson & Johnson, *Hospital Product Evaluation Workshop Manual* (New Brunswick, N.J.: 1976), pp. B2–B3.

Figure 7-2 Request for Product Standardization Review Form

PRODUCT: ______________________________

DESCRIPTION: ______________________________

____

MANUFACTURER OR SUPPLIER: ______________________________

WILL THIS PRODUCT REPLACE OR SUPPLEMENT PRESENTLY USED STANDARD ITEM?
IF SO, PLEASE COMMENT: ______________________________

____

REASON FOR REQUEST: ______________________________

____

WILL THE REQUESTED PRODUCT:

- ☐ BE A PATIENT CHARGE
- ☐ BE CONSIDERED AN URGENTLY NEEDED ITEM
- ☐ BE CONSIDERED A NECESSITY
- ☐ BE CONSIDERED AS NICE BUT NOT NECESSARY
- ☐ PROMOTE BETTER PATIENT CARE
- ☐ PROMOTE COST CONTAINMENT OR COST AVOIDANCE
- ☐ OTHER, PLEASE BRIEFLY COMMENT: ______________________________

____

IN YOUR OPINION, SHOULD AN EVALUATION BE CONDUCTED? ____YES ____NO

IF SO, WOULD YOU BE WILLING TO PARTICIPATE IN THE EVALUATION? ____YES ____NO

SHOULD THE MEDICAL STAFF BE AWARE OF THIS REQUEST BEFORE ACTION OR AN EVALUATION IS CONDUCTED? ____YES ____NO

SIGNATURE OF REQUESTING PARTY: ______________________________

DEPARTMENT OR AFFILIATION: ______________________________

____

DATE: ______________________________

any necessary further information, and discusses all aspects of the potential use of the new product. The possible committee actions are as follows:

a. Outright product acceptance
b. Outright rejection of the product with reasons; or
c. An evaluation period of 30, 60, or 90 days, depending on the ramifications considered by the committee.

If the committee is not completely sure of the necessity or usefulness of the item, it generally will ask that an evaluation be performed under supervision at the expense of the manufacturer or supplier (Figure 7-3). It must be pointed out that the evaluation is not done until the item has been submitted for total review by the Standardization Committee. No item, unless in a bona fide emergency, should gain entrance into the hospital utilization process under any circumstances without the awareness and approval of the committee. Once an item has been reviewed and rejected, it should be the policy of the committee not to consider it again for at least a year, unless there is a price or product change. This will prohibit abuse of the open selection process and save much time.

The standardization process should include products and items from all departments with possible exceptions being pharmaceuticals and perishable foods. Pharmaceuticals are excluded because they are usually supervised and regulated by the Pharmacy and Therapeutics (P&T) Committee of the medical staff. Certainly, all types of forms and printed matter should be reviewed and approved by the Standardization Committee, as should capital equipment.

After it has been decided to make an item the standard, other factors must be considered. In many cases, items are ordered without regard to their effect on the expense-revenue picture, an anathema to good management practices. Criteria determining whether there will be a patient charge must be established and a referral mechanism initiated for new items. Before the standardization review, the item information should be submitted to a patient charge review process for charge differentiation before further decisions are made regarding its purchase. In many cases, knowledge that a certain item will be charged directly to the patient will have a definite effect on whether or not it is accepted.

After the decisions have been made concerning standardization and patient charge, the item is sent to the requesting department for preparation of a written product utilization procedure. Finally, the product must be thoroughly demonstrated to all those who will use it—a function which can be performed by both hospital staffers and sales representatives. Only after these four factors have been thoroughly reviewed should the product be accepted as a

Figure 7-3 Product or Equipment Evaluation Summary Form

ITEM:______________________________

MANUFACTURER OR SUPPLIER:______________________________

BRIEF DESCRIPTION:______________________________

____

DATE EVALUATED: FROM____________________TO____________________

REASON FOR EVALUATION:______________________________

____

UNDER WHAT CONDITIONS WAS THE PRODUCT EVALUATED? (BRIEFLY STATE HOW YOU CONDUCTED THE EVALUATION: UNDER CONTROLLED CONDITIONS, WITH ASSISTANCE FROM THE SALES REPRESENTATIVE, ETC.______________________________

____

____

EVALUATORY REMARKS:______________________________

____

____

YOUR RECOMMENDATIONS ARE:______________________________

____

____

NAMES OF HOSPITAL AND MEDICAL STAFF WHO WERE INVOLVED IN THE EVALUATION:

NAME	DEPARTMENT OR AFFILIATION

EVALUATION CONDUCTED BY:______________________________
(SIGNATURE)

DEPARTMENT:______________________________

NOTE: THIS FORM MUST BE SUBMITTED TO THE APPROPRIATE MEMBER OF THE STANDARDIZATION COMMITTEE TEN (10) DAYS BEFORE THE MEETING AT WHICH THE PRODUCT IS BEING CONSIDERED.

standard for the hospital (Figure 7-4). The following formula represents the entire process of proper product standardization acceptance: PRODUCT ACCEPTANCE = PRODUCT STANDARDIZATION REVIEW + PATIENT CHARGE DETERMINATION + WRITTEN PRODUCT USE PROCEDURE + PRODUCT ORIENTATION.

Figure 7-4 Form to Record Results of Standardization Review

THE PRODUCT____, WHICH YOU REQUESTED BE REVIEWED, WAS CONSIDERED BY THE STANDARDIZATION COMMITTEE ON ____________________________.
(DATE)

THE COMMITTEE RECOMMENDED, AND IT WAS SUBSEQUENTLY APPROVED BY ADMINISTRATION, THAT THE PRODUCT BE:

☐ APPROVED AS A STANDARD ITEM

☐ NOT APPROVED

☐ EVALUATED FOR 30 DAYS

☐ EVALUATED FOR 60 DAYS

☐ EVALUATED FOR 90 DAYS

☐ OTHER:____________________________________

THE COMMITTEE REQUESTS THE FOLLOWING ADDITIONAL INFORMATION:

☐ PATIENT CHARGE DATA

☐ PRODUCT USE PROCEDURE

☐ PRODUCT ORIENTATION SCHEDULE

☐ OTHER INFORMATION:______________________________

____

____

☐ NO FURTHER DATA IS NEEDED

THE COMMITTEE EXTENDS ITS SINCERE APPRECIATION TO YOU FOR YOUR CONSIDERATION, COOPERATION AND PARTICIPATION IN THIS VERY IMPORTANT HOSPITAL PROGRAM.

THANK YOU,

____
(CHAIRMAN)

STANDARDIZATION COMMITTEE

It is not suggested that products be accepted in an indiscriminate manner or that an open entry-review standardization process will result in an influx of new products. It has been demonstrated that just the reverse is true, and that such a standardization procedure should result in an acceptance rate of no more than 15 to 25 percent. It must be remembered that an important task of the chairman of the committee is to remind the members of the art of saying "No."

Interface of the Standardization Committee with Other Committees

It must be general knowledge throughout the hospital, and especially among medical and hospital committee chairmen, that if an item or product is to be considered for purchase or evaluation, it must be referred to the Standardization Committee. When a particular committee deals with products, as well as policies and procedures, part of its task is to make the appropriate recommendation and statement to the Standardization Committee about an item its members wish to consider. Then the Standardization Committee introduces the item to the entire review process and reports its findings and actions back to the initiating committee. (Figure 7-5). Inevitably, there are attempts by individuals and even committees to bypass this process, but if standardization is to have credibility, this must never happen.

After the entire standardization procedure has been followed and the product accepted and purchased, the committee still should be responsible for some type of retrospective review and ongoing product evaluation. For example, what impact has the acceptance of this new product had on patient care, patient cost, hospital per diem costs, etc. Each product should be followed for at least six months to a year to audit its use.

Product Evaluation Procedure[2]

The following six sections deal with basic functions of the Standardization Committee. The material included in these sections, as indicated by the reference notes, was drawn directly from the *Hospital Product Evaluation Workshop Manual*, prepared by the Professional Relations Department of Johnson & Johnson.

Once the Committee has reviewed and approved a product for evaluation, the following procedures should be carried out:

1. Select an area within the hospital for a pilot study.

[2]Johnson & Johnson, *Hospital Product Evaluation Workshop Manual*, pp. B6–B10.

Figure 7-5 Interface of the Standardization Committee with Other Hospital and Medical Committees.

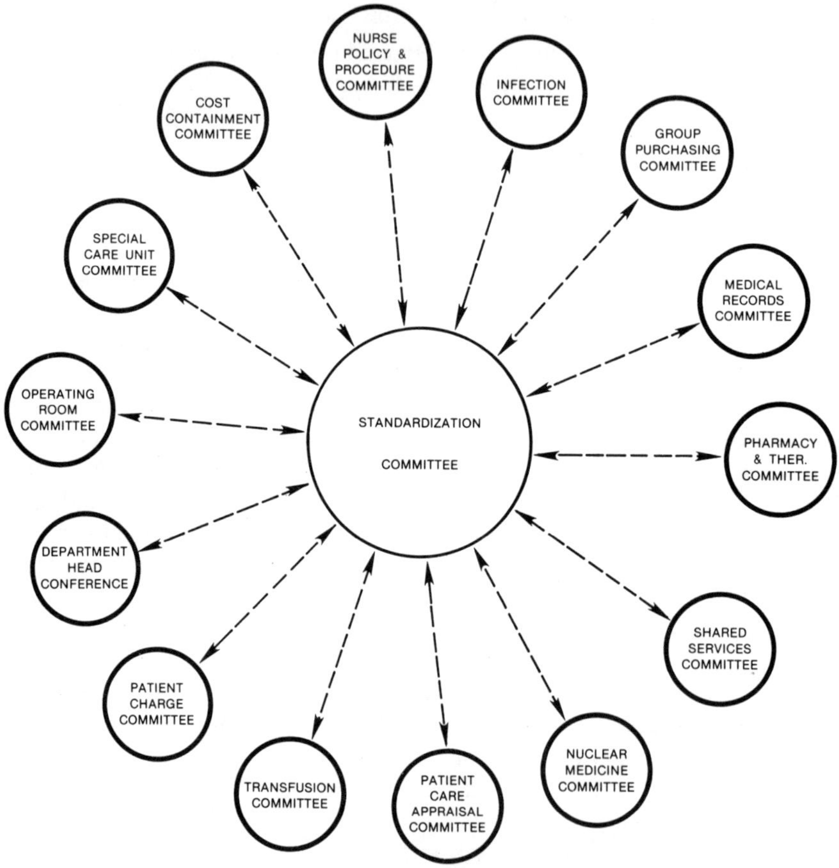

2. Determine the length of time required to properly evaluate the product.
3. Forward a request for product samples through the Purchasing Department to the manufacturer.
4. Prior to use, introduce the product to all three shifts in the pilot area. An inservice trainer should fully explain how the product functions and how it is used. Introduce the hospital staff members who will be involved in the pilot study to the survey questionnaire and tell them what they will be asked about the product. These staff members should be well informed regarding the evaluation points. Such information will

minimize queries when the questionnaire is filled out at the conclusion of the pilot study.

Take advantage of inservice instruction and support by the use of manufacturers' representatives. Such instruction can materially reduce hospital personnel requirements and facilitate the communication of specialized knowledge and techniques.

5. Carry out the product evaluation at the conclusion of the pilot study. This evaluation is done by the participating hospital staff members and it may be accomplished by a written report (see Figure 7-3). The report, specifically designed to structure the information required, will assure that all major criteria are covered and will help in the preparation of the written report.
6. Allow for disposition of "old" product stock. The materiel management representative can offer such guidance to the Standardization Committee.
7. Establish criteria for product evaluation. The following categories of criteria should help establish a basis for product evaluation decisions:

   a. Price—A special criterion: It is certainly reasonable to list price as the number one criterion just as long as you read price as "cost effectiveness" and "value for money." These factors should make price the final consideration after all other criteria have been weighed.

      Factors associated with the price criterion raise related questions:

      1. Quantity requirements and quantity discounts; i.e., is there an opportunity to reduce unit cost, purchase orders, and handling?
      2. Contract flexibility and price term commitment: Is there a purchase contract? Does it offer any flexibility? Is there a term for price commitment?

   b. Product Quality: As appropriate, these criteria may help determine product quality:

      1. Safety—If sterility is a prerequisite, is the product sterile with satisfactory sterile storage life? Does the product permit sterile transfer from package to use site? Is the product free of mechanical and systemic hazards to the patient? Does the product satisfy fire hazard regulations?

2. Storability—Is the product easily handled, stored, adaptable to inventory control systems, logically and legibly labeled?
3. Disposability vs. Reusability—Which is preferable? Concerning disposability of disposables, is there an environmental problem?
4. Effectiveness—Does the product satisfy claims for what it is supposed to do?
5. Quality—Do the product materials, design features, and benefits meet sufficiently high standards so that the product can be called a quality product?

c. Product Service: These criteria measure the service-related aspects of products:

1. Availability—Is the product readily available or in back order? Are basic raw materials in free supply?
2. Waiting Time for Delivery—How long is the period from purchase order to delivery?
3. Inservice Support—Is quality inservice support available from the manufacturer?
4. Servicing and Repair—Is adequate servicing and repair available for reasonable maintenance?

d. Product Comparison Guidelines: These criteria provide a basis for comparison:

1. Other Hospital User Experience—Is this information available? From whom can it be obtained?
2. Competitive Product Comparison—How does the product compare with competitive products?
3. Independent/Company Studies—Are these studies available?
4. Impact of Medical/Hospital Staff Recommendation/Approval—What are the preferences?
5. Other Product Specifics—Are there special considerations?

e. Submit an Evaluation Report: At the end of the pilot study evaluation period, a written report summarizing the results of the questionnaire survey is submitted to the Chairman of the Standardization Committee.

Communication—During the study it is essential to obtain information from concerned staff members. If staff members who are to use the product are not given a chance to voice their opinions during the pilot study, there may be later difficulties, such as poorer utilization of equipment or waste of product/money.

Consistency—Be consistent whenever possible. Many times certain physicians want to use specific brands of products which the majority of hospital members do not like or want. In this instance be flexible to accommodate a particular request. However, recognize that it is very difficult to please every physician and nurse yet be consistent at the same time. The emphasis should be on consistency.

Requesting Samples—Several points of protocol are worth emphasizing. Requests for samples should always go from the Committee through the Purchasing Department. This process is facilitated when the Materiel Manager or Purchasing Agent is a member of the Standardization Committee. For the most part, manufacturers are more than willing to provide samples either free of charge or on a very reasonable basis when the request is in connection with an evaluation program. Although most manufacturers have trial-use programs, which in some instances are part of their contract purchase agreement, it is always sound practice to be aware of what specifically is involved.

Assign Responsibility to Evaluate Information Feedback—The responsibility for handling both the pilot study and the correlation of feedback data is assigned to the Standardization Committee member who requested the product evaluation or who is assigned the product review. The Committee member may delegate this responsibility to the Head Nurse or other applicable persons of the hospital unit in which the study is being conducted.

It is the responsibility of the Committee member concerned to make the evaluation report to the Committee. This report should call either for approval (general or broader use of the product in the hospital) or for disapproval. If the recommendation is for disapproval, the alternatives are: continue use of the present product and/or procedures, reevaluate the need for change, request an extension of the pilot study evaluation time, or review other products. It is the Committee's responsibility to select one alternative; following that decision, the action is directed to the specific member concerned. If the product is approved, the ordering process is coordinated through the Purchasing Department.

How to Measure Product Performance[3]

In measuring product performance three key areas must be emphasized: first, preliminary evaluation review by the Standardization Committee; second, a pilot survey in a particular patient care unit or department; and third, evaluation of the survey and final recommendation by the Standardization Committee. The principal product evaluation criteria are *safety, efficacy,* and *quality*. Let's look at each.

Safety—

While "price" should be considered as the final criterion, safety is unquestionably the most important criterion. If a product is in any way unsafe to use on a patient, it is seldom worth the risk of any potential patient benefit. Safety is a primary factor in terms of patient care.

If the product is intended for use in the operating room or in any other patient care area, the principal safety factor is that it be sterile—and the product is either sterile or it isn't. The nosocomial infection rate can certainly be controlled and monitored if we can rely on product sterility, whether it be provided through the hospital's Central Processing Department or by a manufacturer. Regardless of source of supply, the product package must be designed in such a way to permit sterile transfer from the package to the site of use. We should also have complete assurance about the product's sterile shelf life if it is to be stored for any length of time. We should have a knowledge and understanding of sterilization procedures, product packaging and its relative effectiveness for maintaining sterility over a given period of time, storage conditions, and methods of product handling prior to the product's actual use in the hospital. In addition to being sterile at time of use, a product must be free from mechanical and systemic hazards to the patient.

For example, surgical drapes must provide a sterile moisture barrier which prevents the possible transmittal of micro-organisms which could contaminate the surgical wound site. Drapes must also be free from dust and lint which, even though sterile, could cause a

[3]Johnson & Johnson, *Hospital Product Evaluation Workshop Manual*, pp. C1–C3.

pyrogenic reaction in an incision. Plastics used as moisture barriers must be hypoallergenic with no sharp edges or rough seam lines which could cut or abrade the patient. Although these considerations are directed to disposables, the concept of safety should apply to any product used in any patient care unit.

Another important mechanical consideration essential to safety is: does the product satisfy all fire hazard regulations? This consideration applies particularly to disposable products.

Efficacy—

In addition to being safe, a product must be effective. It must satisfy the claims made for it; it must do what it is supposed to do and do it easily and well. If instructions for use of the product are clearly stated and reinforced by inservice training and visual training aids, the effectiveness of the product will be improved.

For example, I can remember when our hospital changed from the old method of open urinary drainage bags to the closed drainage bag system. The representative from the manufacturer, in collaboration with our inservice education staff, provided indepth orientation for all levels of personnel—including the physician—on all shifts. The transition to a new product was made easier because of this information.

Quality—

The product design elements which contribute to safety and efficacy and the actual materials used in its manufacture are elements to consider in measuring the quality of the product. Therefore, the Standardization Committee must evaluate product quality by checking the manufacturer's claims against satisfactory quality specifications which, it is hoped, have already been established by or for the Standardization Committee. This check is usually provided by the Materiel Management Department's representative on the Committee. What does the manufacturer claim for its specifications? Obviously, it is the responsibility of the manufacturer to maintain the highest practicable levels of quality control. However, the product's design and performance should also be compared with competitive products. The combination of these investigations will help determine the quality of the product.

These three areas of concern—safety, efficacy, and quality—are the keys to measuring product performance. The application of these criteria must provide you with favorable answers to the following questions:

a. Is the product safe to use?
b. Are precautions prohibitive?
c. Does the product perform its intended function to meet your requirements?
d. Does the product meet your standards of quality?

The answers to these questions must be reflected in the evaluation results and eventually in the decision as to which product will best suit your needs in giving quality patient care in your hospital.

How to Summarize Evaluation Results and Make Decisions[4]

Gather Feedback; Tabulate Results—

The following information should be helpful in considering how best to tabulate pilot study results on which the purchase decision will be made. Actually, there are really only two techniques which have general applicability: one is structured and the other is unstructured. Let's consider both in order to determine which might best suit your hospital's product evaluation situation.

Feedback Techniques
Structured—

a. Self-administered Questionnaire: The structured feedback technique uses a questionnaire which is generally self-administered but which is often supplemented by a personal interview. While it is usually desirable to use a self-administered questionnaire by itself, you assure yourself of better correlation if the person or persons in charge of the evaluation survey lists the results in conjunction with a personal interview. (The pilot survey to which we referred earlier is seldom so large that this interview-tabulation process becomes unwieldy. Despite the possibility of interviewer bias, it is often worth the additional and confirming information the interview provides—particularly with regard to qualified responses.) The questionnaire, always tailored to elicit specific responses concerning the product, can be of two

---

[4]Johnson & Johnson, *Hospital Product Evaluation Workshop Manual*, pp. D1–D6.

types. The first type uses questions which are structured. That is, the response is quantified based on a scale which may use numbers of pre-determined values such as "excellent," "very good," "good," "fair," or "poor." In hospital situations where shades of difference in clinical evaluation are of special concern, the value scale—as in this example—is often slanted toward the range of acceptability. That is, the degree of unacceptability is really not of much interest or meaning.

b. Open-ended Questionnaire: The second type of feedback technique uses questions which are open-ended. Examples of these questions are: "How did you like the product?" "What was the patient's reaction to the product?" However, to maintain study consistency, it is essential to work from a pre-determined list of open-ended questions, *all* of which are asked in the process of evaluating the product, and *all* the answers to which are recorded during the interview. It is the answers to these open-ended questions that permit the study to obtain the qualified judgments directly concerned with the product's performance and its desirability for use. It is these judgments that are then submitted to the Standardization Committee.

Unstructured—

The unstructured type of feedback technique is generally used with a panel of people who may or may not be "experts," as the situation requires. The person conducting the panel and responsible for analyzing the results of the study works from a general outline concerned with the areas of interest in the product rather than from a structured questionnaire. In this kind of situation, the members of the panel will all have been involved in working together in the pilot study evaluation. In eliciting responses the panel moderator (probably the Standardization Committee member responsible for the study or the head nurse of the hospital unit in which the study is being conducted) can work either with individual panel members or with a group. In contrast to the open-ended questionnaire, there is no predetermined set of questions. Questions are based initially on the general outline of areas of product study interest; the questions asked later most often stem from the previous responses. Obviously, in working with a panel (as compared with the structured technique of questionnaire and personal interview), the problem of control is both more difficult and time consuming. To be effective in producing results which are readily tabulated requires handling by a highly-skilled person. For this reason, the technique is more often used when outside consultants are called into the hospital to help conduct the study. The strong advantage of the panel technique is in providing in-depth qualitative responses. The procedure is usually a preliminary step used to generate hypotheses where there is a small or nonexistent body of information. The procedure is also particularly useful in establishing values concerned with physical sensations, as compared with providing specific units of measurement.

In our earlier reference to feedback techniques, we mentioned the use of a written presentation. This is perhaps the least satisfactory feedback technique because it relies heavily on the respondent's ability to express himself or herself in writing, and with little or no guidance to cover all of the essential areas of product interest. It is also difficult to correlate, tabulate, and evaluate the information in this kind of report.

While the Standardization Committee can choose its own feedback technique, it would seem that for product evaluation studies (whether they concern products used in the Operating Room or in other parts of the hospital) that the structured technique; i.e., the self-administered questionnaire which uses both structured and open-ended questions in combination with a personal interview, offers the most comprehensive and manageable feedback. And one very strong bit of advice: spend all the time necessary to develop the questionnaire so that you are as sure as you can be that it will elicit the scope of response you seek. It is not at all facetious to say that if you ask the right questions you will get the right answers. Clear, full information makes the process of tabulating results much easier and the results themselves considerably more meaningful.

These feedback techniques are equally applicable to use during any follow-up evaluations such as after the product has been approved and is in use but is still being monitored.

Make Recommendation for Purchase—

At the conclusion of our discussion of "Steps to follow for Product Evaluation" we said that after the Standardization Committee approved a product for use in the hospital, the ordering process is coordinated through materiel management. Now it is evident why a representative of the Materiel Management or Purchasing Department must be a member of the Standardization Committee.

Determine Product-Usage Factor and Source of Availability—

Before the order is authorized, the Standardization Committee determines, with the help of the Materiel Management representative, a product-usage factor and the source of the product's availability within the hospital.

Product-Usage Factor—

The product-usage factor tends to vary in terms of whether the product is an "in-use" product or a "new" product which is being brought into the hospital for the first time. For example, if the product is in use, such as urinary drainage bags or suction catheters which are being changed for a price/quality reason, the usage factor can be calculated readily by developing a forecast of requirements based on actual use in previous years. If it is a "new" product, that is, something which has never been used in the hospital such as disposable O.R. or dressing packs, determination of the usage-factor is somewhat more complicated. However, knowledge of product usage can be facilitated if the Committee wants to take advantage of a service offered by the product's manufacturer. The company is willing to provide a chart which the hospital can use to keep track of the number and type of procedures—current and projected—which can be used to determine pack-unit estimates. The Materiel Management Department can then use these estimates in conjunction with unit costs—which may vary for different quantities—to develop a total dollar value for the order over any period of time.

Source of Availability Within the Hospital—

In addition to developing the product-usage factor, the Standardization Committee also makes a recommendation or request to the Materiel Management Department concerning the product's source of availability within the hospital. Source of availability is determined by whether the product concerned is for general use or whether it is a specialty item. If the product is for general use, e.g., adhesive tape, it will be available through the Purchasing Department, from the Storeroom or Central Supply. In this case the product is generally designated by a Storeroom catalog number. If the product is a specialty item, such as one of the O.R. packs, it becomes a floor item and is usually kept in a special supply room near the O.R. Specialty items are charged directly to the specialty service or department concerned.

Once the usage factor has been determined and product availability location is recommended by the Standardization Committee, authorization to purchase the product may be conveyed directly to the Materiel Management Department either verbally by the Committee or its Chairman or by written memorandum; authorization may also be conveyed indirectly through distribution of the Committee's minutes which indicate the purchase was approved. Using the information generated by the Committee's product evaluation report, the Materiel Management Department processes the order and charges the appropriate budget.

Additional Considerations—

The procedure just described seems generally applicable to hospitals of any bed size. There are no special provisions that are particularly applicable either to small or to large hospitals. However, some additional points should be considered in the product evaluation decision by the Materiel Management Department. These involve consideration of various methods of purchasing such as: direct from the manufacturer vs. dealer supplier, group, consignment, cooperative or contract, and any number of variable terms which may affect the ultimate product price. The Committee's contact with the Materiel Management Department should provide the recommended action.

Considerations for Infection Control[5]

From the infection control aspect, product evaluation is significant. The evaluation of all types of products utilized both directly or indirectly in the care of a patient should include a review of the infection control implications. Continuing problems with the control and prevention of hospital-acquired infections have led to the scientific investigation into the cause of these types of infections by the Center for Disease Control and by Infection Control Nurses and Operating Room Supervisors.

Patient care products and biomedical devices have all too frequently contributed to the cause of infections. These products have been implicated either because they do not fulfill their product claims or they do something that contributes to the possible cause of infection. For example, in recent years, I.V. solutions and equipment have been involved in epidemic-type infection situations. The causes have been faulty sterilizing processes by the company or improper handling and management of the equipment by medical and nursing personnel. Biomedical devices such as transducers, pacer wires, inhalation therapy equipment, anesthesia equipment and urinary

---

[5]Johnson & Johnson, *Hospital Product Evaluation Workshop Manual*, pp. E1–E4.

catheter equipment have frequently been traced as the source of nosocomial infections.

Inadequate sterilizing cycles and the manner in which items have been wrapped, handled and stored within the hospital have also been identified as sources of contamination and possible causes of infections. The manner in which prewrapped, presterilized items are packaged is also important. Are all products in this category packaged to allow for sterile presentation? Or are they easily contaminated because of poor package design? These are just a few examples of how products have been identified in the cause or potential cause of hospital-acquired infections.

The basic question arises: How should products be evaluated for infection control? The logical answer would seem to be that the Standardization Committee should be the responsible agent receiving specific input information from the Infection Control Nurse who functions as a liaison between the Infection Control Committee (ICC) and the Standardization Committee. The O.R. Nurse should also review products for infection control aspects. The I.C. Nurse and the O.R. Nurse should work as a team.

What types of products used in the hospital should be specifically examined for their infection control implications? A few examples are:

1. I.V. Solutions and Equipment
2. Urinary Catheters and Equipment
3. Sterilizing Devices and Solutions
4. Disinfectants
5. Antiseptics and Soaps
6. All Bio-medical Devices
7. All Packaging Design for Sterile Delivery and Sterile Containment
8. Inhalation Therapy Equipment
9. Suction Equipment
10. Housekeeping and Cleaning Solutions and Supplies
11. All items utilized in the O.R., D.R.
12. Procedure areas, isolation units and ICUs; these items include:
    a. procedural O.R. packs
    b. surgical gowns
    c. masks
    d. headcoverings
    e. gloves

Surgical dressings utilized in and outside the O.R. area: There are many types—non adhering—medicated and others. When evaluating these and other products for infection control aspects, the ICN and O.R. Nurse must specifically be examining the safety and effectiveness of each. Of course, all other aspects of the product evaluation process are important, but these two aspects are significantly important to infection control.

How can you be assured of the safety and efficacy of the products you must evaluate? Consider the following:

1. Manufacturer Support: Does the company have clinical data to document product claims? Can these claims be supported in demonstration or trial use of the product? This is not always possible or necessary and depends on the product category, demonstration should be requested when applicable.
2. Literature Searching: Check for new studies and new products that may improve patient care from the infection control aspect. There are many professional journals that include this type of information.
3. Consulting with Experts: In product evaluation such organizations as CDS and FDA have developed many criteria on which to judge products.
4. Communications: The sales representative or detail man (the manufacturer's representative) can give you the direct information you need to assist you in your product evaluation. Usually large well-established companies have representatives who are professional, well trained, and helpful.

You will want to look into all of the areas of evaluating infection control. Ask questions such as:

a. Is this a closed urinary catheter system you are using?
b. Are the antiseptics and soaps which are being used effective against gram-positive and gram-negative organisms, fungus, etc.?
c. What is the efficiency rate of the face mask used?
d. Can the bronchoscope considered for purchase be easily cleaned and sterilized after use?
e. Are all of the sterilizing devices biologically monitored in the proper manner?
f. How easily is the inhalation therapy equipment cleaned? This question also includes its bacterial filters.
g. Do written nursing and medical procedures exist to include the use of new product changes?

h. Are you doing enough reevaluation of products and follow-up teaching in the area of infection control?
i. Should you be a member of the Hospital Product Evaluation Process and/or Committee?

Ask the following questions and think about: What are the differences in the competitors' products, their claims, clinical data, inservice material and support? Actively evaluate and reevaluate all products for the infection control implications. This activity is an important function of the Nurse Epidemiologist and O.R.N. and the Infection Control Program of your hospital. Through sound product evaluation this group can help prevent nosocomial infections.

Financial Considerations[6]

Value Analysis; Value Engineering; Value Improvement—

Three terms that are used popularly today to describe the process of product evaluation are: value analysis, value engineering and value improvement. While the terms generally mean the same thing, they have a somewhat different application. Value engineering is best applied to industrial applications. In hospitals, value analysis is what it's all about. The term covers the broad spectrum of value in each distinct area ranging from the raw materials that are used in manufacturing through to product efficacy.

To many of you this probably sounds much like the old cost reduction routine. Well, you're partially right. What we are going to try to do, however, to shed some new light on this not exactly new subject, is to suggest how value analysis can be achieved and some of the reasons that value analysis is so important today.

Value analysis, or the value technique, first calls for a clear definition of the purpose for which the product or procedure exists. So first, the very need for the function of the product is challenged. Second, alternate ways or methods to perform the same function are explored. Third, cost studies are performed.

Now, if an acceptable alternate method is uncovered that can accomplish the same end but an improvement is identified in terms of efficiency, technique or cost, then a change action is proposed. The Standardization Committee recommends such a change to the department supervisor.

---

[6]Johnson & Johnson, *Hospital Product Evaluation Workshop Manual,* pp. G1–G8.

Reasons for Value Analysis—

Let's look for a moment at some of the reasons for employing value analysis.

1. Advances in Technology—The first and most obvious reason for employing the technique is an advance in technology. The aluminums, polypropylenes, polystyrenes or fiberglass products being developed are looked at continually as new possibilities for use in the modern hospital.
2. Periodic Function Analysis—The second reason to use the technique is the need for periodic function analysis to assure that the original design or requirements for materials are not outdated. This includes testing for actual vs. intended use.
3. Safety—Finally, the third reason is the need to investigate the safety of materials and equipment which can range from step-ladders with locking feet to products with shatter impact. Changes in the area of safety regulations occur almost from moment to moment. Witness the recent release from the FDA Commissioner regarding the already popular use of plastics in packaging intravenous solutions:

> "There is evidence of vinyl chloride migration when polyvinyl chloride is used in packaging materials for products containing alcohol. There have also been reports of the possible migration of polyvinyl chloride container ingredients to non-alcoholic products as well. Because of this, it is necessary to give special study to such packaging material to determine if it is safe for its intended use."*

4. Cost Reduction Factors and Quality Determination—In addition to these reasons, experience has shown that value analysis, properly applied, successfully reduces costs and frequently provides added benefits which will improve quality, reliability, productivity and performance. Of these, the primary concern of the analysis is that of quality determination. The quality level of a product should be determined by the function to be filled. Purchase of material below or above the level required is wasteful, such as the purchase of top quality surgical instruments for general nursing use. For example, while standards

*Research News, May 1974, Volume 21, Number V.

for asepsis may be uniform throughout a given medical institution, the criteria for products used in surgery may differ from those used in nursing or clinical areas such as the need for control of static electricity in the operating room.
Therefore, the standards adopted by manufacturers for products supplied to hospitals for use in the O.R. should not only meet the criteria for aseptic technique but should have U.L. approval and meet the OSHA requirements as well.

In summary, the specifications describing the quality of a product also have the effect of standardizing the terms of a bid invitation. A bid invitation is a purchasing tool. It is a price request for items whose quality is defined in terms of upper and lower limits, both for performance and material.

In considering pricing there are many variables other than quality that have a less obvious but as important effect. Storage, deterioration and cost of capital are some variables. These factors can be grouped under a term called "cost-in-use."

Cost-In-Use:

Six factors can be considered as contributors to cost-in-use. They are:

1. *Storage Space*—Such space can generally be figured at about $5 per square foot per year. Inventory varies from 5 per cent to 25 per cent of dollar value stocked, depending upon type of material and number of personnel required to manage the inventory.
2. *Deterioration & Obsolescence*—Although often avoided through good management, deterioration and obsolescence, spoilage of stock, and damage and pilferage must also be considered as major cost factors.
3. *Acquisition Costs*—This includes the cost of placing orders, expediting, receiving, inventory control and accounting activities.
4. *Quality Level of Source of Supply*—In determining the best source of supply for a product, there is also another group of factors for consideration. The manufacturer or distributor must provide not only a quality product but must assure quality control during the manufacturing process.

5. *Delivery*—After source of supply, we come to delivery. The manufacturer must deliver the product on a scheduled basis allowing for unforeseen increases in demand.
6. *Service*—The next consideration is service. What service can the manufacturer provide? Is an inservice program available? Immediate response must be available in problem situations. Policies covering such areas as "Return Goods" must be available to offer immediate solutions for overstocking and obsolescence. There must be assurance that adequate stock levels of backup supplies will be maintained.

Thus, the total cost to a hospital involves not only finding a source of supply but the administrative costs of purchasing the item, its receipt, storage, use and final disposition. The value of the material, however, must be judged on product performance, availability, obsolescence and the possibility of hidden costs.

Standardization and Cost Reporting—
What we have said so far assumes that there is a degree of standardization within a hospital. However, we know this is not always true. The New Jersey Hospital Association through its Management Engineering Cost Control Service has found that unless there is a good deal of standardization, a system of accurate cost reporting cannot be implemented. I'm sure many of us can think of at least several stock items that are essentially duplicates.

Ways to Reduce Cost-In-Use—
Price can be reduced by eliminating a variety of small-quantity items and consolidating the type of item in larger orders of the same product. Quantity discounts are a major result of such an effort.

Cost-in-use can be reduced by planning orders and developing economic standards for shelf levels. Such standards can reduce storage and handling costs. By reducing inventory levels, the hospital will reduce its required working capital.

Working capital is the amount of money the hospital has paid for services such as linen processing and maintenance and for salaries and products. This capital will not be recovered until the patient, or a third party, pays the bill. If a hospital has 120 days of working capital, this amounts to the average cash paid out per day times 120 days—a substantial amount! Since most hospitals are not considered cash-rich, this means the hospital probably has borrowed the money and is in effect paying interest on the capital as well.

Let's review how the hospital receives its money. Hospitals receive what is referred to in the industry as a per diem. The per diem is based upon an established annual budget and is an estimate of hospital costs per patient day. It is not real costs. The real costs for rendering patient care are not determined until the year has been completed. During the following year, a cost report is submitted to the relevant third parties for the preceding year. Generally, it takes about two years before the hospital receives any adjustments due from the third parties. The difference between the estimated cost and the real cost, if it is a negative figure—and it almost always is—must be financed through working capital.

Reduce Working Capital—The amount of working capital necessary can be reduced by:

1. Standardization
2. Maintenance of an economic inventory level for all items
3. Kindness to the patient. By being cheerful and kind to the patient, there is a good chance that he will make every effort to pay his bill as fast as possible, and will be less likely to bring litigation against the hospital over small incidents.

Impact of Government Controls—

Up to this point we have seen how the technical aspects of value analysis can affect costs, how the practical aspects of cost-in-use can affect costs, and finally, how cash flow works. The last item that has a great impact upon costs is government controls.

We have all seen how, in 1974, Phase III limited hospital costs, not to exceed 5 per cent of labor and 2½ per cent of material costs over those allowable for the prior fiscal year. Later, Phase IV provided an elective consideration for hospitals based upon patient census increases. Length of patient stay also is figured in this formula.

Basically, if an institution has an established procedure, labor and supply costs cannot exceed the established charge even though supply costs and labor might have risen dramatically. During the last year we have seen increases such as 40 per cent for textiles, 100 per cent for heating oil and 50 per cent for electric power. As you can see, this poses a definite threat to the financial position of the hospital. Public Law 92-603 may have enough strength to reinstate several aspects of Phase III and IV controls. If not, even though it may take several years, the state Medicare and Medicaid agencies may adopt the spirit and control systems which have been initiated by the Cost of Living Council. In addition, under President Carter, National Health Insurance legislation is probably not too far distant.

On the other hand, the concept of hospital cost containment has been introduced federally for some of the following reasons. For many people who are not covered by Medicare, Medicaid, Veterans programs and other forms of health insurance, health care is not accessible. These people are generally too poor to afford routine or emergency health care. For many persons covered by health insurance, the coverage is often inadequate. In most cases there is a limit which falls far short of covering the major and more expensive illnesses.

Additionally, there is a lack of any central coordinating and planning system for the health care industry. Up to now, each hospital has acted independently.

Summary—

Now, let's draw all this information together.

First, we now know many of the reasons behind the need for value analysis: products must be safe, effective and cost-efficient.

Second, we have seen what makes the hospital's cash-flow cycle operate. A new awareness of the very real need to reduce costs should serve to remind us of the serious implications of cost in the daily professional setting.

Third, we are aware that there is a procedure that can help us put into perspective all the various aspects for a program of continuing improvement.

Inservice Training Programs[7]

When it came to considering how manufacturers' programs could facilitate managing product evaluation decisions we found an excellent article by Mary Barrett, RN, and Robert W. Pike, which appeared in the 1973 January-February issue of the *Journal of Continuing Education in Nursing*. The paper endorses the concepts we have been discussing concerning support for inservice training. What follows now is largely an edited version of the Barrett-Pike article, "Another Educational Resource: The Manufacturer."

Manufacturers' Programs—

One of the best ways to obtain expertise on new products is from

[7]Johnson & Johnson, *Hospital Product Evaluation Workshop Manual*, pp. H1–H10.

the people who make them. We have reached a stage of technical sophistication where it is no longer safe to assume that a new product introduced into hospital routine will be self-explanatory. Even though it comes packaged with the most careful instructions, there is no guarantee that the instructions will be read (especially in emergency situations). If the product change is a subtle one rather than a genuinely revolutionary change, it can sometimes be more disconcerting. Teaching an old dog new tricks is easier than trying to change his old tricks, because of the attitudes that have built up around them. To introduce innovation without adequate explanation, plus demonstration, is to court error, dissatisfaction and frustration. The purpose of this discussion is to review items which must be considered if the hospital is to get the most out of manufacturer-provided inservice education programs and materials.

Inservice Training—

It Starts With Evaluation—For a manufacturer to be involved with inservice education, the product must obviously have been examined and accepted—however conditionally—by the hospital's Standardization Committee or its equivalent. It is really here that inservice planning should begin.

When the Director of Inservice Education is a member of the evaluation team, inservice training can easily be part of the trial period and then built into the product-introduction package. Indeed, the necessary training can be and should be made part of acceptance.

Pre-trial training for those involved in the test period is recommended in almost all cases since new products must be understood to be fairly evaluated.

This works both ways. In the case of a new disposable, pre-filled syringe for emergency medications, it was the manufacturer who stressed the importance of preparing the staff to use the product. The product is extremely simple to use, and virtually foolproof, yet so radically different from standard types of injectable medications that inservice training was considered an absolute necessity.

An interesting footnote is provided by an experience this same manufacturer had at a nurses' convention, where a nearby exhibitor asked to use some of the syringes in connection with a coronary-care demonstration. Asked if he understood the way the new syringe worked, the other exhibitor said he did, but it later developed that this was a false assumption, and the nurses who used it in the demonstration found it baffling and unsatisfactory.

Yet when the product was properly demonstrated and explained, the nurses were able to have the syringe ready to use within 10 to 15 seconds instead of the minute and one half required with the old approach.

They had seen the objective—to get the medication into the patient faster—but the process had to be learned.

An Exchange of Views Between Hospital and Manufacturer—

Another reason for including the inservice director at the evaluation stage is to provide an opportunity for an exchange of information with the manufacturer's representative. Each may be helped by seeing the other's point of view. The structure of inservice programs varies widely from hospital to hospital and the sales representative should be prepared to fit into the environment as he finds it. The inservice director can be of valuable assistance in the process of adopting a new product.

Who Gets Involved?—

Who should participate in equipment-related inservice education programs? The answer: *everyone* who will be involved with the product. When it is appropriate to include physicians, every effort should be made to enlist the cooperation of the Director of Medical Education.

The backgrounds of the people who will receive the inservice education help determine the type of program developed and who gives it. If for example, aides and LPNs are the primary participants, instructor selection should be based on the experience of the instructor working at that level.

What should the actual inservice training include? Where should the emphasis be placed? To what extent, if any, should already familiar areas be reviewed? The answer depends on the impact of the product on hospital procedures as well as on the target audience.

In instances where the equipment changes but the nursing procedures remain basically the same, inservice programs will most likely concentrate on the equipment only. When, however, the change in equipment is significant enough to affect nursing procedure, it can often be valuable to offer a refresher in relevant physiology or anatomy along with new product information. Here, hospital personnel and manufacturer's representative may collaborate in the teaching role with nurse-instructors handling the basic science review.

New products sometimes represent minor, but important, alterations in old ones or substitutions. Stimulating the adjustments of long-established habit to cope with this kind of change can often be more difficult than teaching something radically new. It was found, for example, that pre-coronary care ambulance emergency medics learned to use the new pre-filled disposable syringes in a shorter time than nurses experienced with other types of syringes.

Depending upon the complexity of what must be learned and the number and variety of personnel who require inservice training, the decision may be made to give primary instruction to a selected core group and then let "each one teach one." Or it may prove more practical in the long run—as it did, for example, in the case of the disposable syringe—to set up continuous, round-the-clock sessions to cover everyone concerned in a short period of time. However, don't forget the weekenders.

Orientation for Sales Representatives—

Some representatives will be better equipped than others to offer inservice training. Almost without exception, the representatives know their product well; but some have the advantage of special training and materials supplied by their company, while others provide the service without this formal backing.

Whether a salesman is able to call on a reserve of audio-visual and print resources or whether he is pretty much on his own, he will need the help of the inservice director to do the best job. And it is to the director's advantage to provide necessary orientation for the sales representative, since by conducting inservice sessions he is saving inservice staff time and at the same time providing a welcome change of pace for those attending.

What help should he be offered, then? Most importantly, the representative should be able to present his product in "before-and-after" terms. Therefore, he must be totally familiar with products and procedures currently in use—and the types of personnel using them.

Let him visit the unit, talk with those who work there, observe procedures. The more openly hospital personnel can discuss the product with him, the more effectively the representative can help them get the most from the product he is introducing.

The Success of the Program—

Some guidelines can help to insure the success of the inservice training program, and to most representatives experienced in the field these guidelines are well known—but check.

A new product is a tangible item—so people should be encouraged to touch it. More than that, they must have opportunity to use it, get the feel of it, see for themselves how it works rather than rely on a "lecture" explanation. For example, in the case of the disposable suction unit, representatives brought not only the product to the sessions, but a variety of tubing, brackets, adaptors, and even suction machines. Most of the questions raised about the new product by the operating room and special-unit nurses who would use it could be answered by actual demonstration.

Person-to-person communication, on an individual or small-group basis, makes for successful equipment training. This is not to say that visual aids do not have their place; they do, for reinforcement. But they must never be relied upon completely.

Audio-visual presentations, where available, can be used in conjunction with "live" teaching. Again, tapes and slides may be extremely useful for the hospital to have to use for several days as a refresher for those who attended the sessions, to inform those who may have been absent or to orient new personnel. Such a presentation can be a valuable tool for unit supervisors or other representatives who might attend a program and return to the floor and teach staff.

Showbiz—

While people don't come to a session expecting to be entertained, it is important to remember that the greatest teachers—even in the most traditional type classroom—have a good understanding of showmanship.

Like all good showmen, the inservice instructor knows when enough is enough. A half-hour is about as long as the presentation section of any session ought to last (if there are questions that prolong it, fine, since that is the audience's choice). One way to keep it short is to be ruthless about cutting out redundancy; if somebody does miss a point along the line, it will turn up either in question-and-answer periods or in try-it-yourself demonstrations.

Perhaps the most important point to share with the representative, however, is that in conducting inservice programs we are dealing with adults—adults who have, in an official sense, "completed" their education. To "re-teach" professional people requires consummate tact.

We must recognize the value of the background of each RN, LPN, aid, technician, and orderly. Together they are making significant contributions daily—even if they aren't up-to-date on every new product or technique. In inservice education we are seeking to change behaviors and skills, which, in many cases, have become habitual. In short, learning a new procedure can be upsetting unless the instructor—nurse or salesman—approaches the situation with understanding. That means not talking down, but treating the "students" as equals which they are.

Follow-up Procedures—

After a few days a fairly standard routine will usually be established. At this point the representative may decide to have a meeting at the end of the day to discuss the product's use with all who have been involved. By then, however, most of the problems and questions have already been ironed out. When the supervisor feels that the staff is fully able to handle the product, the educational portion of the company support program is concluded.

After the introductory phase has been completed, the representative should arrange a follow-up program. This permits him to complete any aspects the hospital feels require attention.

Interviews with the Administrator, the Director of Nursing, Central Supply Head, Controller, and anyone else are arranged to inform them of the progress of the program.

By this time the Controller will have seen the initial invoice for the trial order; it is important to explain that during the first 30 days of the program costs may be disproportionately high. Experience has shown that costs run much lower once a definite use pattern has been established. It is particularly important that the Controller be aware of the distinction between cost and "cost-in-use." It sometimes takes a shift in mental gears to think in terms of "cost-in-use" rather than in terms of actual purchases when a new product is installed. Usually the use-practice period takes about 90 days.

The representative should also follow through in areas such as Central Supply, Housekeeping, and Laundry to be sure these departments are taking advantage of the labor-saving possibilities. He is in a unique position to offer valuable suggestions because of his experience in other institutions. The representative should also check with the Purchasing Department and Store and Supply rooms to be sure that inventories are at sufficient levels for the trial period.

After initial inservice, what?—

Once a new product is no longer "new" in the hospital, there may be a tendency to forget that many hospital personnel *are* new.

How do new employees become familiar with products and procedures they may not have encountered elsewhere?

There are several ways to acquaint them. One is to integrate the new product or equipment in the general nursing orientation given by the hospital. If the product is likely to be in general use in a number of hospital units this procedure would make good sense.

Long-term Follow-up (About 90 days)—

This period covers the time between installation and transition to routine use. The objective is to demonstrate the effectiveness of the product so its use becomes routine.

The representative should maintain at least weekly contact with the involved supervisors either in person or by phone. Finally, he should make arrangements to be on call to the supervisors in case they need his assistance with any problem in the future (this would extend beyond the 90-day period).

Inventory and Supply Continuity—

These two areas are a very important part of the general follow-up period in order to assure inventory level and maintain a continuity of supply. Once this usage factor has been determined, the product can usually be introduced into the hospital ordering cycle. The introduction can be worked out even when the use of a product is cyclic. Most manufacturers can provide guidelines for the Materiel Management Department in setting up special arrangements for inventory control systems. In the process, the representative should make arrangements for returning dead stock of products that will not be used routinely in the future.

Continuity of supply should not be a problem if you are dealing with a reputable manufacturer, unless there is a shortage of basic raw materials—and then everyone is affected.

To some degree the hospital can build in protection for continuity of supply as well as arranging for a more stable price structure through purchase agreements or sales contracts with the manufacturer or supplier. This should be handled directly between the Materiel Management Department and the supplier.

Today there is much concern about cost containment in hospitals from hospital associations, government, and third parties, even to the extent of recommending that hospitals should establish and maintain cost containment committees. However, it should be stressed that the Standardization Committee can be strengthened in scope and authority to include supervision of all cost containment efforts since many cost containment efforts relate to supplies, purchased services, and equipment. In fact, the management supported Standardization Committee can serve as the standardization effort, the pharmacy and therapeutics review, and the cost containment program.

In reference to product standardization, I am reminded of the chicken and the pig in the barnyard talking one morning. The chicken was saying that he felt that since Farmer Brown, their owner, had provided them with the best of food and shelter, Farmer Brown deserved the finest. In turn, the chicken said that they should give Farmer Brown bacon and eggs every morning for breakfast. The pig was quick to retort, "Chicken, for you it would be fine, because for you it would only mean participation; but for me it would mean total commitment!" The product standardization process, similarly, should mean total commitment on the part of hospitals.

REFERENCES 1, 2, 3, 4, 5, 6 and 7 granted through the permission and courtesy of Johnson & Johnson, New Brunswick, New Jersey. References were taken directly from the *Hospital Product Evaluation Workshop Manual* prepared by the Professional Relations Department of Johnson & Johnson, October, 1976.

Pertinent Points to Ponder

1. In your opinion, why haven't standardization committees been successful in the past from the standpoint of containing costs?
2. Should it be mandatory for hospitals to demonstrate supply effectiveness through results-oriented standardization committees? Why or why not?
3. Why do you think third parties have not insisted on product standardization programs heretofore?
4. Who should be the chairman of the committee and why?
5. Who should keep the minutes of the proceedings and why?
6. Do you think that sales representatives should be on the committee? Why or why not?
7. What should be the role of the hospital administrator in the standardization process?
8. How can you get physicians to become enthusiastic about product standardization?
9. Can the standardization process be effective without the participation and support of the medical staff?

10. How can you keep product evaluations from becoming strictly subjective?
11. Could the Standardization Committee be effective without the materiel manager or his designee being a member?
12. Can the committee have too many members? Why or why not?
13. Does a product standardization review always save the hospital money? Why or why not?
14. Should the committee be primarily concerned with costs? Why?
15. Should printed forms be brought before the committee? Why?
16. What should be the action of the committee if the purchasing agent buys an item without consulting it? Why?
17. Should capital equipment be reviewed by this committee? Why?
18. Can drugs be effectively evaluated by the Standardization Committee? Why?
19. Should the Standardization Committee be concerned with lease-buy considerations? Why or why not?
20. Should a patient be a member of the product Standardization Committee? Why or why not?
21. How often should the Standardization Committee meet?
22. Is it important to take minutes of the standardization proceedings? Why?
23. How should product data that has been reviewed and acted upon by the committee be referenced and filed?
24. What if a sales representative takes issue with a committee decision? What is his recourse?
25. Should the committee keep a record of savings or losses created by decisions that it made? Why?

Chapter 8

Distributing the Goods the Right Way*

Recently, there has been an increasing interest in the development and implementation of materiel management in hospitals. This burgeoning interest is mainly the result of efforts to contain costs in the materiel area through the reduction and better use of personnel, supplies, paperwork, and inventory. Certainly, an effective materiel management program can achieve these respectable objectives and much more.

Simply stated, materiel management represents the management and control of supplies and equipment from acquisition to disposition. Moreover, the concept constitutes a continuum that encompasses a myriad of important supply functions (Figure 8-1). Important among these functions is the effective and efficient distribution of supplies and equipment throughout the hospital. For the materiel manager, there are few objectives that are more crucial or more difficult to achieve than this one.

Getting the right supply to the right place at the right time in the right quantity is a tremendous task to perform even under the most ideal conditions. However, the distribution process is hampered by such things as differing supply needs, a variety of systems that must connect at or about the same time, traffic patterns, and structural barriers within the hospital. Furthermore, there might be three or more integrated steps in the purchase-storage-use cycle, and distribution may be repeated many times before the ultimate disposition of the supply (Figure 8-2).

---

* Reprinted, with permission, from *Hospitals, Journal of the American Hospital Association,* (Vol. 51, No. 12, June 16, 1977, pp. 103–105).

Figure 8-1 Distribution Recurrence in the Materiel Management Continuum

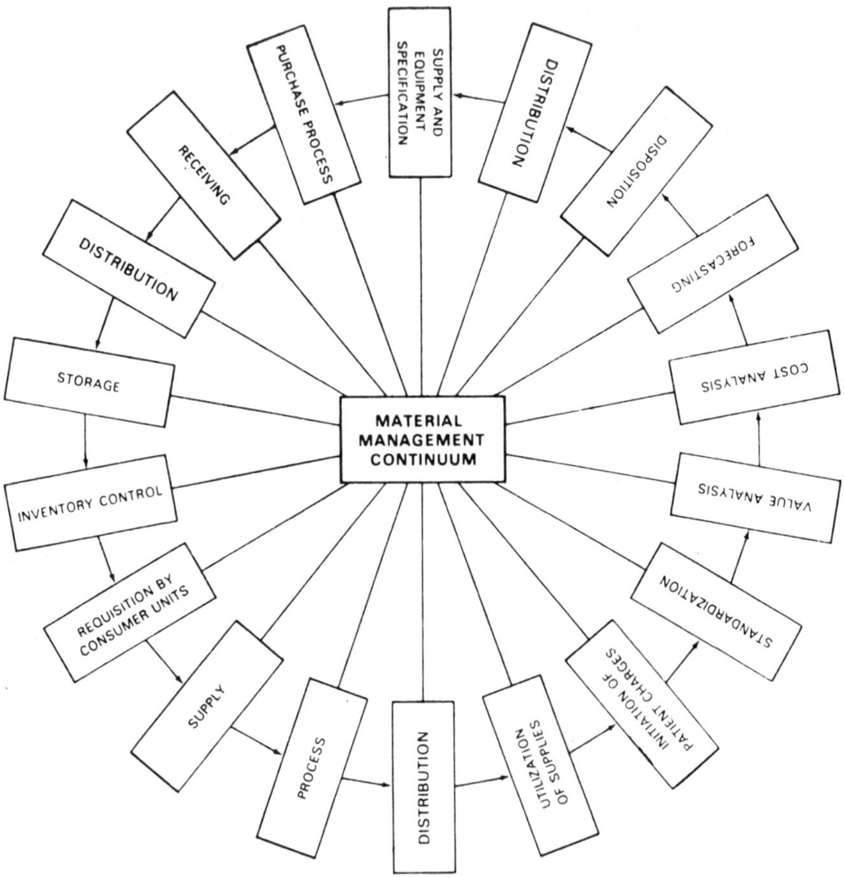

Requisition System

One of the oldest methods of supply distribution is the requisition and delivery system, sometimes referred to as "fetch and carry." Under this arrangement, someone on the nursing unit or in the nursing department has the responsibility for maintaining an adequate level of supplies, for making out a requisition for all needed items, and for physically taking the requisition to central stores for processing. Central stores then will fill the order and deliver the requested items on a supply cart to the destination for appropriate personnel to make proper disposition. This entire process

Figure 8-2 Distribution Alternatives in the Purchase-Storage-Use Cycle

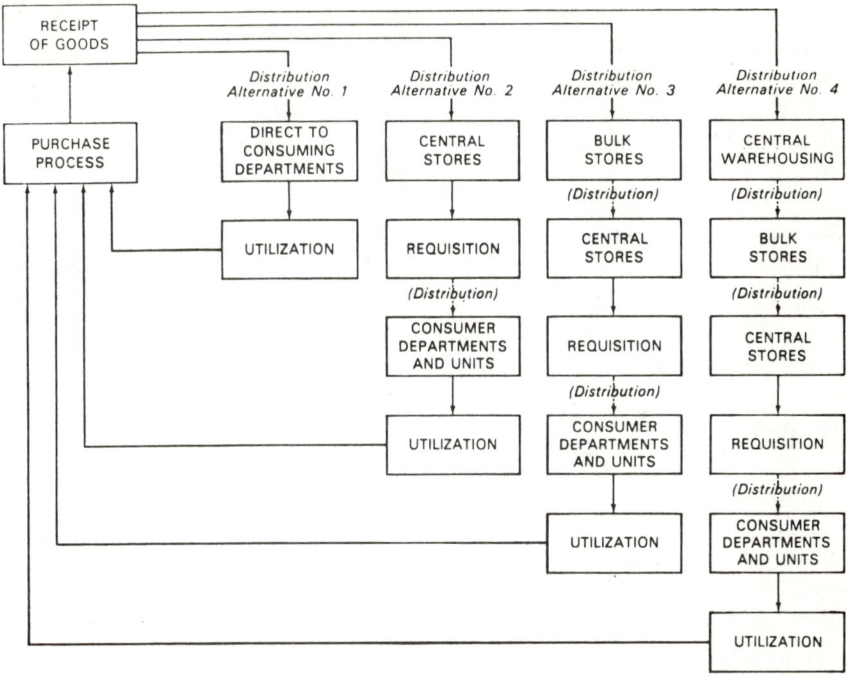

may be repeated at regular intervals several times a week by all of the consumer units and departments.

The distinguishing advantage of this method of distribution is its simplicity; however, there are many disadvantages. Taking inventory before each requisition is time-consuming. Nursing and other departmental personnel must take time from their busy schedules to handle supply chores, and the salaries of these individuals are generally somewhat higher than the salaries of those usually involved in the supply process. Furthermore, the entire burden of supply forecasting is placed on the nursing personnel on each unit. This method also often results in expensive duplication of inventory, which takes up valuable space. Despite its disadvantages, this method still is used in some hospitals.

Par Level Transfer System

Another interesting system of supply and distribution is commonly referred to as the par level transfer system. Using this method, each department continues to use the same storage space that it did when ordering from central stores. However, a quota for each supply item is established, and this quota is maintained by central stores. An attendant from central stores generally makes the rounds of all of the nursing units and departments at frequent intervals, approximately two to three times per week. He uses a large transfer cart to replenish all of the stock back to "par" levels.

The one redeeming feature of this system is that nursing and other departmental personnel are not involved on a day-to-day basis with supply duties. Unfortunately, the replenishment process is extremely slow with this method, because it is performed in departments where fluctuations in use often are the rule rather than the exception. As a result, the attendant usually must return to central stores several times in the replenishment process to restock his supplies. With the par level transfer system the hospital also still must maintain costly storage cabinets and costly additional space in each department.

Exchange Carts

Another mode of distribution that is winning wide acclaim is the total supply cart exchange system. Hospitals have been experimenting with and developing this system over the past 10 years, and the results have been good. The supply cart exchange system works best when carts include all items used by a nursing unit or department, from paper clips to intravenous solutions. Supply quotas should be established in conjunction with each department, and, to be effective, these quotas should be reviewed and updated at least quarterly, because practicality and credibility on the part of the user are of utmost importance with this supply system.

The total supply cart exchange system has proven to be one of the best, if not the best, methods of supply distribution for most hospitals regardless of a hospital's individual characteristics, because it is practical, flexible, dependable, and uncomplicated. This system can be implemented in small as well as large hospitals, old as well as new hospitals, vertical as well as longitudinal hospitals, specialized as well as the general hospitals, and so on. It has been established that it saves time, paperwork, steps, personnel, inventory and money. For the effective, results-oriented materiel manager, there are no real barriers to its development and success.

The total supply cart exchange system serves five integral functions: Supply forecasting, distribution, supply, control, and patient charge accountability. Foremost among these is the function of forecasting. Because a supply shortage can be anticipated 24 hours in advance of the time the item is needed, the materiel manager has adequate time to prepare and make the necessary steps to procure or substitute for an item. Accurate forecasting is imperative, if the total supply cart exchange system is to work. In order to ensure accurate forecasting, all other storage space on the nursing units, such as cabinets, drawers, and storage closets, must be eliminated.

Materiel Manager's Role

Dependability and reliability are essential, if the system is to gain the confidence of the various hospital departments. Ensuring reliability is the responsibility of the materiel manager. Carts should be checked for quality and quantity before being distributed. The cart system also must operate on a 24-hour, seven-day-a-week basis. At least quarterly, there should be a conference between the materiel manager and each of the respective using areas to adjust quotas and to discuss any problems either party is experiencing. A complete orientation to the purpose, functions, and benefits of the total supply cart exchange system should be given to all personnel, including the materiel management department, at least twice annually.

The size of carts should be carefully considered before purchasing them. A cart must have the capacity to hold approximately 200 different items and more than 1,000 items in total. Thus, the larger the cart the better, because the chances are good that there will be a need for more items than expected, not less. No more than two carts should be used per exchange, and they should be covered in storage and distribution to ensure clean, fresh supplies.

There are many other applications for the cart exchange distribution system. It is an excellent system for supply and distribution of pharmaceuticals, linens, and dietary items. Isolation techniques and surgical case pack quotas also can be facilitated by the system.

Automated vs. Manual

Although the supply distribution system of the future will probably be built around a cart, the best method for distributing these carts will continue to be debated. There has been much discussion regarding the advantages and disadvantages of both manual and automated systems. System flexibility is one of the principal considerations, because the type and number of supplies and methods of distribution are always in a state of flux. The manual system offers more flexibility, because one can remain open to change and improved methods without having to justify the costs that would be incurred if adjustments were made using an automated system.

Automated distribution systems usually are expensive. The cost of acquisition and installation alone has been estimated by some to be as high as 10 percent of the total building costs. Another important consideration is that such a high installation expense may not be justified for a system that operates no more than two or three hours per day. Furthermore, automation only pertains to the distribution of the carts and not to their replenishment. To rearrange, clean, inventory, and replenish a supply cart takes an average of 40 minutes. However, to distribute a cart manually only takes an average of two minutes per cart. Thus, the most time-consuming tasks still have to be "people-processed." These are just some of the factors that need to be weighed before selecting either a manual or automated distribution system. The decision is difficult, and it must be made carefully.

Summary

Distribution is an integral part of the supply process; a product or supply has little value until it is in the hands of those who can use it. The traditional "reverse distribution process," in which nursing or other departmental personnel go down to central stores to pick up any needed materials, results in a costly, inefficient use of manpower. When choosing a supply system, one of the foremost considerations that a hospital should keep in mind is how the supply or product will be delivered to where it can be used.

Pertinent Points to Ponder

1. Is distribution really a function of the materiel manager? Explain.
2. Why have high salaried personnel such as nurses been involved in the distribution of supplies and equipment?
3. What is the meaning of "reverse distribution"?
4. Can the requisition process be phased out? Explain.
5. How many times does distribution occur in your materiel cycle before the product is reordered?
6. Enumerate ways in which the distribution process can be reduced.
7. How does the par level method of distribution work in practice?
8. What is the difference between a par level system and a total supply cart exchange program?
9. What are the advantages and disadvantages of the par level system?
10. Do totally automated cart systems actually exist? Explain.
11. Why is it important to review and update supply quotas at least quarterly with the consumer department personnel?
12. How can an automated cart system be "tested" before purchase?

Chapter 9

A Supply Cart System: Highlights of a Ten-Year Study

STAGES OF A MAJOR PROJECT

1. *Enthusiasm*
2. *Disenchantment*
3. *Panic*
4. *Search for the guilty*
5. *Punishment of the innocent*
6. *Decoration for all those who took no part*

Anonymous

For the materiel manager, few functions are more difficult to achieve than the efficient distribution of supplies and service within the hospital. Recently, the concept in vogue is the use of a supply cart exchange system to solve these distribution problems. To examine the process for initiating such a system, we will use the example of Saint Anthony Hospital, Columbus, Ohio, one of the pioneers of the total supply cart exchange system.

Approximately ten years ago, Saint Anthony Hospital was in the preliminary drawing stages of a $10 million building and expansion program, which was completed in 1971. Naturally, there were many considerations concerning finance, equipment, and systems, including those in the rapidly growing area of materiel management. In a hospital composed of buildings constructed in 1890, 1955, 1964, and 1971, what would be the most efficient and most economical method of supply and distribution of goods and services? At that time the hospital was using the traditional requisition and delivery system of getting supplies from central stores to the nursing units. This process inherently had many problems associated with it: excessive time delays, expensive duplication, lack of forecasting, shortages complications, reverse distribution, etc. One thing was readily apparent—there had to be a better way!

A Pilot Program Is Recommended

Members of the hospital's management team were intrigued by the possible use of the cart system. After many trips to other hospitals, it was found that carts were being used to fragment instead of augment the supply and distribution systems. Some hospitals used their carts only for trays, others for intravenous solutions, and others for chargeable items only. Therefore, in addition to their antiquated and expensive requisitioning method, their supply departments were forced to cope with still another means of requesting and distributing. In a study of methods of requisition and distribution of supplies, it was found that no distinct and effective pattern existed. Within the same hospital, the supply department was being bombarded by a myriad of procedures at the same time—unit requisition of supplies on a certain day of the week, emergency orders, walk-ins, partial cart systems, and par levels.

It was apparent that a total supply cart exchange program would solve many problems on the nursing units if it were practical, and that the best way to find this out was to invest in a couple of large mobile carts and use them in a feasibility study. So the administration decided to conduct a total supply mobile cart exchange study on a medical unit for a 90-day period and to thoroughly document this experiment.

Members of the Materiel Management Department and a nursing unit, conferring at length on this matter, came up with a complete supply list with corresponding quotas for a 24-hour period. Included was everything from intravenous solutions to forms and paper clips (Exhibit 9-1). Materiel management personnel selected a cart and furnished it with the requisite kind and number of supplies. At the end, with the exception of a few minor complaints that quotas were not sufficient, the experiment was deemed to be an overwhelming success. At the summation conference, it was particularly noted that the new system would have the energetic support of the nurses, who found that it relieved them of the burden of performing several nonnursing functions.

After the favorable 90-day study, an administrative decision was made to implement the total supply mobile cart exchange program on all nursing units. Since quotas had already been established for a medical unit, all such units initially were supplied using this same inventory supply standard.

Exhibit 9-1 The total supply cart can easily accomodate hospital forms in a minimum of space.

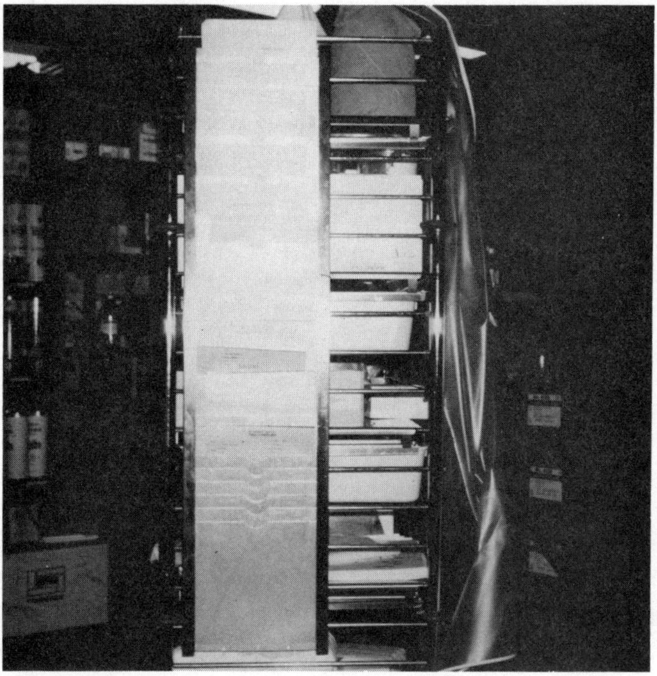

Following the same manner, separate quotas were jointly agreed upon by materiel management and nursing service for all surgical units. It is to be stressed at this point that all nursing units varied according to patient mix and supply needs, therefore each nursing unit was given a supply cart with an individualized quota. For each 32-bed nursing unit, one cart was to be in use on the unit and another to be in central stores being repleted. The carts were exchanged every 24 hours (Exhibit 9-2).

The delineated objectives of the total supply mobile cart exchange program were:

- To provide the nursing units with a total medical-surgical supply system. This meant always providing the right supply item at the right place and time and in the right quantities.
- To relieve the nursing units and other related departments of all non-nursing functions of keeping inventory, requisitioning, recording, delivering, and processing supplies.

Exhibit 9-2 The supply cart can carry a 24-hour supply of all items needed to operate a nursing unit.

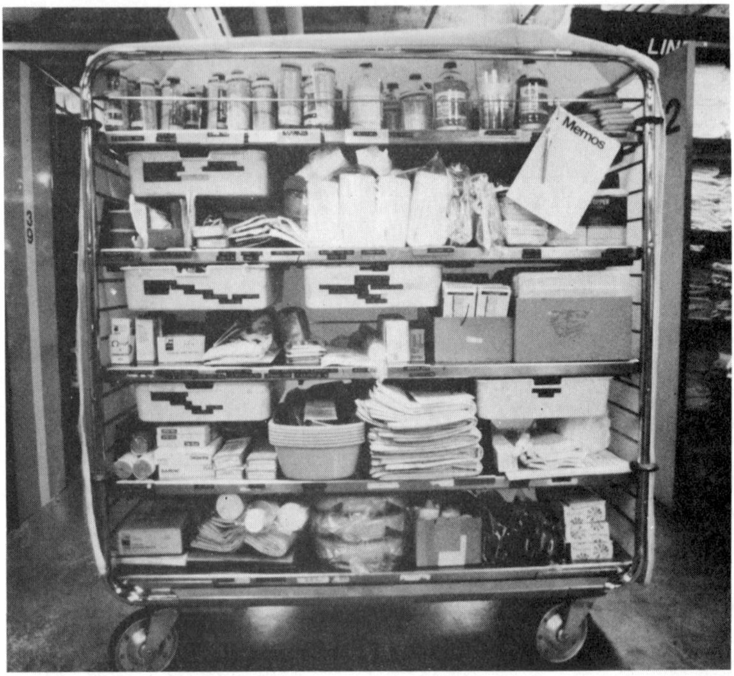

- To effectuate a practical system of controlling "unofficial" inventory that had already been dispensed to the various units.
- To place full responsibility and accountability in the Materiel Management Department for the functions of supply, process, and distribution.
- To implement a system of accountability for patient charges.

Form Follows Function

After the conclusive and convincing pilot program, members of management and the architects decided to design the nursing units with the supply cart as an integral and functional part of the design. Since a cart with the dimensions of 5′ x 6′ x 2½′ was sufficient for the medical and surgical supplies, all other storage was to be eliminated from the nursing units. Certainly, it is evident by now that this maneuver resulted in a savings of hundreds of thousands of dollars in the initial construction costs of the new building. It also had a very important secondary advantage of preventing a situation in which a duplicate stash of expensive supplies is squirreled away on the unit. The enhanced control and use of supplies that resulted was so convincing that even the cupboards and cabinets in the nursing units in the older building were ripped out and replaced by the total supply mobile cart.

Although the supply system changed drastically on the units, there was an even more pronounced metamorphosis in the stores area proper. The former storeroom in the old building became a center for all supply, processing, and distribution functions in the new building. The entire area was planned around the total supply mobile cart exchange program (Exhibit 9-3).

Initially the cart was kept in one place in the old building, and the stores personnel carried the individual items to it. This procedure again represented much duplication of time and effort. Under the new arrangement this duplicative procedure was eliminated, as the depleted carts enter into the rear of the logistics center where the cart is cleaned and all items are rearranged in the appropriate order. At this juncture, the cart attendant takes an inventory of all charge and noncharge items. Using the color-coded preinventory

Exhibit 9-3 The supply, process, and distribution center is set up to process supply carts.

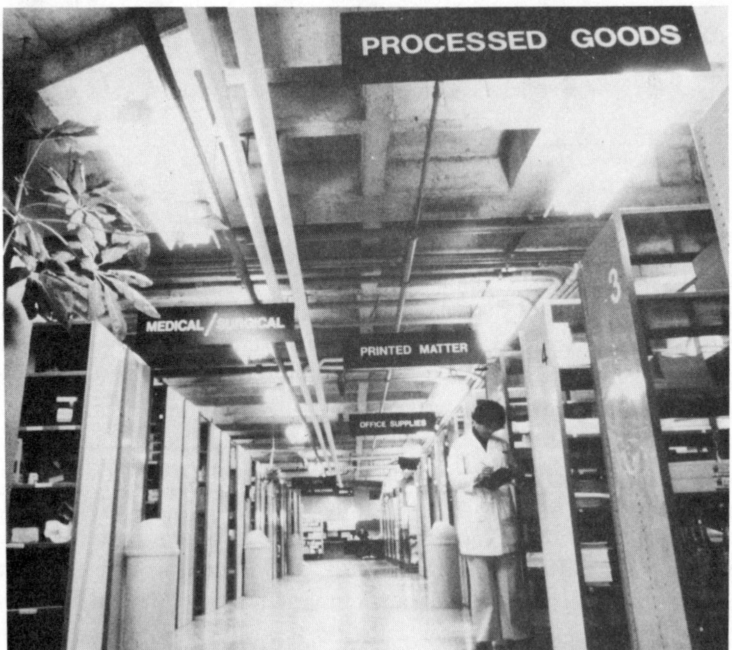

Exhibit 9-4 The assembly line process begins when the depleted cart is delivered to the cart processing area.

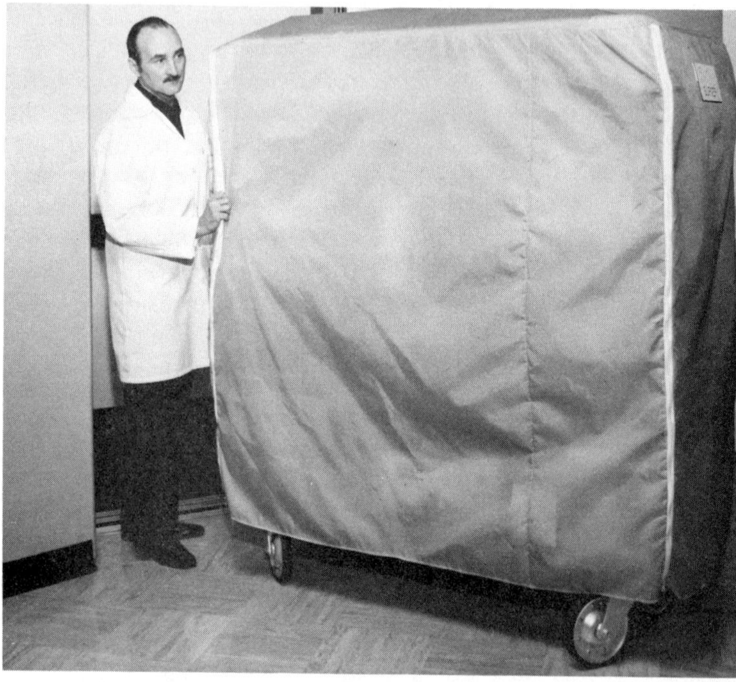

check list, the attendant then computes the difference between the cart inventory and the established quota for that unit. As the attendant pushes the cart down the center aisle of the logistics center, he uses the check list to replenish the necessary items in a sequential order (Exhibits 9-4 to 9-9).

By the time the cart reaches the end of the processing area, it has been completely replenished and is ready for distribution to the unit the next morning. Time and motion studies of the assembly line show that on an average it takes 40 minutes to fully process a depleted cart, after which it is moved to the distribution area where the cart coordinator performs a quality and quantity control check (Exhibit 9-10). Experience has revealed that this simple maneuver is an essential factor in maintaining the integrity of the system by ensuring that the user will find the right item at the right place at the right time.

Depletion—Repletion Cycle of Distribution

As has been stated, the two carts for each nursing unit are exchanged each day between 5:00 a.m. and 7:00 a.m., in an exchange which takes approximately two hours. Time and motion studies performed to determine the most efficient movement of the carts have revealed that 35 percent less time was spent in the cart exchange if the deliveries were made beginning with the nursing units farthest away from the logistics center (a finding which has to do with use of the service elevators). Furthermore, it was found that there was a waiting time for elevators of three minutes per unit for the complete exchange cycle, which became even more critical during the later hours of the day.

Since the cart contains all the medical-surgical supplies for each nursing unit, it is imperative that it be inventoried daily. Each cart carries 200 different supply items of which approximately 100 are not chargeable to patients and 100 are chargeable. It has been found that a cart attendant can inventory

---

Exhibit 9-5 The color coded cart cover is neatly folded and placed on top of the cart.

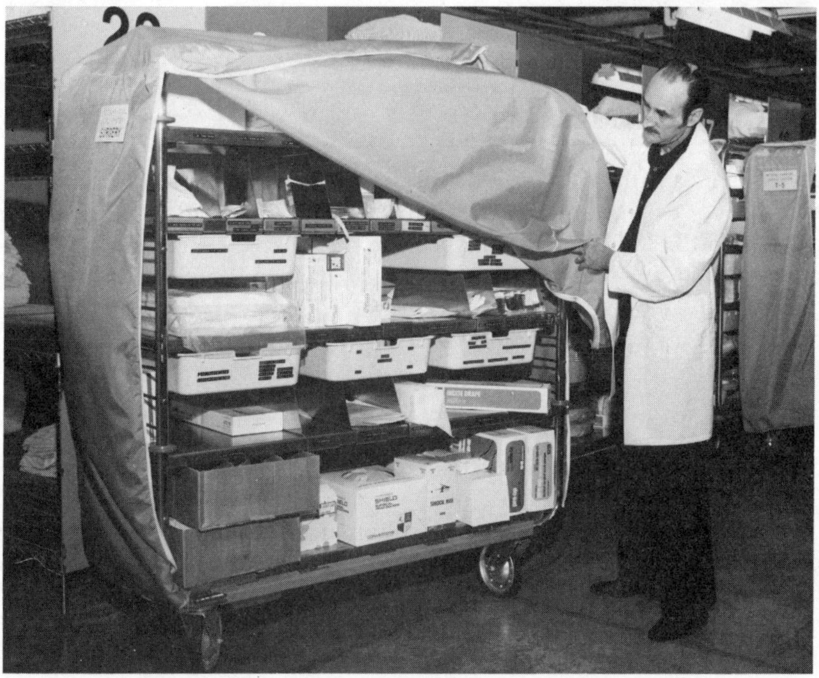

Exhibit 9-6 Items are rearranged according to their original order. The supplies are in disarray after the cart has been on a nursing unit for 24 hours.

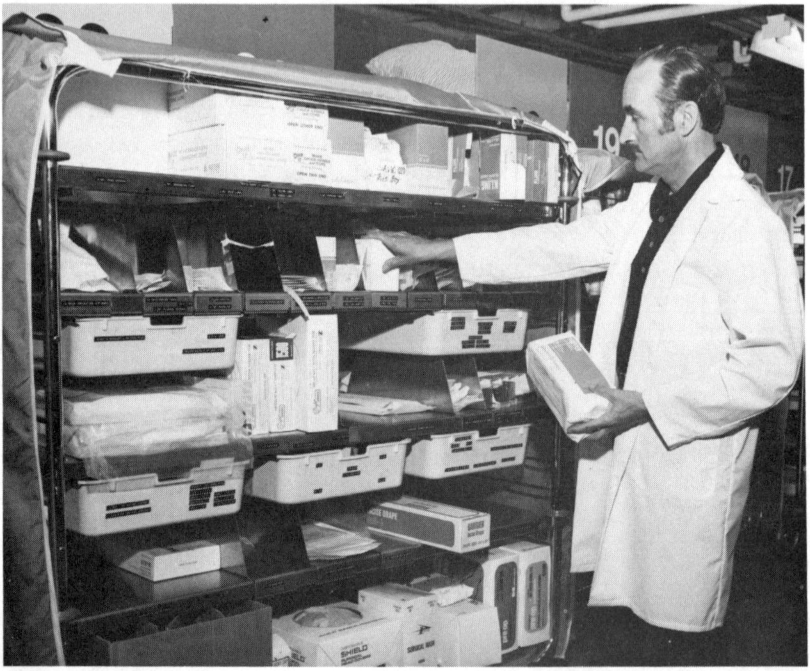

the entire cart with the same efficiency and in the same amount of time as it takes to do a partial inventory of only the charge items. The supplies are charged to the individual units when they are placed on the cart, but these expenses also are reviewed and controlled daily by materiel management personnel (Exhibit 9-11). At Saint Anthony Hospital, over $9,000 worth of supplies are exchanged every 24 hours in a process which has proven to be more effective and efficient than the conventional unit storage and requisition system.

A Patient Charge Mechanism Is Built In

In addition to total supply and distribution, the cart functions as a means of obtaining patient charges. Every item for which the patient must pay has a preprocessed tab card attached to it in a conspicuous place. This tab card, created by logistics center personnel, includes all information needed to process the patient charge with the exception of the patient identification, i.e., item, description, quantity and hospital item number (Exhibit 9-12). Accordingly, when a nurse takes a patient charge item from the cart, she needs only to stamp the tab card with the patient identification (Exhibit 9-13). The tab card then is put in a container which is collected when the carts are exchanged.

When the cart system was initiated, the supply items did not include tab cards and the nurses were required to make many value judgements concerning supplies. Is this a patient charge item? If so, what is it? Also, is the item preprinted on the form or is it to be written in? These questions, which should not concern the nursing units, are of paramount importance to materiel management and accounting. But after a month-long pilot study demonstrated that it was feasible, the tab cards were attached to the items.

Prior to the cart system, the hospital was plagued by lost charges and decreased patient revenues, made worse by the fact that no one could know what charges were not being processed since there was no idea of exactly what and how many items were on the unit. Furthermore, most lost or overlooked patient charges occurred on the evening and night shifts where the personnel were not usually as familiar with the established system and

Exhibit 9-7 The carts are carefully cleaned.

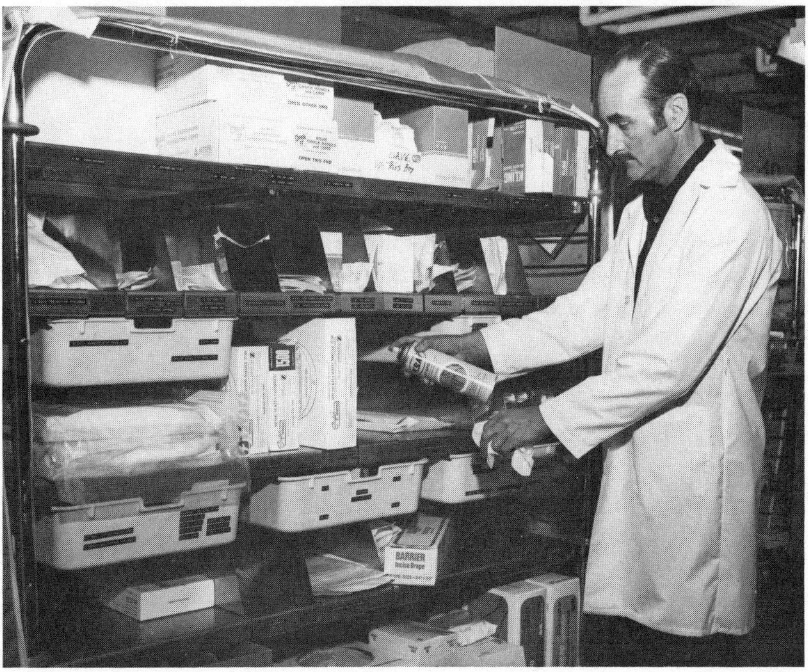

Exhibit 9-8 Next, a complete inventory is taken of all items remaining on the cart.

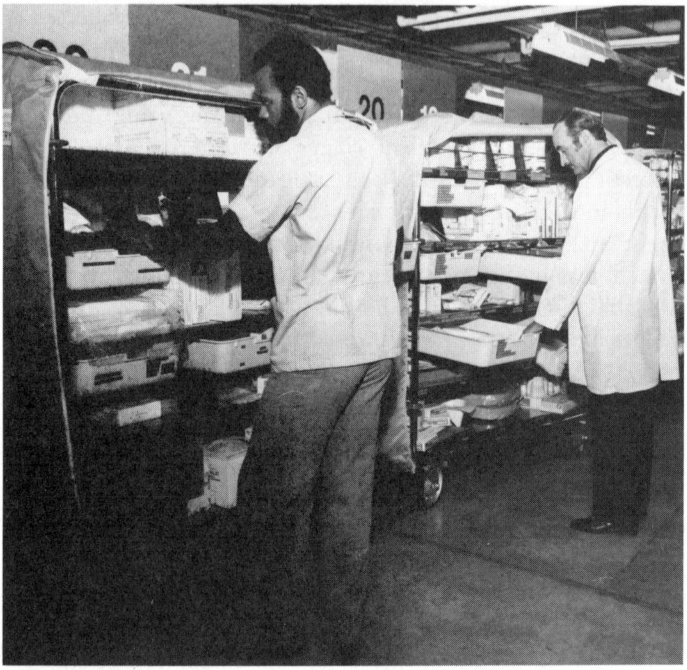

methods. Fortunately, this mess was eliminated by the installation of the controlled total supply mobile cart exchange system. The attached tab card is a constant reminder to the user that this patient charge item must be handled accordingly. Should a required charge not be made, materiel management personnel become aware of this oversight within 24 hours. The cart coordinator then goes to the unit and determines the disposition of the missing item by whatever steps are necessary, even reviewing the charts.

Ten Years Later

Ten years after Saint Anthony Hospital began using the total supply cart exchange system, it can be concluded that the program (distributed manually) is one of the best methods of supply distribution for today's hospitals. It is practical, flexible, dependable, and uncomplicated, and can be initiated in the small as well as the large hospital, the old as well as the modern one, and the vertical as well as the longitudinal. It is an established saver of time, paperwork, steps, manpower, inventory, and money. For the effective and results-oriented materiel manager, there are no real barriers to its development and success. Experience has also shown that there is no such thing as an automated cart system. Given that it takes an average of 40 minutes to rearrange, clean, inventory and replenish a supply cart, and only 2 minutes to distribute the cart manually, there seems to be no good reason to consider automating the system.

Accordingly, after much study and deliberation, the management of Saint Anthony decided to utilize a manual method of cart distribution for the following reasons:

1. System flexibility was the foremost consideration. With supplies and method of distribution always in a state of flux, the manual method seemed to provide the most flexibility. With a manual operation, it is always possible to change procedures without running into the costs involved in altering an automated system.

Exhibit 9-9 The carts are assembly-line processed in the supply, process and distribution center.

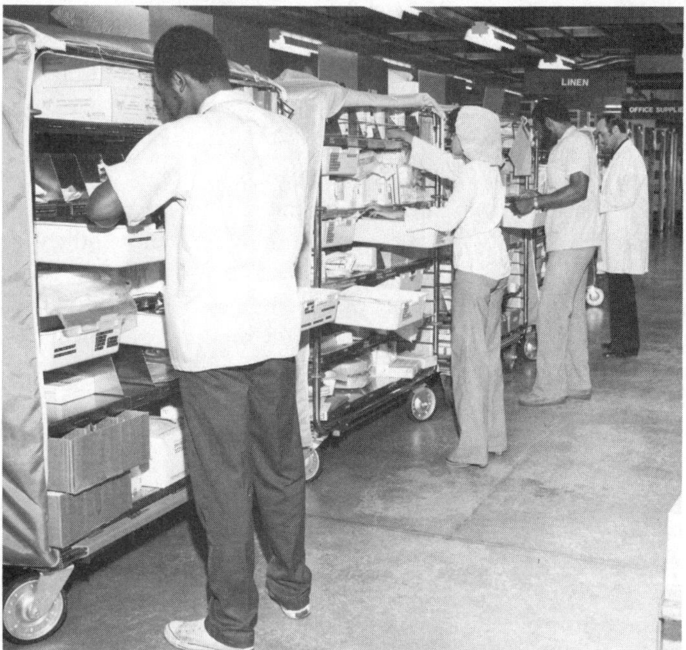

Exhibit 9-10 After the cart has been replenished, the cart coordinator performs a quality and quantity check.

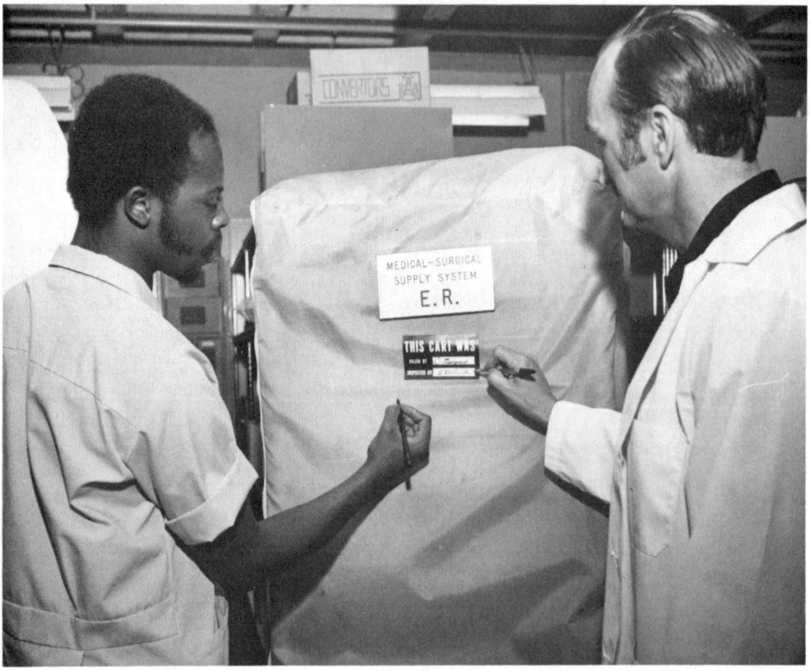

---

2. Automated distribution systems are expensive, especially in acquisition and installation costs. This cost has been estimated by some to be as high as ten percent of the total building costs. Another important aspect to consider is that all this expense is for a system which should operate two or three hours per day at most. At Saint Anthony Hospital, it takes less than two hours per day for total distribution of the carts. The work is performed by semiskilled personnel and costs about six dollars per day, less than the cost of electricity alone for some of the larger automated systems. Additionally, automation only pertains to distribution and not replenishment of the carts, so that the most time-consuming tasks still have to be performed by people.
3. Times when the machinery is down and expensive maintenance costs are usually associated with automated systems. In the past ten years, however, there has never been a day at Saint Anthony when the carts were not distributed to the nursing units. It is interesting to note that the backup for automated systems is manual distribution.

4. The manual cart exchange program has much flexibility and can be totally relocated if necessary. If the location of the materiel processing center should change, the manual cart program could be altered with a minimum of time, effort, and expense. It is difficult and expensive to expand and add on to automated systems.

Functions of the Total Supply Cart

The total supply cart exchange program serves five integral functions: supply forecasting, distribution, supply, control and patient charge accountability (Figure 9-1). Foremost among these is the function of forecasting a supply shortage at least 24 hours before the item will be needed. This gives the materiel manager adequate time to procure or substitute for the item.

The credibility of the cart system depends on responsible and responsive materiel management. That is why the carts are checked for quality and quantity before being distributed. Furthermore, there should be a conference

Exhibit 9-11 The cart coordinator checks to see that all supplies are charged to the appropriate unit or department.

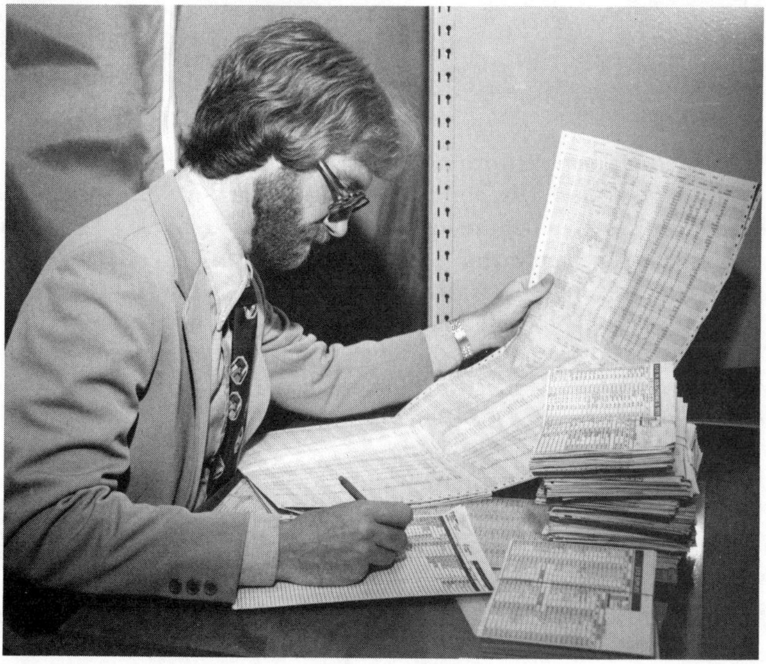

Exhibit 9-12 Patient charge forms are completed with the necessary charge information before being placed on the items.

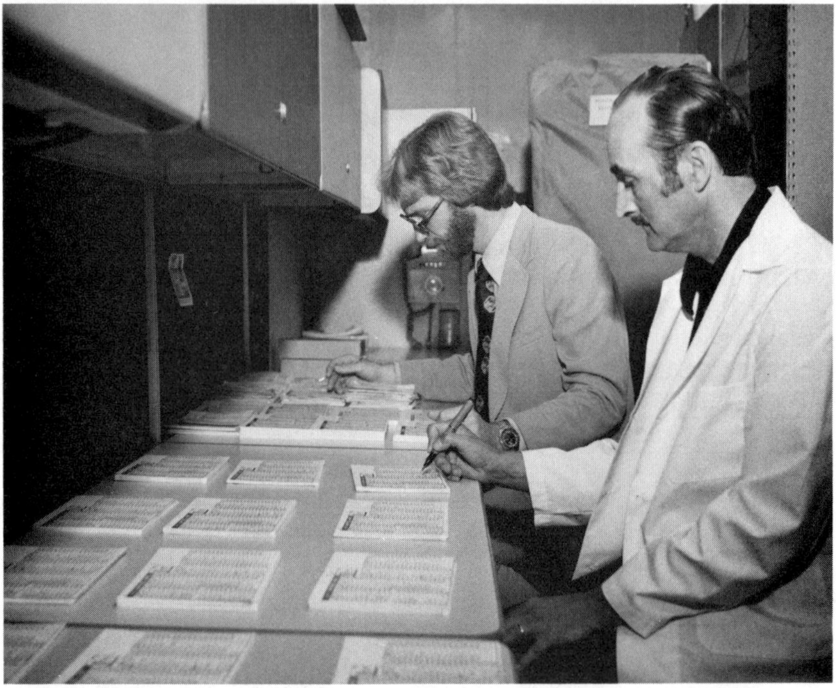

at least quarterly between materiel management and staff of each user area to adjust quotas and discuss any problems either party is experiencing.

Of the many other applications for the use of the cart exchange program, it is excellent for supply and distribution of linens, pharmaceuticals, and dietary items (Exhibit 9-14). Isolation technique, code blue boxes, and surgical case pack quotas also can be facilitated by the system.

Therefore, one can see that the total supply cart exchange program cuts across many disciplines effectively and economically. It is truly the supply and distribution system of the future.

Pertinent Points to Ponder

1. What is meant by a total supply cart exchange program? Explain.
2. What are the major differences between a par level and a cart exchange system?

3. Why have hospitals initiated mobile cart storage programs instead of having built-in storage?
4. In reference to the mobile cart exchange program, rate the five major functions in order of importance in your hospital.
5. Is the exchange cart mainly a vehicle of supply or a function of distribution? Explain.
6. Can all supplies in all hospital areas and departments be maintained via the exchange cart? Elaborate.
7. In your opinion, what would be the most difficult area to convert to the exchange cart program? Why?
8. Why are many hospital materiel managers under the misunderstanding that cart exchange programs are expensive?
9. In your hospital, what area would be the easiest to convert to the cart exchange program? Why?

Exhibit 9-13 Each cart carries the reminder that patient charges must be made when the applicable items are used.

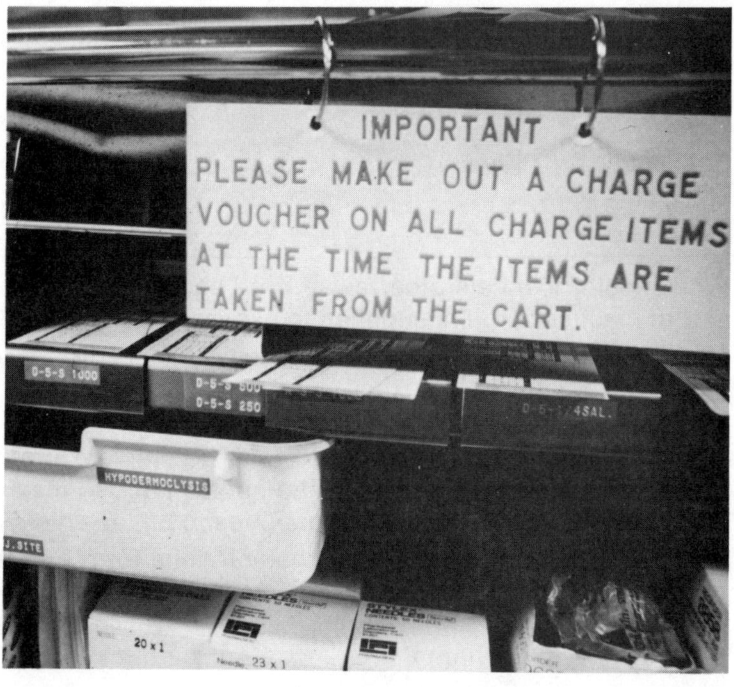
IMPORTANT
PLEASE MAKE OUT A CHARGE
VOUCHER ON ALL CHARGE ITEMS
AT THE TIME THE ITEMS ARE
TAKEN FROM THE CART.
D-5-S 250
HYPODERMOCLYSIS

Figure 9-1 Important Functional Roles Are Met by the Cart System

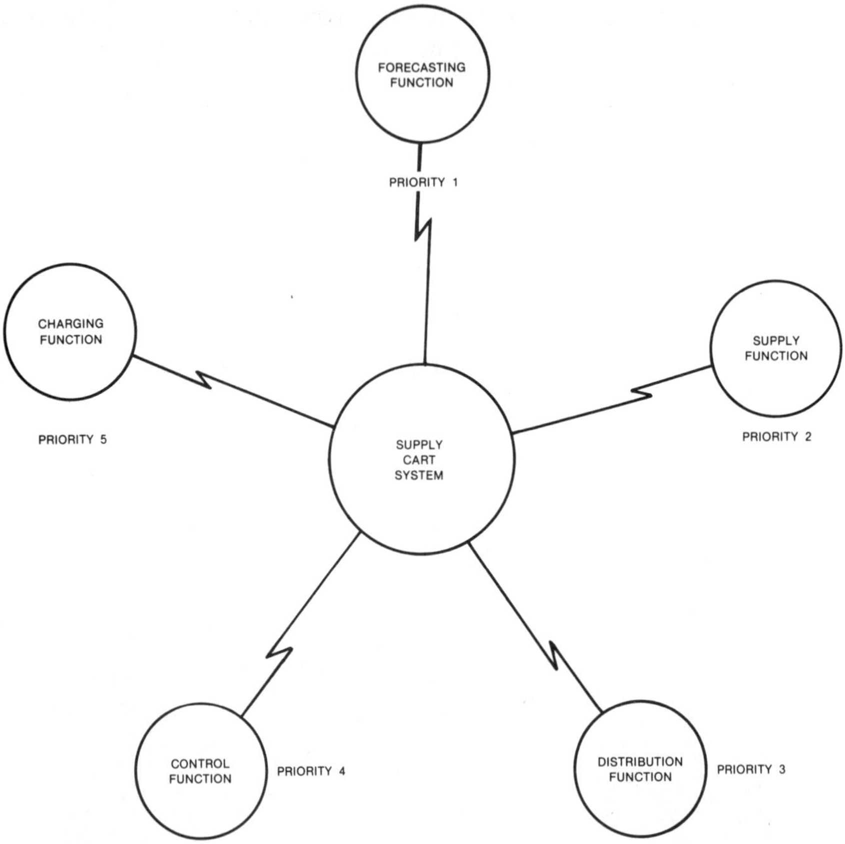

10. Why should hospitals steer away from having more than one cart of medical-surgical supplies to exchange daily?
11. Must the materiel manager or purchasing agent first get administrative approval to experiment with the total supply cart exchange program? Explain.
12. Why is it highly recommended to take a complete inventory of all cart items daily and bring the quotas back to maximum instead of just guessing at the quantities to be replenished?
13. If you were to point out the key characteristic for the success of the cart exchange program, what would it be? Explain.
14. Is it feasible to steam wash the supply carts daily or even weekly? Why or why not?

15. Make an exhaustive list of the possible applications for the exchange cart.
16. Make a comparison of the wire supply cart and the total metal cart. What are your conclusions?
17. How does the exchange cart program enhance the patient charge procedure?
18. It is highly recommended that the supply carts be exchanged on the night shift between 2:00 a.m. and 5:00 a.m. In your opinion, why?
19. Can the exchange cart program still be effective if the nursing units are allowed to keep their storage cabinets and cupboards? Explain.
20. What is the mix of patient charge and nonpatient charge items in your hospital?
21. Why is it extremely helpful to perform time and motion studies on the distribution of carts?

Exhibit 9-14 Surgery is supplied a daily quota of linen packs via the cart exchange program.

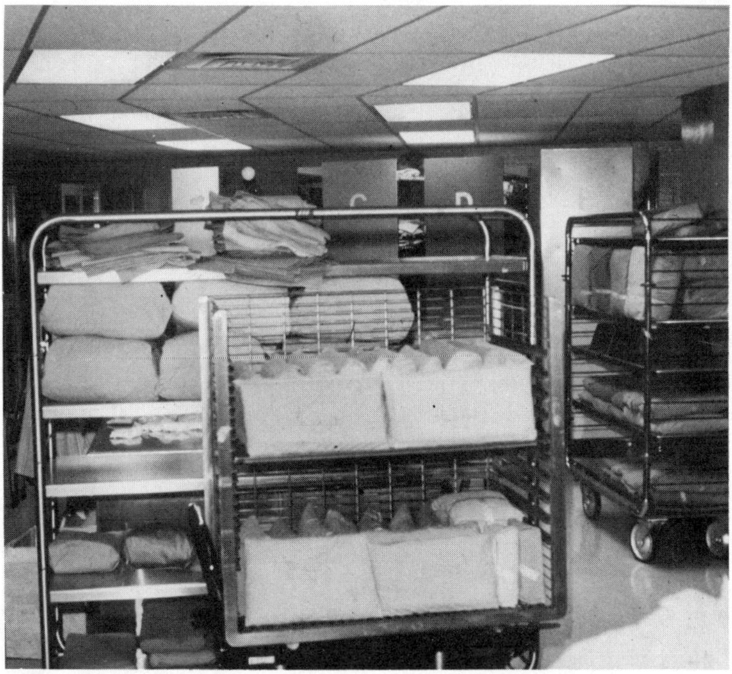

22. It has been stated that a total supply cart exchange program will literally pay for itself in at least 12 months. How?
23. In your opinion why haven't more hospitals converted to the total supply cart exchange system if it is so great?
24. Can an automated cart distribution system ever be justified in terms of costs? Explain.
25. How often should spot cultures be made on a supply cart and why?

Chapter 10

Inventory Reduction Is a Financial Must*

With today's double-digit inflation, hospitals are faced with budgets that do not balance, prices that are not stable, and costs that are not controlled. In this atmosphere, the hospital management is faced with the alternatives of lowering the quality of care or devising a way to cut the cost of providing care at the current level. Should it choose the latter, the materiel manager can play an important role.

There are three major categories of costs under the manager's supervision—personnel, supplies, and inventory. Salaries are usually controlled by top management, and supplies negotiated through prime suppliers, group purchasing endeavors, and bid contracts. Inventory, therefore, is the culprit in the problem of controlling costs of materiel management. To date, too much time and too many words have been expended talking about cost containment, which at best will only maintain the status quo. Inventory reduction, on the other hand, offers the most effective way to reduce hospital costs with minimum side effects. In fact, there will be no repercussions from the medical staff, nursing staff, patients, or administration if stocks are cut skillfully. About the only observable evidence of inventory reduction will be more cash flow and less headaches for the materiel manager.

A Different Philosophy

As never before, our society is turned on to the idea of security in numbers, or if one of an item is good, two is better, and three is best. This trend

---

*Reprinted with permission of DIMENSIONS in Health Service, Journal of the Canadian Hospital Association.

must be reversed if hospitals are to contain costs. I maintain that the hospital with a $250,000 inventory is less efficient than the hospital with a $50,000 inventory, and that materiel managers must adopt an attitude of doing more with less. I have often stated that materiel managers should take a complete physical count of all stock every week to become aware of the trouble and costs of maintaining an inventory. He would certainly find that inventory concerns take much of his time in the purchasing, counting, issuing, controlling, rehandling, and restocking of it. He would also realize that if he doesn't have it, he doesn't have to count it.

What is inventory? True inventory is the sum total and costs of all supplies, official and nonofficial, wherever they may be stored, that have not yet been used. The responsive materiel manager should have control and be responsible for all supplies, whether they be located in the storeroom, central supply, radiology, dietary, pharmacy, surgery, and/or on the nursing units.

I subscribe to the philosophy that inventory is a liability and not an asset. First, most hospital inventory cannot ever be sold for face value. I conjecture that if a hospital needed to rid itself of all medical-surgical inventory within a short period of time, it might recoup 50 percent of its initial investment. Second, inventory has to be controlled and counted continuously, so that the more there is, the more time and effort are expended managing it. Third, excessive inventories breed costly duplication and needless expiration of goods. Accordingly, I conclude that there is no reason for a hospital to become a supply warehouse, and that the art of reduction of inventory should be practiced by the materiel manager at the earliest possible moment.

What Actually Constitutes Inventory?

According to Webster, inventory is defined as "the quantity of goods or materials on hand." As relates specifically to hospitals, inventories can be classified as official and unofficial. Official inventory is that which is brought into a storage space or unit, counted, and controlled until it is dispensed to a using department. It is assigned to an inventory account number, and when it is dispensed the inventory account is relieved of the appropriate amount, which is then charged to the receiving department. There is usually a running total or perpetual inventory of this stock with predetermined minimums and maximums required for reordering. Moreover, the official inventory is counted physically at least annually and the amount is given to the auditors for the hospital annual inventory. This figure is verified by the auditing firm and is entered into the operating statement as an asset. There is also a bona fide attempt each year by the hospital accounting department to reasonably balance the official figure of inventory on hand as of a certain time with the purchases minus the issues.

So that there is some uniformity among hospitals' reporting systems, the official inventory can be broken down into the following categories:

a. Central stores: This should include all items that have not been dispensed to departments upon receipt, but have been stored for distribution and use at a later date, such as:
   1. Medical-surgical items;
   2. Dressings;
   3. Intravenous solutions and sets (Note: Some hospitals include this category under the pharmacy.);
   4. Linens (if an inventory is kept);
   5. Housekeeping items (if an inventory is kept);
   6. X-ray supplies (if an inventory is kept);
   7. Laboratory supplies (if an inventory is kept);
   8. Maintenance supplies (if an inventory is kept);
   9. Office supplies and stationery;
   10. Forms (if an inventory is kept);
   11. All processed and sterile supplies (These items might be found in the central supply if there is a separate area.).
b. Pharmaceuticals: All drugs and like items that are normally kept in the hospital pharmacy for use by the various consumer departments and units.
c. Dietary: This category includes staple foods, unused silverware, china, and related products. (Note: It does not normally include perishables.)

The unofficial inventory is those supplies that have been expensed and dispensed to the various departments and units, where they are stored until used. Most hospitals never count or rarely control this stock. However, considerable concern has begun to be expressed over the unofficial inventories because they can approximate three to five times the amount of the official inventories. In addition, they are usually a complete duplication of the official inventory.

Unofficial inventory exists in all supply-consumer departments such as nursing units, emergency rooms, clinics, surgery, anesthesia, cast rooms, radiology, laboratories, disaster storage, maintenance, dietary, administrative offices, physical therapy, physician offices, recovery rooms, print shops, and special care units (Exhibit 10-1).

Exhibit 10-1 Nursing units can have thousands of dollars tied up in unofficial inventory.

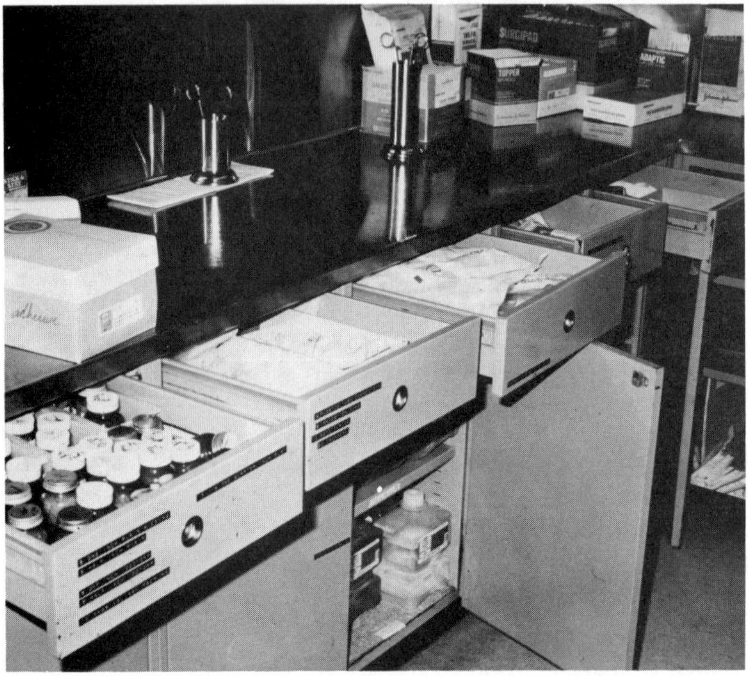

What Is a Responsible Per-bed Inventory?

Inventories will vary according to the type of hospital, its teaching programs, its size, its accessibility to suppliers, etc. But in the long run, all these factors average out, and definite projections per bed can be made. The following rating scale compares inventories per bed to materiel management effectiveness.

INVENTORY CATEGORY	POOR	FAIR	GOOD	EXCELLENT
A. Central Stores	Above $300/bed	$300/bed	$200/bed	$100/bed and under
B. Pharmaceuticals	Above $250/bed	$250/bed	$225/bed	$175/bed and under
C. Dietary	Above $ 45/bed	$ 45/bed	$ 30/bed	$ 25/bed and under

The scale is based on certain assumptions, the first of which is that hospitals should have definite objective-oriented inventory reduction programs. Also, hospitals should strive to avoid duplication of supplies in the central stores and the departments, but should, instead, adhere to the concept of stockless purchasing. Furthermore, hospitals should not stock unused linens and expensive forms since effective agreements with suppliers can be negotiated to avoid duplication of such costly commodities. An effective formulary should also be operational.

On the other hand, since the objective of the materiel management department should be better and tighter controls on departmental inventories, a policy of taking unofficial inventories no less frequently than semi-annually, and more preferably every quarter, should be established. Also, an administrative policy should be delineated to limit departmental inventories to a maximum two-week supply. Therefore, the materiel manager can review each departmental supply budget and divide it by twenty-six to indicate the inventory target for each department.

Some Disturbing Characteristics of Supply Inventories

- Maintaining a supply inventory is similar to keeping one's savings tucked away at home and not investing it. The major difference is that unlike money, supplies become obsolete, outdated, outmoded, appropriated, and mislaid. Anyone who has ever tried to sell a hospital supply inventory knows there is not much future in it.
- The very existence of inventory suggests duplication and backup. This duplication would be alright if hospitals kept only an emergency supply of all items in stock. Unfortunately, the fact is that duplication may be 100 to 500 times the amount needed. Furthermore, no one person really knows where all of the duplication is at any one time. While the official inventory is departmentally controlled, issued to the using departments as needed, and counted and reviewed at least annually by the hospital's auditors, the unofficial inventory is subject to little, if any, control. As Dean S. Ammer suggests in his book *Hospital Materials Management: Neglect and Inefficiency Promote High Costs of Care,* the average U.S. hospital maintains an average estimated official inventory of $630 per bed.[1] Furthermore, his fairly recent survey indicates the following breakdown:

[1]Dean S. Ammer, *Hospital Materials Management: Neglect and Inefficiency Promote High Costs of Care* (Boston, Mass.: Northeastern University, Bureau of Business and Economic Research, 1974), p. 31.

Drugs and pharmacy	$193.00
Medical-surgical supplies	144.00
Sterile supplies (central supply)	77.00
Office supplies—stationery	55.00
Housekeeping linens	49.00
Food and dietary supplies	46.00
Maintenance	37.00
Laboratory supplies	31.00
X-ray, radiology supplies	28.00
TOTAL ESTIMATED INVENTORY/BED	$630.00

This table suggests that the average 500-bed hospital has an official inventory of $315,000. Dr. Ammer estimates that the actual amount of cash tied up in inventory is probably at least $1,000 per bed, which indicates an unofficial inventory of $370; this author suggests a figure of $1,500 per bed, or an unofficial inventory of $870.

- It is easier to increase inventory than to decrease it, and the tendency to do so is omnipresent. If there is a question of having a large quantity or being out of an item, the materiel manager will choose the former every time since he becomes the center of complaint when there is a shortage, but is never admonished when supplies are overstocked.
- Inventories must be counted. There is nothing more distasteful to the materiel manager or purchasing agent than having to take inventory as required by most hospitals at least annually. As a rule of thumb, an official inventory that takes three people more than a day to count is too large. In addition to this annual physical count, there is also a perpetual inventory system which must be constantly updated to reflect changes in the stock levels and which is nearly always incorrect.
- Inventories must be controlled. This effort takes staff to man the stockrooms at least eight to sixteen hours per day. The more the inventory, the more the cost of control will be.
- Maintaining large inventories does not necessarily mean fewer stockouts. The smaller the inventory, the easier it is to check on shortages by the eyeball method of maintaining inventories. Moreover, the smaller the inventory, the less the need for costly data processing of inventories (Exhibit 10-2).

Inventory is truly a liability to the materiel manager, and it is to his advantage to devise an affirmative action plan to reduce it. Such a program can free large sums of money that were formerly tied up in stock, reduce personnel, and cut unnecessary paperwork.

Exhibit 10-2 The storerooms with too much inventory can never be assessed by the eyeball method.

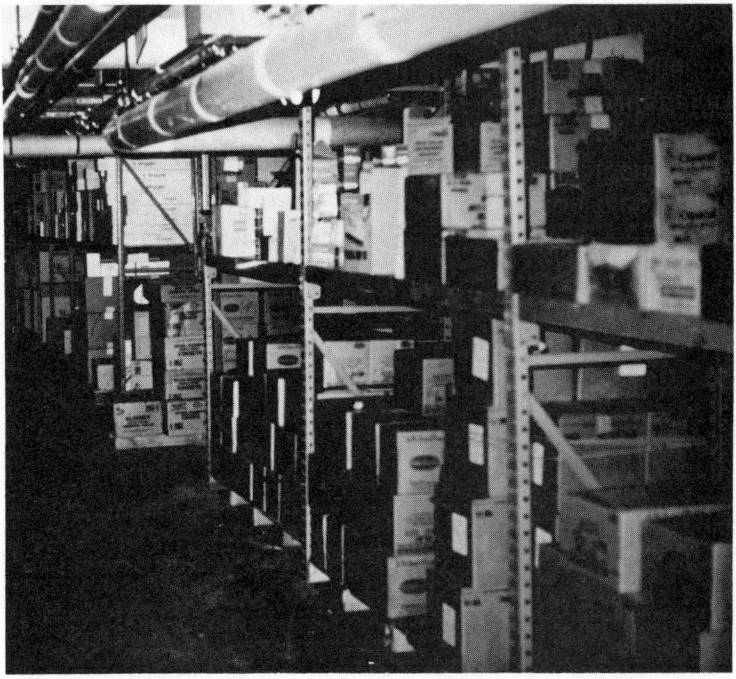

Plan To Reduce Unnecessary Inventories

1. Formulate administrative policies in regard to inventories and define certain responsibilities.
   a. Inventory control will be a function of the Department of Materiel Management, assisted by all pertinent departments.
   b. Control of both official and unofficial inventories is the responsibility of the Department of Materiel Management; inventories will be physically counted no less often than semi-annually.
   c. Each department will maintain no more than a two-week supply of unofficial inventory. Each department's stock will be based upon the annual approved supply budget divided by 26. Furthermore, each department head is to requisition from materiel management a two-week supply of operational inventory on the first and fifteenth of each month. These supplies are to be stockless purchases. For example, x-ray films are to be requisitioned and

purchased twice per month, with no film being kept in central stores. This means that all departmental supplies are to be ordered, expensed, and used in the same month.

   d. All purchases are to be made by the Department of Materiel Management.
   e. The combination of official and unofficial inventories shall not exceed $600 per bed.

2. Formulate and implement pertinent materiel management policies.
   a. All nursing and related units will be part of a 24-hour total supply cart exchange system (or another comparable program).
   b. Stockless purchasing will be practiced for all departmental purchases whenever possible.
   c. The prime supplier approach will be practiced for all major supply categories and reviewed accordingly.
   d. In reference to the prime suppliers, the necessary lead times are reviewed and approved periodically by the materiel manager.
   e. A multidisciplinary Standardization Committee will meet at least monthly to review and approve all new items prior to purchase.
   f. Appropriate item substitutes will be made when the supply of the standard item is delayed or becomes nonexistent.
   g. Certain large dollar volume items, such as orthopedic and cardiac implants, will be purchased on a consignment basis.
3. Combine all supply, process, and distribution functions under the supervision of materiel management.
   a. Central sterile supply will be a processing unit, not a source of supply items.
   b. Supply quotas are to be reviewed and updated with the pertinent using departments at least quarterly.
4. Perform a timely performance review for all prime suppliers and consumer departments and nursing units within the hospital by the Department of Materiel Management.
5. Develop and use timely administrative reports by the Department of Materiel Management.
   a. Vendor usage report
   b. Vendor performance report
   c. Departmental purchase report
   d. Nursing unit usage reports
   e. Shortage reports, by dollar amounts
   f. Standardization report.

Obviously, there is a necessary amount of inventory for the smooth functioning of the hospital. The key question is, "How much is necessary?'' As we have seen, the necessary level for most hospitals is many times less than the quantities now kept. If administrative and managerial attention is given to this area immediately, monumental costs savings and a more efficient materiel management program can be the rewards. In reference to inventory, remember that more than enough is wasteful and costly.

Fifty Ways to Reduce Your Inventory

1. *Don't gorge, George.*
2. *Recycle, Michael.*
3. *Don't replete, Pete.*
4. *Take it down hill, Jill.*
5. *Put it on a cart, Bart.*
6. *Start a formulary, Gary.*
7. *Reduce, Bruce.*
8. *Clear the aisle, Kyle.*
9. *Don't increase, Maurice.*
10. *Get it down today, don't let it stay, Kay.*
11. *Don't let the pressure get you moody, Rudy.*
12. *Make it sane, Wayne.*
13. *Take it to zero, Flo.*
14. *Change the way you think, Link.*
15. *When one will do, don't order two, Lou.*
16. *Use a prime supplier, Ira.*
17. *Don't reorder, Porter.*
18. *Don't carry, Larry.*
19. *Don't loada, Rhoda.*
20. *Keep it slim, Jim.*
21. *Motivate, Kate.*
22. *Check the expiration date, mate.*
23. *Take it to a few, Andrew.*
24. *Think thin, Ben.*
25. *Don't buy, Guy.*
26. *Create a void, Boyd.*
27. *Let the people wonder where it went, Brent.*
28. *Keep inventory low, Joe.*
29. *Drop ship, Skip.*
30. *Don't purchase many, Lenny.*
31. *Dispose, Rose.*
32. *Plan ahead, Ted.*
33. *Send it back, Mack.*
34. *Don't look back, Jack.*
35. *To centralize is your duty, Trudy.*
36. *Let it be, A-B-C, Genevieve.*
37. *Keep it clean, Charleen.*
38. *You won't get hurt, Bert.*
39. *Let it reach the min, Ken.*
40. *Don't cram, Sam.*
41. *Make it work, Kirk.*
42. *Keep it lean, Jean.*
43. *Think less, Bess,*
44. *Don't order a barrel, Carole.*
45. *Let the stock get bony, Tony.*
46. *Don't jam, Pam.*
47. *Standardize, guys.*
48. *Don't remember back when, Gwen.*
49. *Save a buck, Chuck.*
50. *Don't tarry, Mary.*

Pertinent Points to Ponder

1. What is your definition of supply inventory?
2. What are the differences between official and unofficial inventory?
3. Why aren't all supplies just charged off at the time of receipt, eliminating the need to put them into inventory?
4. Do inventories per bed differ in volume in the large hospital as compared to the small one? Why?

5. Which will tend to have the larger per diem inventory, the large hospital or the small hospital? Explain.
6. What elements are involved in inventory holding costs?
7. What percentage of the costs per annum are for inventory holding?
8. Why are physical counts taken of official inventory at least annually?
9. In the average hospital, why isn't a physical count taken of the unofficial inventories?
10. In what ways can the materiel manager work with the supplier in inventory reduction?
11. Is distribution a factor of inventory costs? Explain.
12. How does one account for pilferage in the inventory procedure?
13. For best results, how frequently should official inventories be taken?
14. Name ten ways to reduce official inventory.
15. When taking physical inventory, how does one count broken packages and outdated stock?
16. In your estimation, how much inventory is on an average nursing station in your institution?
17. Should the supplier ever be allowed to take physical inventory of stock? If so, under what conditions?
18. What unit or department is most likely to account for more inventory than any other in the average hospital? Why?
19. How can the actual physical inventory be made easier?
20. Why is it that most materiel managers and purchasing agents dislike taking inventory?
21. After the physical inventory has been taken, what should be done with the results?
22. In the modern hospital, who is most interested in the results of a physical inventory? Why?
23. Should linen currently in use be inventoried? If so, how often?
24. If you had a $100,000 inventory and needed to sell it within a week, what would be your asking price? How much would you probably get? To whom would you sell it?
25. What procedure is used to inventory equipment that is in use? Why is this done?

Chapter 11

Stockless Purchasing Makes Dollars and Sense *

Traditionally, hospitals have used central stores to back up all supplies that are used in every department. A typical hospital storeroom could contain as many as 3,000 different stock items exclusive of the thousands of different kinds of pharmaceuticals and foodstuffs. In addition to central stores, many hospitals have established bulk stores and even off-the-premises warehousing. In contrast, a far better approach would be to initiate, develop, and fully implement the concept of stockless purchasing, or the buying of supplies for direct use by the departments without accumulating an inventory in the central stores.

According to the concept of stockless purchasing, central stores should consist of only standardized items that are used by several consumer units or areas. An excellent example of such items is intravenous solutions. They are used by every nursing unit in the hospital including the emergency room, recovery room, and surgery. Consequently, the ideal central store should be able to provide for a minimum supply of an item to adequately handle a maximum number of consumer units or departments. If this idea is fully implemented, the entire stock in central stores should approximate an average inventory of $75 to $100 per bed and should be completely turned over 26 to 50 times per year. The new concept of central stores is also applicable for pharmaceuticals, especially since the rapid turnover does not allow for much accumulation, obsolescence, or pilferage. With the nursing units consuming approximately 50 percent of expendable supplies on a basis of rapid turnover, it is equally important to implement a system to purchase and control the

* Reprinted with the permission of DIMENSIONS in Health Service, Journal of the Canadian Hospital Association.

other 50 percent that does not turn over so rapidly and uniformly. These supplies are usually unique to one department. The following departments and items are prime examples of areas in which stockless purchasing should be implemented:

a. Radiology
b. Laboratories (hematology, chemistry, blood banking, etc.)
c. Surgery (sutures, implants, disposable packs, etc.)
d. Plant and maintenance
e. Respiratory therapy
f. Housekeeping
g. All capital equipment
h. Dietary (staple foods and perishables)
i. Linens
j. Forms

In most cases, these areas purchase and store supplies that require special handling, such as laboratory reagents and serums which need refrigeration: X-ray films which should be stored with attention to light, humidity, and temperature; dietary items that require refrigeration; and forms which must be kept in a dry place. To replicate these conditions by stocking such items in central stores would be costly from many perspectives.

Stockless purchasing thrives best when the concept is supported and promulgated in writing by top management. The administrative policy should spell out the areas to be involved and certain time parameters. Ideally, the inventory to be kept in the stockless area should be approximately a two-week supply, which can easily be determined by dividing the current supply budget by 26. If a quarterly physical inventory indicates that the department is substantially over the two-week supply, then the materiel manager should assist the department director in bringing the stock into conformance. Reordering for stockless items should be done on the first and fifteenth of each month so that the cost, expense and revenue from the supplies can be appropriately recorded and charged.

The most crucial and challenging aspect of stockless purchasing is the specification and delineation of appropriate departmental quotas. This takes time, effort, expertise, and cooperation from both the materiel manager and the respective department directors. The initial quotas that they establish must be flexible and subject to change with little notice to assure that if a quota is incorrectly set, it can be changed without too much protocol.

With stockless purchasing more responsibility is placed on the department head for effective supply utilization, cost containment, and supply specification. Consequently, the materiel manager should begin implementation of stockless purchasing with a department that has relatively few items so that quotas can be clearly quantified. It is further suggested that the new concept be perfected in the pilot department before another department is approached, since nothing gets results like good results.

Of course, advertising aside, establishing realistic quotas is the entire key to the success of the program. The quota-setting phase must encompass such important issues as lead times, supplier backup, turnover ratios, and peaks and valleys in the supply cycle. After these factors have been carefully considered and appropriate quotas established for all of the stockless items in the department, then a preprinted department stockless supply requisition is developed with complete supply descriptions and quantified quotas for a 14-day period. There should also be a section on the requisition for comments from the department head since he may want to increase or decrease the quota for that order period. Immediately upon receiving and verifying the quantities, the materiel manager or purchasing agent initiates the purchase process. If functioning correctly, this process will be repeated time and again with little effort and splendid results both for the department and the ma-

Exhibit 11-1 The laboratory is an excellent area in which to implement stockless purchasing.

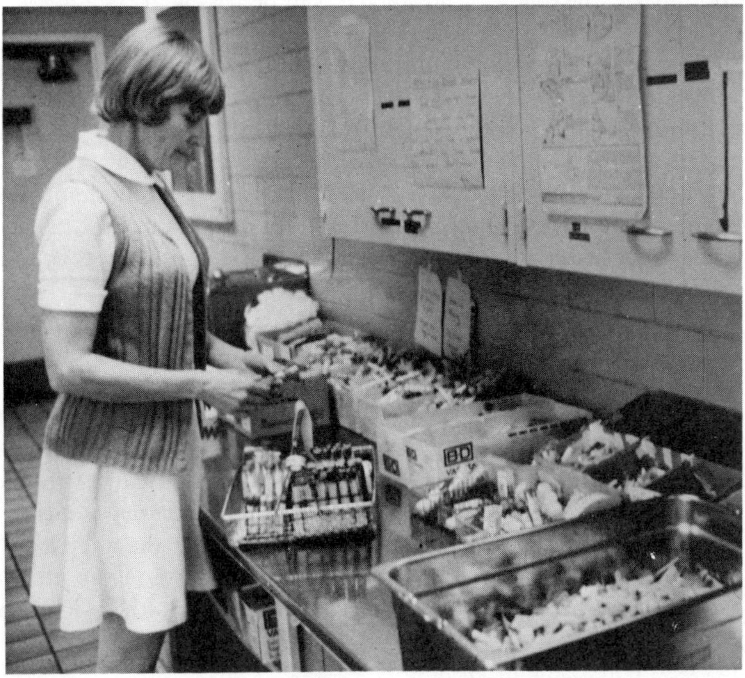

teriel manager. After the successful development, the materiel manager is ready to begin implementing stockless purchasing in another department. It is suggested that no more than one department be involved in this change-over at the same time, so that the materiel manager can consider and approach each department with a new set of values and expectations.

I am often asked which department is the easiest to convert to stockless purchasing. Even though each institution and situation is different, in most cases the best department to begin with is the one with the best supply specification and/or the least amount of items. Consequently, radiology may very well be the best starting point. On the other hand, there are some departments that have a track record of being difficult for one reason or the other. Surgery is difficult because of the myriad of supplies and suppliers. Maintenance supplies are usually difficult at first because of the lack of specifications and the rather technical nature of the products. Laboratory supplies, despite the number of items involved, are not to difficult because almost all of them can be purchased through a prime supplier (Exhibit 11-1). Fortunately, no department presents insurmountable problems that prohibit implementation of stockless purchasing.

Stockless purchasing is the catalyst which will cause other things to happen along this continuum of functions called materiel management. If implemented properly, the following advantages will be readily discernible:

- Stockless purchasing creates a supply discipline and philosophy that will permeate the entire institution. It brings the materiel manager face to face with the entire management structure, and quickly sets the tone for professional development of the materiel management endeavor.
- Stockless purchasing eliminates at least one level of costly supply duplication, thus saving the hospital thousands of dollars annually.
- It allows for better and more efficient use of the central stores by freeing space and eliminating congestion.
- It drastically reduces holding costs, conservatively estimated to be at least 25 percent of the total inventory investment on an annual basis. In other words, if a $100 item remains unused in stock for one year, its cost will appreciate to $125.
- Stockless purchasing results in less handling which means less man-hours for the receiving and supply functions. For example, many of the stockless departmental supplies can be accounted for by central receiving and be taken directly to the consumer department by the supplier. This eliminates the function of receiving the supply, storing it in central stores, processing a requisition, then distributing it to the using department.
- Stockless purchasing means less paperwork.

- It promotes the prime supplier approach to purchasing.
- Stockless purchasing greatly reduces supply shrinkage.
- It provides for more control over unofficial inventories.

Stockless purchasing does not in any manner interfere with the concept of centralized purchasing, but instead it supplements and reinforces it. The philosophy of stockless purchasing is truly representative and characteristic of a well developed materiel management effort.

Pertinent Points to Ponder

1. Why are hospitals reluctant to initiate stockless purchasing?
2. In your opinion, what is the supplier's attitude toward stockless purchasing? Why?
3. In your hospital, what department or area would be the most reluctant to implement this concept? Why?
4. How does stockless purchasing differ from perpetual inventory?
5. Why is it important to get administrative support before implementing this concept?
6. In your opinion, what department or area would be the least resistant to stockless purchasing?
7. Would it ever be possible to eliminate all official stores inventory? Why or why not?
8. Who has the most responsibility for making the concept work? Why?
9. In your opinion, what item of supply is the most duplicated throughout the hospital? Why?
10. How should the concept of stockless purchasing be introduced to the departmental directors?
11. Why is it a good idea to charge and pay for an item the same month?
12. In your opinion, what is the future of stockless purchasing? Why?

Chapter 12

Creating a Buyer's Market*

Recently the materiel manager has added some new words to his vocabulary—contract purchasing, systems contracting, and prime supplier. These three terms, essentially the same, indicate that entire categories of supplies are purchased from a single source on negotiated terms of quantity, quality, price, and time. Although they describe a situation which on the surface eliminates competition and creates a supplier monopoly, it seems that this arrangement may be the best for the hospital in both the short and long range.

For years, hospital purchasing agents have done their buying from several vendors because they felt that this process protected the hospital from exorbitant prices. Consequently, the vendors became familiar with this technique and adjusted their salesmanship tactics to it. In counter-response, hospital materiel managers must now become innovative in their purchasing approaches and create a buyer's market instead of competing in a seller's market. This is especially pertinent since hospital purchasing practices in the next few years will be reviewed and scrutinized by many concerned parties, including government, insurance companies, and accreditation commissions.

The Great Fallacies of Hospital Purchasing

Some distinctly discernible ideas and philosophies have permeated the art of hospital purchasing for many years. These "Great Fallacies" of Hospital Purchasing" will be described in the following section.

---

*Reprinted with the permission of DIMENSIONS in Health Service, Journal of the Canadian Hospital Association.

Fallacy Number One

Hospitals are doing a good job in the area of purchasing. As Dean S. Ammer states:[1] "Competent purchasing and inventory control can reduce aggregate hospital charges by at least $1,000,000,000 per year, but improvement is not likely without active encouragement of third party payers." This statement alone should provide the impetus for hospital materiel managers to upgrade and dignify the art of purchasing.

Fallacy Number Two

Anyone can purchase. This statement is substantiated by the fact that many persons in hospitals, including the pharmacist, dietitian, maintenance engineer, and C.S.R. supervisor, are involved with the purchasing of goods and services. Furthermore, purchasing agents usually lack training, education, and experience. This situation must be stopped for the sake of efficiency, effectiveness, and credibility. Centralized purchasing must be initiated and practiced by trained professional purchasing agents who can bring expertise to the hospital setting.

Fallacy Number Three

Basically, purchasing is materiel management. Nothing could be further from the truth. Many hospitals have given their purchasing agents the title of materiel manager, but their functions have remained the same. This ignores the notion that purchasing is a very small function of materiel management. In fact, with the negotiation of contract purchasing, the specific act of purchasing can to a large degree be automated.

Fallacy Number Four

The supplier dictates purchasing policy. In other words, the supplier sets the price, dictates how and when supplies will be delivered, and indicates what supplies and quantities will be kept in the inventory. This has been true in the past, but the hospital management now delineate the purchasing policy, and the supplier should respond accordingly. Purchasing is a symbiotic relationship between hospitals and suppliers, with contract purchasing providing the avenue for hospitals to specify the why, what, how, when, and where of the procurement functions to the supplier.

Fallacy Number Five

Larger hospitals get better prices than smaller ones. Although it seems

---

[1] Dean S. Ammer, *Hospital Materials Management: Neglect and Ineffeciency Promote High Costs of Care* (Boston, Mass.: Northeastern University, Bureau of Business and Economic Research, 1974), p. i.

that because of volume the larger hospital would get the better price, this is not actually the case. Good purchasing is the art of negotiation and the better the negotiation, the better the prices. Contract purchasing enhances the hospital's purchasing power.

Fallacy Number Six

Competitive bidding is a good indicator of proper purchasing practices. By using the bidding process, the buyer attempts to keep the competitive edge, but the result is often confusion, bad will, and mediocre prices. For one, the bidding technique mandates concise product standards, something that has been lacking in hospital purchasing since the beginning. Two, it is very difficult to legislate performance and acceptable quality from suppliers on a uniform basis. Three, traditional bidding is outmoded in the area of supplies, especially since many suppliers refuse individual item bids, so that suppliers may be rather nonchalant in their response to bid. However, if the prize to be gained is supplying all medical-surgical needs, an order which may range into the millions of dollars, suppliers are very responsive and accommodating.

Contract purchasing offers the hospitals this opportunity. It provides leverage for demanding best price, quality, and performance. In addition, since it encompasses all supplies of a certain category—small as well as large volume items, less expensive as well as the most expensive ones—the hospital consistently gets the best overall deal with a fraction of the time and effort expended with traditional purchasing methods.

It should be stressed at this point that the hospital may not realize maximum overall savings during its first year of contract purchasing. Many suppliers are reluctant to give up their profit margins until they know for sure the hospital means business. Therefore, the hospital should make the first year under the system an exemplary one to put all other suppliers on notice that if they don't compete, they won't get any of the business.

Fallacy Number Seven

Hospitals should be in the supply and warehousing business. The primary objective of hospitals is the delivery of patient care, while that of manufacturers and suppliers is supply and distribution. For some reason, though, hospitals almost try to compete with the supplier at his own specialty. Some hospitals pride themselves in large inventories and elaborate distribution systems, which represent misuse of costly square footage, an expensive manpower budget, and much duplication. For instance, the materiel manager who has a supply department which consists of 5,000 square feet of storage space, at an estimated $60 per square foot building cost, is sitting on a $300,000 empire, an estimated $150,000 inventory, and a $150,000 annual salary expense. What is more disastrous, this situation often exists in ten or fifteen other hospitals in the same geographic area that may be served by two or three large supply distributors.

Built into the price of every supply item is a certain percentage for storage and holding for a certain interval of time. If a hospital purchases an excessive inventory of any or all items, the hospital is assuming a costly burden which becomes advantageous to the supplier and detrimental to itself. If, however, hospital managements begin to regard the function of the suppliers as a shared service, much of the hospital space now being used for storage could be converted into patient care areas. These ideas represent the difference between materiel management and mere purchasing.

Fallacy Number Eight

Equal prices are relative. In other words, the same price for a particular item from several companies is comparable. It has been the case, for example, that the highest quoted price for the same item turned out to be the least expensive in the long run. Many factors other than the quoted price have a bearing upon the actual price. For instance, a purchasing agent may purchase a certain supply item at the best quoted price, which then has to be back-ordered from that vendor. This necessitates purchasing a current supply of the item from another vendor, probably at a higher price. The end result is that he ends up paying an average higher price and has an excessive inventory when the original order finally is delivered. Therefore, when considering price, one must consider supply and lead times.

If getting the better price means opening a new account and initiating a new set of books, the decision to go with the new supplier should be challenged. The materiel manager should delineate a cost factor for this maneuver, and it must be considered as part of the price of doing business with that company. In addition, dealing with an additional vendor can result in more deliveries being made, which in turn raises the expense of doing business.

Fallacy Number Nine

Contract purchasing means lack of competition. The major criticism that is proffered against the idea of contract purchasing is that it eliminates competition and puts the hospital in a vulnerable and defenseless position. However, competition in and of itself, means nothing. The materiel manager must always be aware of market conditions, and if contract purchasing does not offer the best overall purchasing power in a certain situation, he can try other methods. Also, the viability of contract purchasing is the understanding that the contract will be renegotiated at a future date. For example, if a hospital enters into contract purchasing for a two-year period and faithfully practices its precepts, the other potential suppliers are even more interested in being involved in the next contract negotiations. Consequently, contract purchasing actually creates a very worthwhile atmosphere of competition.

Methodology for Initiating Contract Purchasing

For those who are still suspicious, it is recommended that contract purchasing be tried on a small scale to investigate the advantages and disadvantages. For example, begin with the hundreds of forms, many obsolete, that are printed in the hospital or bought from outside printers. Most hospitals use several printers, as well as various reproduction machines. The following steps provide a guideline.

STEP 1. Search out all the tangible and intangible costs of the entire forms operation, i.e., personnel, external printing, supplies, service on machines, depreciation, and inventory obsolescence.

STEP 2. Establish performance standards, i.e., quantities of each form to be printed, two-week inventory levels instead of annual bulk quantities, lead times, and capacity to print all forms.

STEP 3. Require that an option be included to have the vendor purchase all of the hospital printing equipment.

STEP 4. Require that the use of existing forms be studied, especially for the possibility of combining several forms and redesigning others.

STEP 5. Prepare a written presentation to be sent to the printing companies delineating the objectives, purposes, methods of quotation, length of proposed contract, etc.

STEP 6. Interview the interested companies and distribute the contract purchasing specifications.

STEP 7. Select a company based upon price, service, and quality. Let the other companies know who received the contract and indicate that this procedure will be followed again at some future time.

STEP 8. Evaluate the performance of the company on a quarterly basis.

This procedure can prove to be very rewarding and will lead to a credible process which will most likely involve the development of more contract purchasing.

Advantages of Contract Purchasing

Based on several years of experience utilizing contract purchasing in many areas, the following advantages can be identified:

1. Large dollar volumes make the hospital a preferential customer, and consequently it gets special consideration in times of supply shortages.

2. A better total overall price is a negotiated result of contract purchasing.
3. Better service is assured since the supplier is competing for total dollar volume of a category instead of just a portion of the business.
4. There are fewer back orders because supply quantities are delineated and assured through the penalty clause.
5. Since price is negotiated on the best volume unit regardless of the quantities ordered, inventory is reduced.
6. The larger volumes under contract purchasing can have a deterring effect upon price increases because of the fear of losing a good customer.
7. Contract purchasing does not necessarily advocate or require standardization.
8. Fewer deliveries are required.
9. Fewer checks are written.
10. Paperwork, including purchase orders, is drastically reduced or eliminated entirely.

Anatomy of the Prime Supplier Concept

There is no magical formula to use when buying hospital supplies, but negotiation is the watchword. In order to promise enough volume to make negotiation worthwhile to the supplier, the prime supplier technique (contract purchasing) is recommended. This is the concept of purchasing 95 to 98 percent of the total dollar volume of a particular category of supplies from one vendor for a specified period of time. This approach is particularly applicable to the following supply categories:

1. Medical-surgical supplies,
2. Indirect pharmaceuticals,
3. Intravenous fluids and administration sets,
4. Staple foods,
5. Laboratory supplies,
6. Radiology supplies,
7. Linens,
8. Office supplies, and
9. All printed forms.

From the materiel management perspective, the anatomy of a prime supplier contract consists of five basic parts: the term of the contract, best quantity price, a negotiated percentage off best quantity price, a penalty clause, and the motivation percentage (Figure 12-1). The prime supplier contract should be negotiated for a period of two or three years with price protection if possible. Next, the price negotiation should begin with the largest volume

Figure 12-1 Factors for Consideration in Negotiating Contract Purchasing

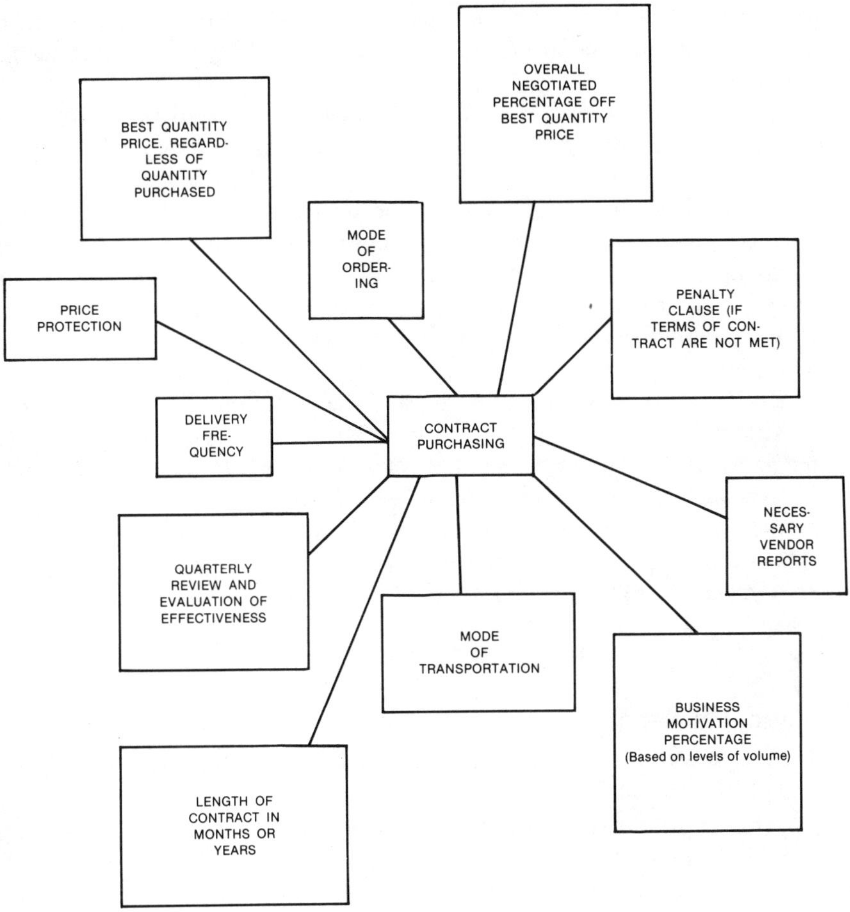

quantity regardless of the quantity purchased so that the unit price for an item to the hospital is always the same.

For obtaining the percentage off best quantity price, the materiel manager must know his institution's purchasing cost profile for at least the past five years. He should know such facts as the average total dollar volume purchased, number of vendors involved, inventory on hand, inventory turnover factor, corresponding admissions each year, number of patient days, inflationary ratio, and the average percentage of increase in supply costs each year. With this knowledge he can negotiate with the hospital's best long-term interest in mind.

Since a prime supplier contract will also assure better service, a penalty clause should be included concerning the supplier's responsibility to meet the normal, established quotas for a particular item. Since most prime suppliers are adept at supply forecasting, they generally are willing to negotiate such a penalty.

Last, but by no means least, a motivational clause based upon projected quantities of total dollar volume is valuable. In other words, a hospital may negotiate a standard percentage discount up to a million dollars and receive an additional percentage of total volume after the million dollar ceiling is reached. This mechanism serves as the motivation for the materiel manager to pass up the "glamour" discounts from other suppliers and practice the prime supplier technique for its maximum effect. This is especially pertinent when a group of hospitals are participating in the prime supplier effort—group purchasing at its best!

While I do not see any disadvantages to the prime supplier concept, some materiel managers seem to feel that it eliminates or reduces the purchasing prerogative by limiting the number of vendors with whom they can negotiate. This is a fair statement, but it describes a situation which I tend to see as advantageous rather than disadvantageous. It is important to remember that if the supplier cannot meet the negotiated commitments, the hospital is free to make other arrangements.

Pertinent Points to Ponder

1. What is meant by a buyer's market?
2. Who should represent the hospital in negotiating prime supplier contracts? Why?
3. Who should dictate purchasing policy—the provider (supplier) or the consumer (hospital)? Why?
4. Which has the best negotiators, the supplier or the hospital? Explain.
5. Why do prices for supplies differ even in hospitals of comparable size in the same locality?
6. What are the differences between contract purchasing and group purchasing?
7. Is contract purchasing a form of group purchasing?
8. Can the means of supply transportation to the hospital from the supplier really be negotiated? Explain.
9. Are most hospitals really practicing contract purchasing while being unaware of it? Explain.

10. In your opinion, what do the suppliers think of contract purchasing?
11. Do all suppliers have the capability of being a prime supplier? Explain.
12. What is meant by the term "corporate prime supplier"?

Chapter 13

Suppliers Can Provide Much More Than Price*

Hospital purchasing agents used to shop for quality, price, and service, in that order. However, times have changed. Today quality is almost taken for granted since so many agencies are monitoring the packaging, sterility, storage, and distribution of supplies. Price is still a negotiable item, but it too has lost some of its power since hospitals have begun purchasing in large dollar volumes through prime suppliers, group purchasing, and shared service endeavors. This leaves service, a commodity which even institutions such as banks and shopping marts are now promoting as a sales point.

For most hospital materiel managers, service is a sought-after commodity which the suppliers have denied to date. However, if the materiel manager is to be effective in the areas of cost containment and inventory reduction, supply service is a factor which can be negotiated in the same terms as price and quality. To do so, he must be able to define adequately the terms of service in writing so that there is no misunderstanding between the supplier and the hospital.

After negotiation of acceptable prices, there are many service aspects that must be carefully considered. Foremost is supply availability upon request. Hospital materiel managers must become skilled in determining supply needs for certain periods of time, and these quotas should then determine supply service. Using these figures, he should bargain with the supplier to keep the necessary inventory of each item for at least a 90-day period. This inventory should be sequestered and protected by the supplier for that hospital.

The terms of this inventory holding should be written into an agreement and backed up by a penalty clause which would provide an incentive for

*Reprinted with the permission of DIMENSIONS in Health Service, Journal of the Canadian Hospital Association.

the supplier to honor the agreement. The materiel manager would be responsible for delineating a preferred list of supplies to be reviewed and agreed upon by both the hospital and the supplier. Given a reasonable time for inventory building of these preferred supplies, the hospital should expect to be able to draw from it upon request. If for any reason the supplier should be unable to supply under the terms of the agreement, he should be required to pay a predetermined penalty. Furthermore, if the hospital has to purchase from another supplier for a premium price, the designated supplier should compensate the hospital for the difference in cost.

This concept drastically reduces the amount of back orders, which should be able to be held to 2 percent or less, and eliminates the costly and time-consuming task of having the hospital purchasing agent shop around for product availability. It also makes the supplier assume the responsibility for supply accessibility. Once put into practice, this entire concept of supplier accountability will lead to greatly reduced hospital inventories, decreased holding costs, and overall increased supply efficiency.

Generally speaking, hospital supply companies are well managed, profit-oriented organizations. They are the professionals in the areas of supply, warehousing, marketing, purchasing, and distribution. Their entire business is supply service oriented, where at best, the supply function in the hospital represents an expensive duplication of time and dollars. Their salespeople are well educated (usually with at least an undergraduate degree), experienced, and astute business professionals who are fully supported by all of the organizational accoutrements of a multimillion dollar corporation.

It certainly seems reasonable for the hospital to use all this talent that is available to it just for the asking. For example, the supplier has a vast reservoir of knowledge concerning future supply trends such as price increases, stock outages, manufacturer's delivery problems, and truck strikes, all of which would be helpful in preparing the hospital's supply and capital equipment budget projections. If the hospital materiel manager schedules semiannual conferences with highly placed and knowledgeable representatives of the major suppliers, he will probably pick up information that will be useful in overseeing the hospital operation. These conferences should be documented and reviewed after a while to determine which sources provided the most reliable data.

Most major companies have computer accessibility and capabilities and should be able to provide the materiel manager with summary product activity reports on a monthly, quarterly, and annual basis. These reports should include all aspects of the purchasing profile, i.e., product and identification, quantities purchased, line items involved, number of line items per order, prices, back-order percentages, and total gross dollar purchases.

Furthermore, most suppliers can provide invaluable assistance in the areas of supply maximum-minimum determinations and economic order quantity delineations, and some can even provide an integral interface between their computer and the hospital's so that the purchasing function can become an automated process.

The supplier also can provide assistance and innovation in the area of purchase ordering. There are several electronic methods of transmission of purchase data which can basically eliminate the paper entry system, and many companies will provide these to the using hospitals at no service charge. Suppliers may even provide the hospital with preprinted purchase order forms at no cost if the subject is broached in an appropriate and timely manner.

Another problem area that can be eased by the supplier is transportation and distribution. A high percentage of supply delays can be directly traced to the transportation source, a factor over which the supplier and the hospital have little control. With a third party providing the transportation, it is next to impossible to schedule the arrival of the shipment, and the hospital and supplier are placed at the mercy of the transporters. But the materiel manager can request that the supplier get into the transportation and delivery act. At present, many suppliers are researching and evaluating their role in supply delivery. If they would accept responsibility for the goods from delivery to receipt, the materiel manager could negotiate for the appropriate delivery date and time. Supply receipt scheduling would be greatly facilitated and lead times could be projected more realistically.

Suppliers are also now seen as having responsibility to provide and participate in good quality, noncommercial seminars and other educational endeavors for the hospitals they serve. Many suppliers are realizing this responsibility and developing or sponsoring excellent educational programs. The materiel manager should, through the local sales representatives, let the companies know of material and topics which would be helpful to him in the execution of his duties.

There are many other ways in which the supplier can ethically come to the aid and assistance of the materiel manager. There is the possibility of having the supplier perform the physical inventory for the hospital. This certainly seems reasonable, since the supplier is the expert with hundreds of thousands of dollars tied up in inventory as a substantial asset which has to be counted on a periodic basis. Furthermore, the supplier can greatly help prevent confusion by adopting a flexible returned-goods policy and allowing the representative to issue immediate on-the-spot credit for returnable merchandise.

The supplier and hospital materiel management must always maintain an ethical and open relationship based upon integrity and honesty. Furthermore, the hospital and the materiel manager should set aside the stereotype of the supplier and the salesman and explore new avenues to increase efficiency and lower overall supply costs to the hospital.

Pertinent Points To Ponder

1. Do the suppliers and the hospital have the same objectives? Explain.
2. Should hospitals perform annual evaluations of their key suppliers? Why or why not?
3. Does the supplier have the last word in supply negotiations? Why?
4. What is meant by "supply service"?
5. Can most hospital suppliers provide quality, price, and service? Why?
6. Should the supplier get involved with the transportation and distribution of supplies from the company warehouse to the hospital? Explain.
7. What is meant by a "full service supplier"?
8. Should sales representatives be allowed to participate in taking hospital physical inventory? If so, under what conditions?
9. What is the function of the sales representative in relationship to the hospital?
10. Have you ever seen a job description of a sales representative? If not, do you think it could be made available to you?
11. How can you get the supplier to be more helpful in your materiel efforts?
12. What factors should be considered in the evaluation of a supplier?

Chapter 14

Capital Equipment Acquisition Considerations*

Purchasing capital equipment differs greatly from buying expendable supplies. First, capital equipment involves a large, single purchase expenditure, normally ranging from a few hundred to several hundred thousand dollars. Second, such an equipment purchase also involves negotiation of a warranty or service contract. Third, this purchase may be from a supplier with whom the hospital does little or no business, and there exists a certain element of risk in not being familiar with the company's credibility, and a certain need to clearly delineate responsibilities. Fourth, the acquisition will probably involve bidding with clearly defined specifications. Fifth, the delivery and installation may take several months to a year, and last, the purchase of capital equipment usually requires administrative and/or board approval. All these aspects can complicate the purchase and require extra attention in writing specifications, ordering equipment, receiving shipments, supervising installation, and giving final approval for payment.

Hospital Policy for Capital Equipment Acquisition

Since there will be special approval considerations, a policy for the acquisition of capital equipment should be delineated for all departments and areas. The following is an example of such a policy:

- Each department head will specify in detail the capital equipment deemed necessary for the forthcoming fiscal year. All recommendations will be

*Reprinted with the permission of DIMENSIONS in Health Service, Journal of the Canadian Hospital Association.

brought to the Hospital Budget Committee for review and approval. Items that are approved are then submitted to the administrator for approval.

- All capital equipment items shall be approved by the administrator and then specified by name, reason for purchase, and estimated purchase cost in the annual capital equipment budget. The administrator shall submit this budget to the board of trustees for review and approval prior to the fiscal year in which it will be effective.
- After the capital equipment budget has been approved by the board, the administration will discuss the capital equipment items with the respective department directors and set a projected date for the purchase of each item. As the purchase date approaches, the department director again reviews the need and justification for the item, and if the purchase is still deemed necessary, submits an equipment requisition to the respective administrative representative. The representative again reviews and discusses this purchase with the department director. If they agree that the purchase is still a necessity, the equipment requisition is submitted to the Department of Materiel Management for negotiation of price, terms of service, warranty, and terms of purchase. This process entails requesting quotations from every acceptable source. The processed requisition is then sent to the administrator for review and disposition.
- If the requisitioned equipment meets all of the above conditions, including a total purchase price of $15,000 or less, the administrator is authorized to approve the purchase. Accordingly, the administrator refers the documentation to materiel management for the assignment of a purchase order number and the regular purchase procedure is initiated.
- If the requisitioned equipment meets all of the criteria, but the total purchase cost is in excess of $15,000, the administrator refers the documentation and recommendations to the Finance and Economics Committee of the board of trustees. After a review, the committee refers the requisition, along with its comments and recommendations, to the board. If approved and signed by the president, the administrator refers the necessary paperwork to the materiel manager for initiation of the purchase process. If unapproved, the administrator will seek another resolution to the matter.
- From time to time, a genuine demonstrated need may arise for equipment which was not included in the annual operation budget. In this case, the same basic procedure will be followed, but all items of this nature in excess of $1,000 will be referred to the board of trustees for review and disposition.
- EXCEPTION: In the event that a piece of equipment or part thereof is damaged or becomes inoperable, and such equipment is essential to the

delivery of patient care, the administrator is authorized to expend capital funds to repair it to normal functioning. At the next scheduled meeting of the board of trustees, the administrator will advise the board of his actions in the matter.

Negotiation Considerations

After the decision has been made to purchase a piece of capital equipment from a specified supplier and the necessary approvals have been given, the materiel manager should begin the procurement clarification process. The more specific are the written understandings, the better the purchase. It is suggested that the hospital's regular purchase order process be used to procure capital equipment and that a list of supplemental considerations, preferably signed by the authorized representatives of the company, be appended to the purchase order.

The following list of particulars should be agreed to by the company selling a piece of capital equipment. While acceptance of these considerations probably will represent many hours of negotiation on the part of the materiel manager or purchasing agent, the hospital will reap the benefits in the long run.

- It should be made clear that the price indicated on the purchase order will be the hospital's total financial commitment for this purchase. Any additional parts or accessories which may be needed to install the equipment and make it operate properly will be at the expense of the supplying company unless otherwise stated in writing.
- It should be fully understood that payment will be made in full upon installation and acceptance of the equipment by the hospital. Many companies will request a partial payment arrangement, but the materiel manager should indicate that it is hospital policy to pay total invoice price only upon installation and that no other payment schedule is acceptable. This policy not only speeds up the delivery, but also gives the hospital the interest on the money for a longer period of time.
- All equipment specified and quoted should meet or exceed all of the necessary city, state, and federal standards and have U.L. approval where applicable. All equipment will be inspected upon receipt by the biomedical engineer or other responsible party and, if found in violation of the delineated specifications, will be returned freight collect.
- Operating manuals, pertinent electrical and mechanical schematics, and current parts list must be received prior to payment of the invoice.
- The equipment should be shipped all at the same time. This negates the possibility of partial shipments and the likelihood of storage loss. If

there is to be a back order of a part or accessory, it is better that the company and not the hospital receive and be responsible for it.

- All shipments either complete or partial are to be f.o.b. hospital. It is imperative to state exactly who has the responsibility for freight in case the company elects to process partial shipments.
- A representative of the company should be responsible for the final equipment receipt checklist prior to the installation. He should determine both from a quality and quantity basis that the specified equipment has arrived and is ready for installation. If at all possible, the hospital should provide a secured room or place for the representative to store the pieces until the installation is complete. Since the company usually notifies its representative of the date and mode of shipment, he can be expected to be available for this task.
- The company selected should be responsible for detailing instructions for equipment layout and installation. This includes specifications for equipment arrangement and the necessary completion details for meeting such requirements as electrical needs.
- All equipment or parts thereof must carry at least a one-year full warranty on parts and labor, endorsed and supported in writing by the manufacturer or distributor. Many companies adhere to a list price, but are open to negotiating the length of the warranty. Aim for a two-year warranty, and if this cannot be accomplished, settle for a cost-reduced maintenance contract. In addition, there is much to be accomplished in the negotiation of a five- or six-year price-protected maintenance contract at the time of the purchase. Remember, too, that the hospital's clout exists before the purchase is made!
- The hospital purchase order number must appear on all pertinent cartons, packages, packing lists, and invoices.
- The hospital should specify that the company has the risk of loss or damage of the equipment until it is properly installed.
- There must be clarification as to the responsibility of the seller in case of an equipment or attachment recall. The total cost of the recall should be borne by the manufacturer.
- If the equipment or part thereof must be returned to the manufacturer because of a fault of the company, it should be at the company's expense.
- A qualified representative of the company is to provide the necessary inservice education to all appropriate hospital personnel.
- The hospital should specify a certain person or office that the seller should contact in case of questions or problems in reference to the shipment.

Capital equipment acquisition is different from routine supply purchasing and should be dealt with accordingly. Since capital equipment usually represents a large outlay of cash and sometimes even outlasts the company from which it is purchased, the prudent buyer should carefully spell out the necessary understandings. The more clearly the equipment acquisition considerations are delineated, the better the company's performance and capabilities can be demonstrated.

Pertinent Points to Ponder

1. What constitutes a capital purchase in your institution?
2. What restrictions are placed upon capital equipment purchases in your hospital? Why?
3. In what ways does a capital equipment purchase differ from that of routine supplies?
4. Should the materiel manager or purchasing agent be involved in the equipment specification and selection phases? Why?
5. To whose budget is capital equipment charged? Explain.
6. Is an order for $10,000 of surgical instruments automatically considered a capital purchase? Explain.
7. What methods are used by hospitals for financing capital equipment purchases?
8. Why do some third party payers require hospitals to submit three-year capital equipment budgets?
9. How does the medical staff get involved in the capital equipment budget process?
10. What is the average depreciation schedule for capital equipment?
11. Is a lease considered a capital purchase? Explain.
12. Is it better for the hospital to buy or lease its capital equipment? Why?

Chapter 15

Effective Reporting Provides Administrative Support*

No one can question the importance of the major managerial functions of planning, organizing, staffing, directing, and controlling. To be added to the list is the new function of reporting or "feedback." In order to get the necessary top management support, the materiel manager must be able to report or feed back pertinent data that will be meaningful to the administration. This is the means by which the administrator can document evidence of the competence of the materiel manager.

From the administrative viewpoint, there is a definite need to know certain information on a regular and uniform basis. Uniformity of reports is necessary because it allows for comparable data to be reviewed on a periodic basis. Format is also important because the administrator needs to be able to read and digest the information in the shortest time possible. Therefore, the reports must be concise, timely, meaningful, and interesting. They should be made on a monthly, quarterly, semiannual, and annual basis.

Monthly Reports

One of the most meaningful reports is the departmental expense and revenue report. It contains information indicating how well the materiel manager is managing his resources and staying within his budget, including

*Reprinted with the permission of DIMENSIONS in Health Service, Journal of the Canadian Hospital Association.

salary, supplies, capital equipment, travel, and education expenses, as well as data from any areas such as pharmacy that may be revenue centers. Operational statistics are necessary for top management to keep abreast of the financial aspects of the total hospital operation, and if any of the areas mentioned are significantly over or under budget, the materiel manager should explain why. This report should also indicate the actual figures for each parameter for the same period a year ago to give the administrator a clear picture of the past and present financial status of the materiel management function.

Prices for patient care items are increasing almost daily, and price protection is practically a thing of the past. Total cost increases for supplies and services are averaging about 10 to 15 percent per year, which is driving the costs of hospital care upward. Not only do the hospitals take the blame from the public, but what is even more devastating is that controls are being placed on hospitals instead of on the suppliers and manufacturers. The administrator needs to have a credible, written record of these happenings so he can document his explanation of why costs are increasing. The role of the materiel manager in this situation is to prepare a monthly Increased Supply Cost Report documenting all price increases with an extrapolation of the net long-term effects. For instance, if a case of XYZ is increased by the supplier by $10.00 per case and the hospital uses 10,000 cases per year, there will be a net excess expenditure of $100,000 that the hospital must cover, probably through increased charges to the patient.

To supplement the report on increased costs, the materiel manager should prepare a monthly Cost Containment Efforts Report to document his efforts to offset many price increases and even cut costs. For example, not all suppliers increase prices on like commodities at the same time, and like products can be substituted for others that have become more expensive. Also, most suppliers will not even consider negotiating annual price protection contracts with hospitals, but the prudent purchaser might request price protection for a shorter period—say six, three, or even one month. Yet another excellent cost containment effort is to reduce stores inventory to coincide with the inflation factor. In other words, inflation could increase the "worth" of an inventory in dollar amount by 50 to 60 percent over a five-year period, during which time the materiel manager should have been reducing the inventory quantity by the same amount. Still another tactic is to make do with less, especially on reusable items. There are many more examples of cost containment, which the materiel manager should both employ and document.

Since there are many departments and units which are supplied monthly, the materiel manager also should prepare a Departmental Supply Expense Report indicating the using department, dollar volume, and account numbers to which all supplies have been expensed. It should compare these figures to those for the same period a year ago. This report serves several purposes. It lets the department directors know that their supply expense is being recorded and that the administrator will review it monthly. It also serves to keep supplies from being charged indiscriminately to departments by materiel management. Moreover, by using these figures to point out any department that is using an inordinate amount of supplies, the materiel manager may detect some pilferage in the process of preparing this report.

The Vendor Report, indicating the dollar volumes purchased from all vendors, can be of utmost assistance to the materiel manager. For example, if only a small purchase is being made from a particular vendor, it may be in the best interest of the institution to combine this order with the purchases from another supplier and thereby reduce the number of purchase orders, negotiation time, checks, and accounting techniques. The report will supply this information at a glance. This same presentation of the information can instantly show the administrator which businesses are patronized by the hospital and pinpoint potential conflicts of interest.

Finally, the materiel manager should be responsible for producing a monthly Product Standardization Report based on the work of the Standardization Committee. This report should contain trade names of all requested supplies, the requesting department or unit, the number of supplies approved for standard use, the number rejected, a computed approval ratio to the number of items rejected, the savings or loss for each approved item, a total savings or loss for the month, and an evaluation of each item selected for standard use.

Quarterly Reports

The frequency with which a report is made usually depends upon the relevancy and urgency of the data it contains. Sometimes trends can best be distinguished by a report that is issued quarterly rather than monthly. For example, the Linen Usage Report can be prepared on a quarterly basis and still give the administrator or fiscal officer the necessary information on a timely basis. This report indicates the number of pounds of linen used by all areas for a certain period.

If the pharmacy is under the materiel management concept, certain useful information can be depicted by a quarterly Pharmaceutical Services Report. This report should contain certain pertinent data such as inpatient line items processed, outpatient line items processed, number of employee prescriptions filled, the number of hyperalimentations prepared, formulary additions, formulary deletions, and number of pharmacist-physician consultations.

The frequency of all reports can be increased or decreased if so desired by the parties involved, but the main factor to be considered is relevancy.

Semiannual Reports

Certain data should be reviewed at least twice per year. If the hospital utilizes the management by objectives approach, then the materiel manager should submit a report on the state of completion of the objectives and the results up to that point. Furthermore, physical inventories should be completed and reported to the administrator and fiscal officer on a semiannual basis. The report should reflect both official and unofficial inventories on at least a three-year comparative analysis with individual departmental inventory goals to be met. A brief explanation of the highlights and efforts involved should accompany the report. The materiel manager should also proffer suggestions for further beneficial developments in this regard.

Annual Reports

A special annual departmental summary report covering such areas as budget accuracy, changes in inventory levels, unusual happenings, and cost effectiveness must be submitted to the administrator. This report should be in the nature of an auditor's statement and be concise, factual, and reflective. It should include a list of realistic, obtainable objectives for the coming year which will function as a vehicle for better communication and understanding between administration and materiel management.

Pertinent Points to Ponder

1. Do administrators usually expect periodic reports from the materiel manager? Why or why not?
2. What are administrators usually looking for in reports?
3. Should the materiel manager keep the administrator abreast of the happenings in the department? Why or why not?
4. In your opinion, does the administrator really care about what is happening as long as there are no complaints? Why?
5. Does the written report negate the need for verbal contact between the materiel manager and the administrator? Explain.
6. Are reports worth all the time it takes to complete them? Why?
7. Besides the administrator, who else should receive materiel management reports? Elaborate.
8. In reference to product standardization, who should make the report, the materiel manager or the chairman of the committee? Why?

9. Should the medical staff get certain materiel management reports? Why or why not?
10. How frequently should the report format be reviewed and revised?
11. How long should materiel management reports be kept on file?
12. What is meant by "exception reporting," and should it be used by the materiel manager?

Chapter 16

Working with the Hospital Committee Structure*

One of the most ubiquitous and controversial devices of organization is the committee—a group of persons to whom, as a group, some matter is committed. It is this characteristic of group action that sets the committee apart from other organization devices.[1] In the hospital, committees are functional at all levels, including board, administrative, medical staff, department head, and supervisory, and they are responsible for the performance of many important functions and tasks.

Since materiel management is an essential function in the hospital organizational structure, the materiel manager must be cognizant of the importance and ramifications of the hospital committee structure. The materiel manager must manage people, systems, money, negotiations, and materiel, and to do so effectively, he must work with and through several hospital and medical staff committees whose decisions greatly influence the materiel management process. The difference between success and failure of the materiel management concept may well be determined by how well the manager works within the committee structure.

The materiel manager must be in a position to influence the committee decision process either as a chairperson, as a member, or as an advisor to any committee that deals with the supply and materiel process since many management decisions are made through group deliberations. Consequently, it is essential that the materiel manager review the entire hospital committee structure and decide which of the 50 or 60 committees he should join. This generally involves participation in no more than 15 of them (Figure 16-1).

---

* Reprinted with the permission of DIMENSIONS in Health Service, Journal of the Canadian Hospital Association.

[1] Harold Koontz and Cyril O'Donnell, *Principles of Management,* 3rd edition (New York: McGraw-Hill Book Co., 1964), p. 340.

Figure 16-1 The Materiel Manager and the Hospital and Medical Staff Committees Must Interact to Fulfill Their Various Functions

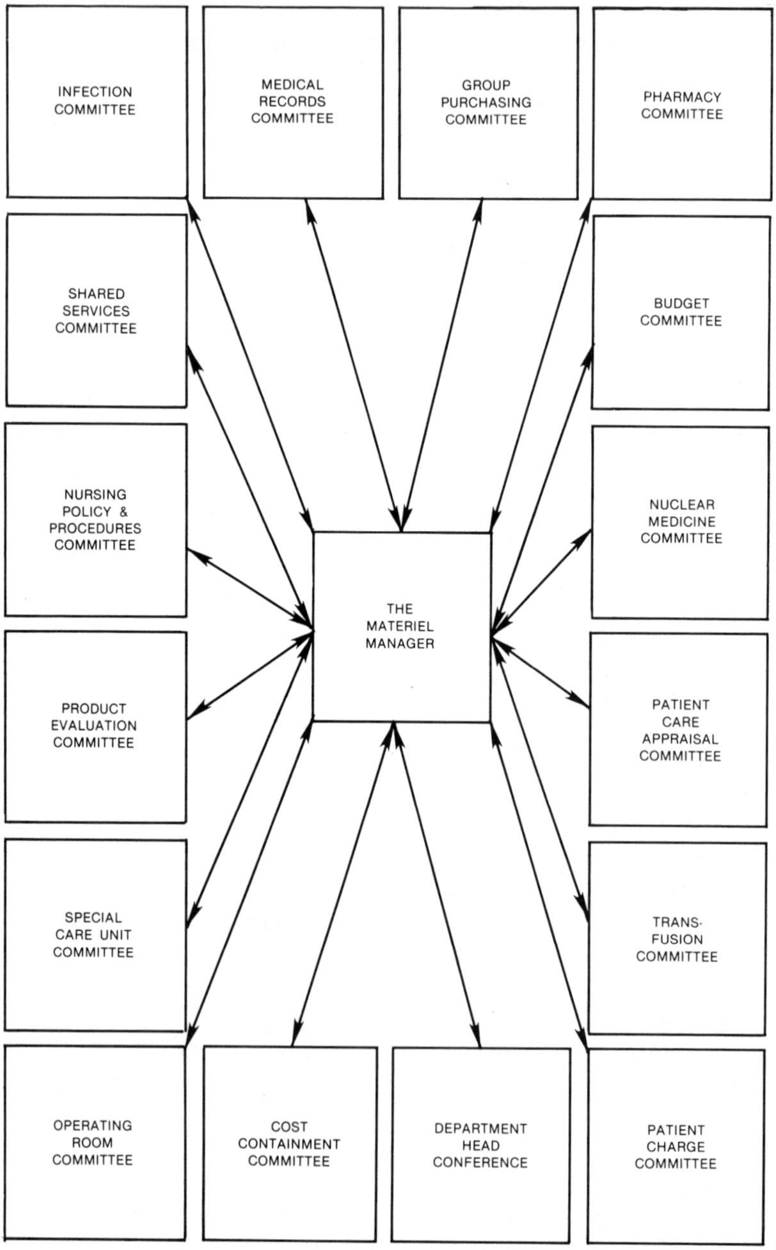

Of all the hospital committees, the most important from the standpoint of the materiel manager is the Product Standardization Committee. The materiel manager should assume a very definite leadership role with this committee, probably as chairperson of the entire standardization effort. He should be responsible for elevating this committee to the stature at which it can be most effective. One way to do this is to insure that physicians be appointed to the committee by whatever process appointments to medical committees are made. Another is to insist that the committee be a multidisciplinary, hospital-wide committee. Both are attempts to provide the committee with the necessary clout, dignity, and continuity to get the task performed with alacrity.

As chairperson of the Product Standardization Committee, the materiel manager must be responsible for providing leadership to the medical staff, nursing, administration, and other departmental managers regarding the standardization process. As previously noted, this process should include products and items from all departments, with the possible exception of pharmaceuticals and perishable foods. All forms and printed matter most definitely should be reviewed and approved by the committee, which is also an excellent mechanism for the review and recommendation of capital equipment. In truth, the credibility of standardization needs to be restored in today's hospitals, and there is no better way than the actual demonstration of its effectiveness. Furthermore, there is no better person to lead this effort than the trained, results-oriented materiel manager.

The Pharmacy and Therapeutics Committee is usually a medical staff committee. However, because it deals with the supply, process, and distribution of drugs and medications, it is recommended that the materiel manager also be a member. He can be helpful in the reduction of inventories of drugs, distribution patterns, development of a formulary, and the selection of sources of supply.

Another medical staff committee of great importance to the materiel manager is the Operating Room Committee. As part of its duties and responsibilities, it evaluates major equipment and supplies and makes pertinent recommendations to administration in this regard. The materiel manager should be a member or an advisor to this committee.

The recent emphasis on the sharing of ideas and services between hospitals has resulted in the creation of a Shared Services Committee and a Group Purchasing Committee. The group purchasing effort usually deals with the purchase of goods and services based on combined volumes. The shared services program deals with group efforts to develop new ideas in such areas as data processing, billing and collections, and continuing education programs. These two committees are usually under the supervision and direction of the hospital's administrative council and include representatives from each of the involved hospitals. Naturally, the materiel manager belongs on both committees.

Another recent effort to show hospital responsiveness to reduction of health care costs has been in the establishment of Cost Containment Committees supported by most hospital associations. Here again, the materiel manager has a very important role because he knows where the costs are and should have ideas for reducing operational expenses. In fact, many of the possible expense reductions are in the area of materiel management, i.e., inventory reduction, more efficient product turnover, reduction of paperwork, and centralization of supply services.

Another medical staff committee that is receiving more attention recently is the Nuclear Medicine Committee. Its important functions include recommending radioisotopes for purchase and receiving and storing these isotopes. The materiel manager can be very helpful in this area if he is knowledgeable of the process, and he should sit on this committee in at least an advisory capacity.

There are many more committees that need at least periodic input from the materiel manager. For example, his knowledge and experience can be helpful to the Medical Records Committee in recommending the type, frequency of use, and volume of forms to purchase. The materiel manager's input to the Infection Committee could prove essential to the sanitation and environmental program of the entire hospital, and his knowledge about costs, expenses, supply utilization, and supply cost increases make his participation on the Budget Committee essential for effective cost and revenue projections.

Pertinent Points to Ponder

1. Why should the materiel manager get involved in the committee process?
2. In which committees should the materiel manager take a definite leadership role? Why?
3. Who usually appoints members to a hospital committee? To a medical staff committee? To a board committee?
4. Why do hospitals have committees?
5. Could the materiel manager be effective if he did not participate in any committees? Why?
6. Name other members of the materiel management team that should have a committee role.
7. Can committees make decisions? Explain.

8. If a committee decided to change a certain product, would the materiel manager have to act accordingly? Why?
9. After a committee makes a recommendation, who makes the actual decision? Why?
10. Could the materiel manager ever be a member of a medical staff committee? Why?
11. Could the materiel manager ever be a member of a board committee? Why?
12. What should determine whether the materiel manager is a member of a committee or not? Why?

Chapter 17

The Materiel Manager's Role in the Budgetary Process*

Budgeting definitely affects the daily operating plans of all managers; however, it has an even greater impact on the materiel manager. Simply stated, budgeting is a managerial maneuver whereby total revenues and expenses are forecasted for a certain period of time, usually for a year. Its two key aspects—forecasting and control—are both key responsibilities of the materiel manager, who must be able to develop a functional budget for the Department of Materiel Management and also act as an advisor in reference to supplies and equipment to all of the other departments. In other words, the materiel manager has both line and staff authority relationships in the hospital budgetary process. Moreover, hospitals are being required by third parties and other regulatory bodies to develop and submit budgets for periods of up to three years. This makes budgeting an even more devastating and intimidating procedure and calls for much expertise and professional polish.

With the centralization of all supply, process, and distribution functions, the materiel manager now has the direct accountability for the personnel component of many departments, units, and functions and indirect responsibility for all supplies and capital equipment. The supply component can account for 20 to 30 percent of the total hospital expense budget and materiel management personnel another 15 to 20 percent, depending on the makeup of the department. Top management should keep this fact in mind when recruiting, evaluating, and setting the salary for the materiel manager.

Before developing his departmental budget or advising other managers on budgetary matters, the materiel manager needs to know what administra-

---

*Reprinted with the permission of DIMENSIONS in Health Service, Journal of the Canadian Hospital Association.

tive policies have been formulated for the upcoming year. They may vary from hospital to hospital, but all will resemble the following:[1]

- What is the projected percentage of occupancy for the coming year?
- What will be the estimated number of patient days?
- Will there be an increase or decrease in the number of available beds?
- What will be the average length of stay?
- How many major and minor operations are forecasted?
- What is the estimated number of emergency room and clinic visits?
- Is there an overall salary increase projected? When and how much?
- Are there any major programs contemplated which will require more manpower or capital outlay?

These questions all will directly affect the materiel manager's budgetary program both in a line and advisory capacity. After these topics have been adequately and thoroughly addressed, he can begin his budgetary planning for the next year.

The budgetary process calls upon all of the managerial functions (Figure 17-1). One of the first principles of budgeting is that the process must not be hurried. Accordingly, it is suggested that the materiel manager begin planning the skeleton of the next year's budget at least six months in advance of its becoming operational to allow enough time to collect and examine at least eighteen months of previous data for trends in supply increases, holding costs, transportation costs, etc.

The next step is to formulate departmental objectives for the next budget year. The effective manager will invite participation from the departmental personnel regarding the following objectives:

- Major reduction of official and unofficial inventories.
- Development of a results-oriented standardization program with multidisciplined representation.
- Centralization of all supply, process, and distribution functions including pharmacy and dietary.
- Computerization of the perpetual inventory system.
- Initiation of a property management or assets management program.
- Research and development of a total supply cart exchange system.
- Research and initiation of a plan to control and standardize forms.
- Initiation of a stockless purchasing program for all direct departments.

---

[1]Charles E. Housley, "Budgeting at the Supervisor's Level," *Hospital Topics* (March, April 1976): 8, 9, 11.

Figure 17-1 The Responsibilities of the Materiel Manager Involve Interface Between Budgeting and Other Management Tools

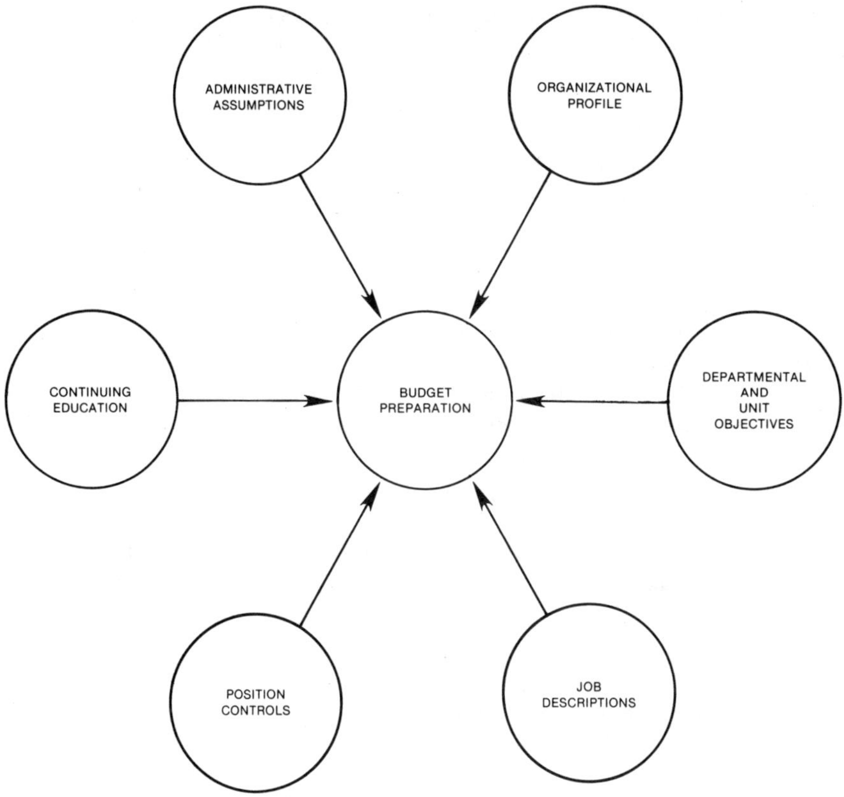

- Simplification of the purchase order process.
- Reduction of the staff by at least two to three persons as a direct result of these efforts.

The objectives should be succinctly and clearly spelled out with target dates for their initiation. Both expenses and savings should be projected for each objective with a specific suggested priority in case some of the objectives are not approved, although most of these goals and objectives will be readily accepted by top management on a cost containment basis alone. It is further suggested that an achievable list of objectives that can be initiated in a 12-month budget period be submitted to administration. Since the list will be the basis of the future budget, it is recommended that it be reviewed and discussed with top management to get at least a tentative approval.

At this point, the materiel manager is prepared to begin the actual budget formulation that will be the basis for future expectations and performance. The departmental expense budget should take on the following profile:

1. The Personnel Component
    a. An actual organization chart (with new positions indicated in red) should be submitted with the budget.
    b. Salaries, with fringes included, will comprise approximately 55 to 65 percent of the total departmental expense budget.
    c. When the materiel manager is confident with the personnel expenses, the budget can be considered at least two-thirds completed.
    d. In preparing this component, the materiel manager should use at least the current past 18 months of experiential data to establish trends and budget effectively.
    e. The materiel manager must involve the department supervisors in this phase.
    f. Before disseminating the necessary budget data, the materiel manager should make sure that all working data are correct and current.
    g. If new positions are requested, the materiel manager must document the need with a brief statement of the need, a complete job description, and a projection of the results in terms of revenue and expense. This documentation is to be submitted with the budget.
    h. In calculating the salaries, use the salary increase percentage as formulated in the administrative assumptions.
    i. Overtime should be delineated as a separate line item, if only for the materiel manager to note it.
    j. At least two to three months of the six-month budget preparation time should be allotted for the complete delineation of the personnel component.
2. The Supply Component
    a. This component represents an area where the materiel manager has both line and advisory responsibilities.
    b. Supplies can approximate 20 to 30 percent of the entire hospital budget and are the most difficult to project accurately.
    c. The materiel manager should perform a review of the past 18 months on the utilization of supplies to determine fairly accurate

projection data. These trends and projections can then be used by the other department heads in arriving at their supply budgets.

d. The supply budget should be projected for each month as the census data justifies it because supply costs will vary month to month as a result of such factors as number of patient days, percentage of occupancy, number of emergency room visits, and number of days in the month.
e. In this area, the materiel manager can win points from all other departmental managers if his projections are true.
f. For all major supply categories, the materiel manager should strive to get price protection for at least the length of the budget period.
g. The materiel manager should spend at least two months of the preparation period dealing with all aspects of the supply component.

3. The Travel and Education Component
   a. As most accreditation and professional organizations begin to require continuing education on an ongoing basis, this category becomes more important to the materiel manager.
   b. Ample funds for good educational programs should be a priority when completing the budget.
   c. The materiel manager should keep a file of each employee's continuing education history indicating the course name, date, cost, and content.
4. Capital Equipment Component
   a. Again, the materiel manager has both line and advisory responsibilities for this category.
   b. In reference to the budgetary projections, the following protocol should be completed on every capital equipment request:[2]

      - A complete description of the item.
      - A complete explanation of the need and demand.
      - An explanation of whether the purchase is for an addition, improvement, or replacement to the capital equipment.
      - A submission of quotations from at least three different manufacturers with price protection for at least 8 months, and a recommendation as to which one to purchase.
      - A recommended date of purchase and probable date when funds will be expended.
      - A classification of the item's priority as to whether it is urgent, essential, economically desirable, or just desirable.

---

[2]Housley, "Budgeting at the Supervisor's Level," pp. 8, 9, 11.

- An indication of the probable outcome of this purchase:

    1. Will it improve patient care?
    2. Will it increase or decrease departmental revenues?
    3. Will it increase or decrease the patients' per diem?
    4. Will there be a charge for its use? If so, how much?
    5. How often will the item be used?

c. The materiel manager can provide an indispensable service in the approval and purchase of capital equipment for all hospital departments.
d. The delineation of the capital equipment component should take at least a month for preparation.

Effective budgeting takes much talent and professional expertise. The materiel manager should develop his/her skills in this regard, and the entire hospital will be the beneficiary in the long run.

Pertinent Points to Ponder

1. What exactly is a budget?
2. What are the purposes of a budget in relationship to the materiel process?
3. What is the relationship between the revenue budget and the expense budget?
4. What is the materiel manager's role in the budgetary process?
5. If the various department directors develop the expense budget, who develops the revenue budget? Why?
6. Can a materiel management department operate without a budget? Explain.
7. How does the capital equipment budget differ from the supply budget?
8. What is meant by staff authority?
9. What is meant by line authority?
10. If a piece of equipment does get approved in the capital budget, does that mean it will be purchased? Explain.
11. What happens if a department's budget does not get approved? Explain the process.
12. Who has ultimate responsibility for the approval of the budget?

Chapter 18

The Pharmacist as a Materiel Manager*

The pharmacist has traditionally been looked upon as a manager of materiel, but not necessarily as a materiel manager. With the expanding role of the Department of Materiel Management in today's hospitals, there is much interest in qualified and trained managers for this critical area. Since there are no formal training programs for hospital materiel management, institutions must undertake the training of their own managers in the empirical setting. As a result, there is no uniformity regarding scope, complexity, function, or type of person filling the position. Generally, however, there are three broad categories of background for hospital materiel management—hospital training, industry training, and pharmacy.

The Hospital-Trained Materiel Manager

Most of the hospital-trained materiel managers have received their experience as purchasing agents, central stores managers, directors of central sterile supply, armed services medical supply officers, or some combination thereof. In fact, in many instances the promotion represents a name change rather than a change in function or responsibility. This is an anathema to good management practice, but since the condition exists, the most should be made of it. It must be emphasized at this point that the entire materiel

---

* Reprinted with the permission of DIMENSIONS in Health Service, Journal of the Canadian Hospital Association.

management concept must be an administrative policy which has the approval and support of top management. Moreover, the responsibility for developing and selling the idea and principles of materiel management belongs to the materiel manager.

If the position is structured and supervised responsibly, there are numerous advantages to the institution with a hospital-trained manager. First, he brings with him a wealth of experiential information concerning supply items, supply utilization patterns, distribution cycles, sales representatives, product lines, prices, etc. Second, he is familiar with the hospital infrastructure, which, in many cases, makes him more acceptable to middle management. Third, with a background in purchasing and stores, he generally has fundamental skills in the art and science of negotiation.

Regarding the limitations of the hospital-trained manager, there is more critical information available than for the other two types of manager because there have been more of them. He tends to think more about purchasing and supplies than about the total picture of patient care—the hospital's primary purpose for being. Furthermore, there are certain established collision patterns between purchasing and other departments, especially nursing, that limit his effectiveness because of his tendency to perpetuate this phenomenon by practicing antiquated methods of materiel management. Another limiting factor is the lack of credibility that exists between purchasing and the majority of the other departments. In order to resolve this credibility gap, the hospital-trained materiel manager must develop a positive attitude through continuing education and personal professional development.

The Industry-Trained Materiel Manager

In recent years, some hospitals have tapped industry for trained materiel managers. The industry-trained manager brings with him a fresh look and a knowledge of industrial engineering techniques to apply to the area of hospital logistics. The industry-trained manager makes use of such industrial management concepts as the queuing theory and regression curves. Additionally, he is more experienced in the art of negotiations and is usually associated with the purchase of expensive items and materials.

With all the advantages, he also has his limitations. Primarily, he lacks familiarity with the hospital. He must create new interdepartmental relationships and begin to build hospital supply contacts. In addition, he is not in a position to use the purchasing policies, procedures, and product specifications with which he has become familiar. Yet even with these limitations, the industry-trained materiel manager has already made valuable contributions to the field of hospital materiel management.

The Pharmacist as Materiel Manager

Traditionally, the graduate pharmacist has been trained to practice either in the retail store or the hospital setting. Over the years, the role of the pharmacist continually has expanded, with the next area of promise being the field of hospital materiel management.

The advantages to such a move are tangible and numerous. Foremost, the pharmacist has long been a respected member of the health care team, and it is now time for this health professional to serve in a greater capacity than the purchase, storage, and disposal of supplies. An integral function of materiel management is the study and evaluation of product utilization, whether it be a medication or a catheter tray. This process can easily be performed effectively by the pharmacist, whose traditional role has been one of service, research, and education. These are admirable objectives for the entire continuum of materiel management.

The pharmacist is already practicing the fundamentals of materiel management. For example, in most cases the pharmacy represents the largest single dollar volume inventory in today's hospitals. The pharmacist usually is chairman, or is at least a member, of the Pharmacy and Therapeutics Committee, paralleling the function of the materiel manager on the Product Standardization Committee. In addition, he interviews sales representatives and is familiar with the hospital purchasing process.

Since the concept of total materiel management encompasses the important area of processing, the pharmacist's knowledge and familiarity with sterile technique and infection control provides him with the necessary credentials to supervise the central sterile supply and surgical linen preparation functions. He has had valuable experience in repackaging and codification practices, and is qualified in the area of distribution.

In reference to limitations, the greatest problem is the pharmacist's fear of losing his professional identity. The pharmacist who may have inclinations toward materiel management has many questions. Who is this materiel manager? How does he fit into the organization? How is he looked upon by the professional counterparts? This very real concern is best alleviated by developing and upgrading the materiel management department to be credible, respected, results-oriented, effective, and professional.

The pharmacist is also reluctant to venture out of his own professional realm and become involved in areas with which he is not familiar. In other words, he tends to favor the pharmacy and neglect the other areas. Furthermore, the pharmacist is technically oriented, and generally is lacking in the critical managerial functions of planning, organizing, controlling, coordinating, and forecasting.

There are no known prototypes of the perfect materiel manager. However, the pharmacist has much to offer to the field of hospital materiel management. With his knowledge of pharmaceuticals, hospital organization, negotiation, supply process and distribution, he enters the arena with excellent credentials. The pharmacist, professionally, legally, and managerially, has the potential for becoming an excellent materiel manager.

Pertinent Points to Ponder

1. Why haven't more pharmacists become interested in the field of hospital materiel management?
2. What is meant by "trained incapacities"?
3. In his present role, is the pharmacist really a materiel manager? Explain.
4. Where do most hospital materiel managers receive their training?
5. Do you feel colleges and universities will be offering degrees in hospital materiel management in the near or distant future? Why?
6. How do hospitals train and orient their materiel managers presently?
7. What keeps more people from becoming interested in hospital materiel management?
8. What is most lacking in the present materiel manager's training and experience?
9. What will it take to increase the credibility of the position of materiel manager in today's hospitals?
10. How can you measure a materiel manager's effectiveness?
11. In your opinion, will the hospital field experience the entry of more industry-trained materiel managers in the near future? Why?
12. What are the advantages and disadvantages of having a pharmacist as the materiel manager?

Chapter 19

Consumer Evaluation of the Materiel Efforts*

In the hospital organizational structure, each department must carry out its duties and responsibilities effectively or the entire institution suffers. The whole supply component is a massive, vital, and somewhat problematical area which must be addressed with concern and finesse. Its functioning should be based on the objective of serving those who serve. If the materiel component is being performed well, the other departments just seem to operate much better.

The materiel management function transverses all interdepartmental lines of authority, communication, and responsibility and should occupy a very credible position in the organizational posture. However, the objective and scope of materiel management must be clearly delineated, promulgated, and enforced throughout the institution. Certainly purchasing is much more than mere buying, and supply is much more than storing. The materiel management function must encompass the entire area from acquisition to disposition.

Since the Department of Materiel Management interacts most frequently with the Nursing Service, there must be a careful and effective interface between them. It is imperative that every individual in both departments is aware that the primary objective of the total supply program is to serve the supply needs of Nursing-Patient Service. Such an attitude will insure maximum cooperation between the departments. If everyone remembers that health care is a service industry and that the objective of the supply system is to see that the patient gets the right supply at the right time in the right quantities for the right price, quality health care will be provided.

---

* Reprinted with the permission of DIMENSIONS in Health Service, Journal of the Canadian Hospital Association.

How does one measure the performance of the Department of Materiel Management? First, certain performance criteria should be drawn up by the materiel manager. This is commonly referred to as the statement of services for the department and should be distributed to all of the supply consumers. The following is an example of such a statement.

Statement of Services to the Nursing Units

a. A total supply cart exchange program for each nursing unit will furnish 95 to 99 percent of the supply requirements for each unit for a 24-hour period.

    1. The supply quotas will be individualized according to the needs of each nursing unit.
    2. These supply quotas will be reviewed and updated at least quarterly.
    3. The carts will be exchanged daily at 5:00 a.m.

b. A 24-hour, 7-days-a-week delivery service will be provided for items that are not on the cart.

    1. If you do not have a supply item for any reason, use the supply hotline for immediate delivery (within 15 minutes) around the clock.
    2. Do not send unit personnel to central stores to pick up supplies.

c. Equipment rounds to each nursing unit will be made twice daily to check such items as suction machines, K-pads, etc. (Exhibit 19-1).
d. Every Monday, a check of the miscellaneous equipment (flashlights, stethoscopes, scales, etc.) will be performed. You are to sign that this service was performed.
e. Every attempt will be made to keep your units supplied with the proper items and equipment. In order to assure this, the central stores supervisor will make daily supply rounds on each unit, Monday through Friday. If you should have any supply, process or delivery problems, please bring them to his attention.
f. A current supply reference catalog is filed on each nursing unit for your convenience and assistance.
   It is our pleasure to provide your unit with total supply service around the clock. Thank you for your considerations.

After the evaluation criteria have been delineated, the most important issue must be addressed: Who should evaluate the materiel management

Figure 19-1 Sample Supply Service Questionnaire

1. Are your supply and linen carts delivered on time (before 7:00 a.m.)? Yes ☐ No ☐
2. Generally, do the supply and linen carts contain all of your needs? Yes ☐ No ☐
3. Cart supply quotas are to be reviewed with you at least quarterly. How long has it been since someone in materiel management reviewed with you your supply needs? ____________________
4. Did you know that only "charge" items have charge tickets and need your attention to process them immediately? Yes ☐ No ☐
5. If the supply is not on the cart, can you use the telephone hotline and receive immediate (within 20 minutes) delivery? Yes ☐ No ☐
6. When you have a supply problem, do you feel free to call someone in Central Stores to get immediate action? Yes ☐ No ☐
7. When you call Central Stores, are the attendants courteous? Yes ☐ No ☐
8. Are they knowledgeable and helpful? Yes ☐ No ☐
9. When you phone Central Stores, what is the average delivery response time: 10–20 Minutes ☐ 20–30 Minutes ☐ 30–60 Minutes ☐
10. Do you ever have to send someone to Central Stores to pick up items? Yes ☐ No ☐
11. Does the linen cart meet your linen supply needs? Yes ☐ No ☐
12. If "No", what needs our attention? ____________________
13. Equipment rounds to check suction machines, K-Pads, etc., are made on your unit 7 days/week at 10:00 a.m. and 2:00 p.m. Did you know this? Yes ☐ No ☐
14. In your opinion, are these equipment rounds effective? Yes ☐ No ☐
15. Also, we check and replace, if needed, items such as flashlights, blood pressure units, stethoscopes, etc., every Monday morning. Did you know this? Yes ☐ No ☐
16. Are these items being maintained well on your unit? Yes ☐ No ☐
17. In your opinion, what area of supply service needs our immediate attention to assist you most? ____________________
18. Generally, how would you rate our overall supply service? Poor ☐ Fair ☐ Good ☐ Excellent ☐
19. If you indicate "fair" or "poor", simply state why in 25 words or less. Please use the reverse side of this questionnaire.
20. Any other comments are welcomed:

---

performance? The most logical choice is the persons who use the service. At least every six months, the materiel manager should request that the consumer departments complete a questionnaire in reference to supply service (Figure 19-1). The information that the materiel manager receives from this activity can be used to provide better services to the consumers and ultimately to the patient.

Pertinent Points to Ponder

1. Why offer total supply service to the departments and nursing units?
2. Should total supply service be the objective of materiel management in today's hospitals? Why?
3. Is materiel management actually a service department? Explain.
4. What is the difference between a service and a professional department?

Exhibit 19-1 Equipment rounds should be made at least twice daily to each nursing unit to check such items as suction machines.

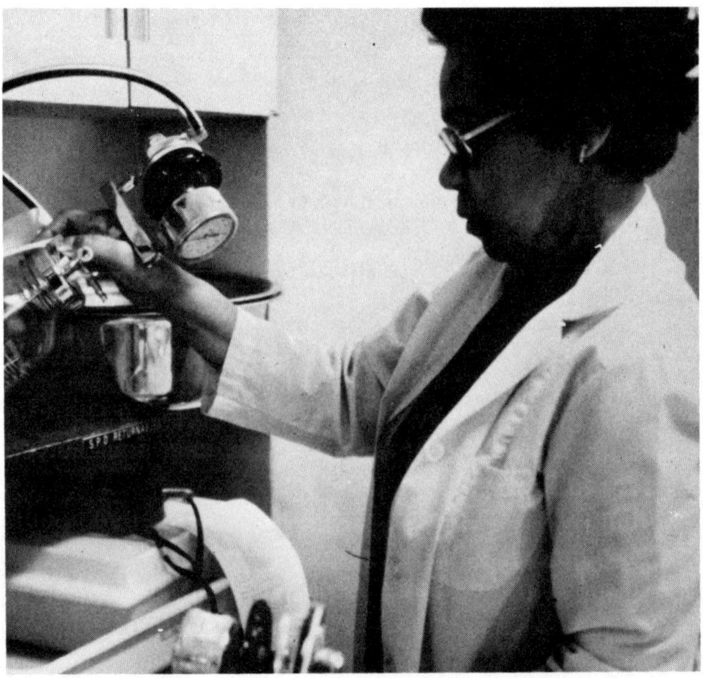

5. Most materiel managers are reluctant to incorporate total service into their efforts. Why?
6. Why has there traditionally been friction between purchasing and nursing service?
7. What can be done to bring about a better understanding of materiel management in the hospital organization?
8. Should nursing or departmental personnel be asked to pick up supplies from central supply and central stores? Why?
9. What is meant by "reverse distribution?"
10. What are the purposes of supply surveys?
11. In your opinion, are they helpful? Why?
12. How can the surveys be made truly objective?

Chapter 20

Telling the Story of Materiel Management*

With the development of materiel management at some level in most hospitals, including the prerequisite centralization of all materiel functions, there is a tremendous need for effective orientation and communication programs to disseminate valuable information to all those who need to know. This task, however, is complicated by the lack of constancy in the field. People, products, equipment, procedures, sales representatives, and techniques change all the time, and decisions are made almost daily at all levels of management that can affect the materiel management picture. There are many examples of this phenomenon. For example, if a new building project is authorized, the materiel manager must be intimately involved with the planners, architects, contractors, and suppliers. For another, if the administration decides to initiate an entirely new service such as a renal dialysis unit, the Department of Material Management will have a very different task to perform. At any point, any one of several thousands of items that are handled by the materiel management department could be eliminated, altered, or substituted.

How are these decisions to be communicated to the materiel manager and all the other people who are affected? Some hospitals have incorporated into the materiel management organization a position similar to that of public relations officer. This person is responsible for communications between the users of products and equipment and the materiel management department. But whether or not such a position exists in a hospital, and no matter how sophisticated the materiel management is in an institution, all effort is worthless unless the consumers know about the product or service.

---

* Reprinted with the permission of DIMENSIONS in Health Service, Journal of the Canadian Hospital Association.

Telling the Materiel Management Staff

There are many barriers to effective communication within the department itself. Because materiel management is a constantly ongoing procedure there are three sets of personnel (shifts) to deal with instead of one. Also, the department is divided into several distinct units with the personnel in each concerned only with their own portion of the task. Furthermore, there are thousands of products and pieces of equipment and numerous procedures that must be followed to the letter by personnel who often do not know how, why, and under what circumstances the supplies and equipment are used. Finally, to complicate matters even more, there is no one common name for most supplies. These problems all make the task of materiel management difficult both from the consumer and the provider points of view. However, there are some very interesting and effective solutions to these problems.

The most knowledgeable persons concerning the total materiel management perspective must be the materiel management staff, all of whom must be ambassadors for the department. However, it is often said that the personnel in this area are not as informed as they should be. This should never be the case. One of the primary responsibilities of the materiel manager is to see that his personnel are knowledgeable and able to communicate all necessary and correct information to the appropriate persons. Therefore, it is imperative that an ongoing communication and orientation program be implemented for the entire materiel management staff. Listed below are some suggestions for the materiel manager undertaking this task.

- All employees in the department should be oriented to the entire hospital upon initial employment.
- All employees should receive a carefully structured orientation to the department and to their individual work units.
- The materiel manager and the supervisory staff should meet collectively with all the workers twice a month to discuss new items, procedures, and problems. The minutes of these meetings should be posted on the bulletin board in the department for handy reference.
- The department should develop its own internal newsletter about pertinent events of interest to all.
- A well organized and current policy and procedure manual, easily accessible to all for ready reference, should be written.
- To the degree possible, all persons should receive training and experience in many areas. This gives each employee a better understanding of the total materiel management function, and serves to provide backup for key positions in case of sickness or vacation.
- A supply locator list should be developed and kept current. This docu-

ment contains a listing of all supplies, equipment, and trays kept in inventory. The supplies are listed in alphabetical order and by bin numbers. The list is a useful tool for orientation of new employees and for reference by part-time, evening, and night personnel.

- A cross-reference of supplies and equipment by all generic, trade, common, and vernacular names should be developed and delivered to the appropriate employees. All departments and nursing units should also be provided a copy for proper ordering.
- The materiel manager should utilize the professional services of the hospital staff development department for providing quality educational programs to his employees on a scheduled basis. This staff department can give expert advice and assistance in special areas such as infection control, sterility procedures, and professional relations.
- The materiel manager should provide an opportunity for his employees to spend time in some of the patient care areas so that they can receive firsthand training in product utilization and problems arising from the use of equipment and supplies in the field. For example, a day on a nursing unit for a cart attendant or processing attendant can be most productive.
- If at all possible, the materiel manager should arrange for a physician to speak to the employees at least once per year. The physician could discuss such issues as the problematical aspects of supply shortage and product substitution for the physicians and the patients.
- All employees should be encouraged to attend at least two educational seminars or conferences annually.

In conclusion, good materiel management starts within the department itself with the development of the employees. Informed employees are the department's most valuable asset.

Telling Nursing and Other Consumer Departments

If the personnel in the various consumer units are knowledgeable about supplies and equipment, the entire materiel management department looks good. However, if one little problem, such as a shortage, develops, the entire materiel management effort looks bad. How do the materiel manager and the department cope with such a devastating and irritating problem? Some helpful suggestions follow.

- An initial orientation for all new hospital employees should be developed to acquaint them with the materiel management philosophy and supply system.

- All personnel involved with supplies in the consumer departments must attend annually at least two materiel management sessions developed especially for them. New methods, techniques, procedures, and items can be effectively put into service in this matter.
- All new equipment and products must have a use procedure written on them and be thoroughly explained to the people who will use them before becoming standard items.
- Key nursing and departmental personnel should be represented on the Product Standardization Committee and be responsible for keeping their employees knowledgeable about current supplies.
- All nursing units and departments should be provided and be familiar with a complete and current set of materiel management policies and procedures.
- The use of supplies in all areas should be monitored, potential problem areas singled out, and employees given further inservice training as needed.
- All consumer departments should be supplied with a current supply cross-reference for proper ordering.
- Educational tours through the entire materiel management area should be conducted periodically to acquaint all supply consumers with the functions, responsibilities, and available services.
- Educational seminars at the hospital (with outside speakers if necessary) should be developed to assist in communicating the philosophy and regimen of materiel management to the entire hospital staff. Continuing educational credits should be given to all who attend. If possible, all departments should be included in the educational endeavors.
- A supply and equipment fair might be held at least annually to acquaint personnel from all departments with the newest in supply and equipment technology.
- An annual evaluation procedure should be developed so that the consumer departments can rate the materiel management performance of the past year according to a set of delineated criteria. The materiel manager should use this information to upgrade the services of the department.
- Management should strive to create an atmosphere of cooperation, professionalism, credibility, and respect for the materiel management philosophy.

Telling the Medical Staff

It is vital that the medical staff support and participate in the materiel management effort. After all, the physicians usually are directly responsible for the ordering of patient care supplies, drugs, and equipment, and there would be no need for hospital materiel management without them. Most efforts in this regard in the past have been mostly by trial and error, but now a bona fide attempt must be made to involve the physicians in the materiel aspects of the hospital decisionmaking process. The following suggestions can produce interesting and effective results.

- Get the physicians involved in the supply selection process. This is done by significant representation on the applicable committees, Product Standardization and Pharmacy and Therapeutics. These physician-committee members should communicate and disseminate pertinent information to the medical staff at large. Medical Staff members should get the same recognition and credit for attending these committee meetings as for the meetings of strictly medical staff committees.
- Initiate a monthly bulletin about supply, drugs, and equipment decisions to be sent to medical staff members on a regular basis. Such a mechanism can bring credibility and respect to the materiel management effort very quickly.
- A descriptive catalog of available drugs and supplies should be placed in appropriate areas such as the physicians' lounge for handy reference.
- Before annual budget preparation, the chairmen of all of medical and surgical sections and departments should be invited to submit suggestions for capital equipment acquisition. A form should be developed for this purpose to include such information as item description, reason for purchase, priority, qualifications for use, etc.
- The materiel manager and his/her staff should strive to create an atmosphere of accessibility and cooperation with the medical staff at all times.

Telling the Sales Representatives

Many problems and misunderstandings can be prevented in this area by some initial careful planning. Sales representatives can be a valuable asset to the materiel manager if they are managed correctly. Ample consideration should be given to the following suggestions.

- Develop a thorough orientation for the new sales representatives and make this fact known to all of the companies with which your hospital does business. If at all possible, try to have the new representative scheduled for this orientation prior to his/her calling on your account.
- Develop and distribute a brochure for all sales representatives. This brochure should incude but not be limited to:

a. A brief statement of the hospital's philosophy toward total materiel management;
b. The hospital's concept of centralized purchasing;
c. All pertinent policies and procedures governing the actions and responsibilities of sales representatives in the hospital, such as visitation to the departments, etc.;
d. Hours the department is open to visitation by sales representatives;
e. Delivery and receiving times;
f. The handling of purchase orders and invoices;
g. Statement concerning the policy on rebates, discounts, etc.;
h. Statement concerning the hospital's position on group purchasing, shared services, and the prudent buyer relationships; and
i. Statement concerning purchasing and selling ethics.

- Initiate an annual evaluation procedure and program of each company's performance and effectiveness as seen from the hospital's point of view. This should include such topics as prices, service, handling of problems, back orders, etc. Then this document and a delineated plan of improved performance should be reviewed with the appropriate representatives of the company on a convenient basis.
- Devise a program for handling complaints and problems of the sales representatives.
- Always strive to create an ethical atmosphere of mutual respect and cooperation.

Telling the story of materiel management to everyone who has a need to know is no easy task. It takes time, effort, and much patience on the part of the materiel manager. It is, however, the only way to obtain anticipated results.

Pertinent Points to Ponder

1. Whose responsibility is it to tell the materiel management story?
2. How do most departments get to know about the services of materiel management?
3. How long should the departmental orientation be?
4. Who should conduct the hospital orientations? The departmental orientations?

5. How can the materiel manager be involved in so much and at the same time stay knowledgeable of the field?
6. Why should an orientation on the materiel management concept be given to the medical staff?
7. How can the medical staff orientation be best achieved?
8. Who orients the administration to the changes and innovations in the field of materiel management? Elaborate.
9. Why is it necessary to spend time to orient sales representatives?
10. What is your reaction to having a full-time materiel management employee perform all inservice and orientations for the department?
11. What is the evidence of good departmental orientation and inservice education programs?
12. Should every hospital employee receive an orientation to the materiel management philosophy on a periodic basis? Why or why not?

Chapter 21

The Many Ways To Contain Costs Through Effective Materiel Management*

Cost containment in the hospital industry involves the utilization of human resources and physical assets in a way that ensures economical delivery of high-quality healthcare. Although the term cost containment is used here because of its wide acceptance in hospitals, in a sense it is a misnomer for cost effectiveness. The true goals of a cost containment effort in a hospital are to evaluate whether the institution is obtaining optimum quantity and quality of goods and services for its money and to seek improved ways of acquiring those goods and services—all within the parameters of the institution's established standards for patient care.[1] It is also quite possible that a cost containment idea may result in better quality or service at or about the same costs.

The function of materiel management can represent a major contributor to the cost containment efforts of today's hospitals. It has all of the necessary ingredients: a fairly large personnel component, an enormous paper trail, systems fragmentation, monumental inventories, and duplications galore. The purpose of this chapter is to point out cost containment ideas with suggested plans of action that are quite feasible and can be implemented by the hospital materiel manager and his/her staff.

Reducing Official Inventory

Reduction of official inventories is a very potent area of cost containment for all hospitals. A recent survey of 500 hospitals of all sizes revealed that

---

*Reprinted with the permission of DIMENSIONS in Health Service, Journal of the Canadian Hospital Association.

[1] American Hospital Association, *Organizing a Cost Containment Committee in the Hospital* (Chicago, Ill.: 1976), p. 1.

even the smaller institutions could reduce their official inventory by at least $100,000, while some of the larger ones could free over $1 million through inventory reduction. Such a buildup of supplies for which the hospital has already paid represents a sizeable investment that pays no dividends. When this stockpile has been reduced, the real money gained can be invested or be put to better use.

Another method that can be used by hospitals to cut inventory is to reduce automatically the amount of supplies by the annual cost increase for those supplies. For example, the costs of supplies have been increasing at the annual rate of 7 to 10 percent, and the hospital could reduce the inventory accordingly to offset this expense. In other words, the hospital that holds its inventory to a set maximum is in fact reducing it by about 10 percent per year. However, this very slow and methodical way of inventory reduction is recommended only after inventories have reached acceptable levels.

The fact is that most administrators and materiel managers do not realize that their inventories are reaching unacceptable levels. Being aware of the costs and disadvantages of inventory is one of the first steps in dealing with it. The second is to take an immediate physical count of all official inventory (central stores, pharmacy, and dietary) and devise an immediate plan of action to reduce it to approximately $300 per bed. For the most part, inventory reduction is painless. Once begun, it should be an ongoing program.

Reducing Unofficial Inventory

Many hospital departments are "fat" with unofficial inventory. Their administrations have, however, generally ignored these supply stockpiles when attempting to contain costs because once this inventory is dispensed, it is officially out of sight. In all probability, the materiel manager should begin the unofficial inventory reduction program in surgery, which normally has an enormous unofficial inventory, and proceed to the special care units and then to the emergency room. Many hospitals can free from $100,000 to $500,000 of capital just in these areas alone.

It is safe to assume that unofficial inventory will be approximately three to five times the amount of the official inventory. Here, too, these supplies have been paid for and represent a nonproductive investment which in the general medical-surgical hospital can amount to millions of dollars. Hospitals must begin to control this area of expensive duplication.

To start, it is recommended that the materiel manager confer with top management and gain their support for unofficial inventory reduction programs. Next, he should organize inventory teams to perform an actual count of all supplies. In a combined effort with all respective department heads, a hard-nosed plan of action should be delineated and initiated immediately. Inventory should be used, sent back for credit, or even thrown away as a last resort. Finally, the materiel manager should establish realistic maximum levels for all unofficial inventories and then take a physical inventory quarterly to ensure that the departments are following the guidelines.

Amalgamating Supply, Process, and Distribution Functions and Areas

Hospital architects are still specifying that the central stores be in the basement, central sterile supply on the second or third floor, and the pharmacy on the first floor. Also, most still recommend that there be a separate central sterile supply department. It is high time we relate to them and to ourselves that these functions are similar and should be located together. As separate areas, they all have their own personnel, supervision, distribution, supplies, and inventories. If the functions are combined or located in close proximity, many of the tasks and duties can be shared.

In most cases, central stores and central sterile supply can be combined and the staff reduced. Pharmacy should be a part of this system, too, so that it can become a part of this one storage and distribution center. Unit dose carts from the pharmacy should be programed to be distributed at the same time by the same personnel as are the medical-surgical and linen carts. Of course, it is hoped that any hospital about to be constructed make plans to combine these functions. Existing hospitals with fragmented functions of supply, process, and distribution could greatly improve their service and costs by taking steps to combine them.

Eliminating Excess Personnel in the Materiel Areas

The materiel manager must always be cognizant of the personnel component because the tendency to increase it is omnipresent. The combination of the supply, process, and distribution functions can always be counted on to reduce the number of personnel by at least one or two in the smaller hospitals and by as many as twenty-five in the larger ones. Also, the purchase of disposables should result in reduction of personnel or their use cannot be justified. Things (systems, programs, equipment) usually are cheaper than people, but a combination of the two is excessively expensive and totally unacceptable from a cost containment point of view.

Using Consignment as an Alternative to Purchasing

With the use of newer and more expensive supplies such as pacemakers and total hips, it is imperative that the materiel manager seek better alternatives to the purchasing procedure. Consignment, the principle of having the manufacturer stock a commodity at the hospital but not charge for it until it is used, seems to be a promising option. This plan benefits the hospital greatly, but recently manufacturers have been reluctant to continue it because of their interpretation of the health devices legislation. Most manufacturers seemed to feel that under its provisions, if they let an item out on consignment, they had no control of the supply but still had the ultimate responsibility. Fortunately, there has been a recent clarification of the principle, and many manufacturers are once again favorably inclined to the use of consignment.

Hospitals and materiel managers should literally insist upon the use of consignment by the manufacturers for these expensive supplies, even to the point of assuming responsibility for the proper storage of the supplies in writing. They have the responsibility if they purchase the supplies outright, so why not have the suppliers provide the inventory free of charge? Consignment can save hospitals thousands of dollars and is an excellent means of cost containment.

Stockless Purchasing

Stockless purchasing can help to reduce both official and unofficial inventories at the same time. In fact, through stockless purchasing hospitals can cut enormous unofficial inventories to a workable level of $300 per bed.

Product Standardization

Product standardization can bring about a materiel discipline that has never before been paralleled. To be the most effective as a means of cost containment, it must be a five-point program: standardization review, patient charge determination, procedural documentation, inservice delineation, and followup. A hard-nosed, results-oriented standardization program should be mandatory for all hospitals.

Buying Special Items Locally

From time to time, most hospitals are in need of unique items of supply that may only be used once or twice every ten years. The cost conscious materiel manager should never think of stocking this type of supply. These kinds of items can best be purchased locally from such suppliers as hardware stores and pharmacies.

Indirect or Wholesale Drug Purchasing

Pharmaceuticals are an expensive supply category and should be purchased with care and concern. For years, hospital purchasing agents have felt that they get the best possible prices by buying directly from the manufacturer. Most manufacturers do give a discount on direct purchases, but usually there is a certain minimum that must be bought; moreover, some drug manufacturers do not give hospital discounts. The prudent materiel manager should be alert to all direct purchase policies and compare them to an indirect drug prime supplier where no dollar minimums are required. In fact, in many cases, it will be to the hospital's benefit to purchase from the wholesaler, especially if the company will give prime supplier volume discounts regardless of quantities purchased. It will always be advantageous to purchase the slow moving or exotic drugs in the smallest quantities possible from the wholesaler. Hospitals should follow the example of the retail pharmacy, which keeps a low inventory worth about $20,000 and greatly utilizes the service of the wholesaler.

In addition, the reliance of hospitals on the hospital discount from the direct drug manufacturer may be at an end. The United States Supreme Court recently put explicit restrictions on the use of drugs bought by hospitals at preferential prices. In the "Portland Case" ruling, the court stated that a pharmaceutical company cannot sell drugs to a hospital at lower prices than they do to retail pharmacies in the area if the hospital uses those drugs to fill prescriptions for outpatients.

In making the final judicial statements in the case first brought about by the Portland, Oregon, Retail Druggists Association against 11 pharmaceutical manufacturers, the Supreme Court made it clear that pharmaceutical purchases by a hospital are exempt from the Robinson-Patman Act's ban on discriminatory pricing when they are dispensed to the following persons:

a. Hospital inpatients or emergency room patients while they are in the hospital or at the time of discharge;
b. Outpatients for use on the hospital premises or to be taken home after their visit; or
c. Hospital personnel or staff physicians for their personal use or that of their dependents.

Accordingly, preferential drug purchases are not exempt if the drugs are dispensed to the following persons:

a. Discharged inpatients or emergency room-clinic patients as refills or repeats;
b. Walk-ins who have no patient status at the hospital; or
c. Hospital or medical staff for use other than for themselves or their dependents.

The likely outcome of this landmark decision will be:

a. Some or many pharmaceutical manufacturers will eliminate hospital preferential pricing from their marketing policies;
b. Hospitals may elect not to participate in any of the nonexempt dispensing activities; or
c. If hospitals elect to participate in nonexempt dispensing activities, they must set up and follow strict recordkeeping practices that differentiate the nonexempt from exempt use.

Since the wholesale or indirect drug companies give discounts based on volume alone, their pricing arrangement is not considered to be in violation of the Portland decision. Therefore, it may be beneficial for hospitals to look to the drug wholesaler as their principal supplier. It is further suggested that the hospital materiel manager negotiate with the wholesalers on a prime supplier basis.

Negotiating Term Instead of Full Service Contracts

Many equipment service companies decide without negotiation what preventive maintenance should be performed and the frequency of the service. Hospitals should take a hard look at all such contracts and demand that their input be considered in setting the service specifications. It may be that the equipment does not need as much servicing as is proposed by the company. There is ample room for modifying most service contracts, and the prudent materiel manager will see to it that the hospital is getting adequate service for a justifiable cost. Even if the service companies have no equal competition, hospitals can contain costs by negotiating the service specifications.

Controlling Forms

In the modern hospital the panacea for all problems seems to be the creation of another printed form. For the most part, forms can be initiated, changed, and redeveloped without the permission or knowledge of anyone in authority. One of the most devastating characteristics of forms is that they are so easy to reproduce, especially since copy machines are located in almost all departments. It is estimated that the average-sized hospital of 350 beds will have some 600–700 different forms in its inventory.

Most hospital materiel managers agree that controlling forms is a definite problem. To deal with this issue, it is recommended that a survey referencing each form by initiating department, quantities used, description, and annual costs be completed. It should also indicate whether or not the form is an inventory item. The forms survey should bring out any duplication by departments and be the basis for the forms control program.

Some hospitals have initiated forms committees which have bringing some organization to this paper chaos as their main objective. However, it seems that the formation of another committee just brings recognition to the problem without solving it. It is preferable for the materiel manager and his staff to review the forms survey and make recommendations as to discontinuing certain forms, combining others, and standardizing them all. After this task has been completed, the materiel manager should refer the matter to the Products Standardization Committee, which should attempt to reduce the number of forms to around 250 by whatever method is possible.

The Product Standardization Committee then should set certain policies such as the following:

1. Any new form regardless of its use must be submitted to the Product Standardization Committee for review and approval before being used in the hospital.
2. If a new form is approved, all quantities of the old form must be used before the new one is used. This policy can save the hospital money and reduce the number of unnecessary new forms.
3. A control numbering system should be initiated to identify the forms for usage and reordering.
4. Many medical staff forms are reviewed by the Medical Records Committee. When a proposed form has been approved, it should be submitted to the Product Standardization Committee for review and recommendations.
5. When a proposed form is submitted for review, it must be accompanied by printing and storage costs.
6. When a standard form is being considered for repurchase, it should be submitted to the Product Standardization Committee for review in case any changes are contemplated on a hospital-wide basis.

The hospital materiel manager should implement the prime supplier approach to purchasing forms. In most cases, forms suppliers, especially at the local level, will work carefully with the hospital. It is suggested that the hospital put their forms out for quotation on a prime supplier basis and make a part of the agreement the condition that the supplier store the printed matter in reasonable quantities, ship to the hospital on an as-needed basis, and bill accordingly. With this relationship with the supplier, there would be no need for the hospital to keep an inventory of forms.

After the individual hospital has gotten some control over this paper jungle, forms standardization on a cooperative basis should be considered. There is no reason why hospitals in the same locale cannot standardize the major patient care forms such as admission forms, TPR sheets, graphic sheets, and doctors orders. For the most part the same doctors use all the hospitals, which makes the reasons for each individual hospital to have its own individualized forms even more absurd. Since group purchasing is very much in vogue, it seems reasonable to standardize and group purchase hospital forms.

Purchasing Copying Machines

In the past, hospitals have had to lease or rent copying machines. However, things have changed and companies now sell their machines along with reasonable service contracts. First, it must be stated that the hospital should exert some kind of reasonable control over forms reproduction. The convenience and accessibility of copying machines have led to a proliferation of forms, often in senseless quantities. By purchasing the machines, at least the hospital is not burdened by a per copy charge. Second, the hospital should review its copying policies and experience in order to decide whether it is in the hospital's best interest to lease or buy.

Sharing Infrequently Used Supplies with Other Hospitals

Hospitals that are located in the same locale should assist each other by stocking infrequently used supplies and equipment at only one hospital. This sharing would contain costs for each one in the group. At the end of a certain period, each would bill the others for services rendered. In this manner, even infrequently used supplies would be available at all times, duplication of supplies reduced, and much paperwork eliminated.

Limiting the Number of Supplies in the Central Stores Area

The materiel manager should review the number of items in central stores and decide whether they are absolutely necessary. Most hospitals can manage very well with 350 to 400 standard items, whereas they now have around 3,000. Reducing this number negates the need for computerization, frees up more space, and cuts out costly duplication. It is suggested that the materiel manager draw up a set of guidelines, specifications, and criteria for stocking an item involving definition of need, number of users, critical nature of the item, cost of the supply, and lead time for procurement. If the hospital has an effective standardization program, the review and decision can be made through the standardization channel. Keep in mind that it does not take too much ingenuity to manage a storeroom with 3,000 items and $300,000 worth of inventory. However, to function effectively with only 300 items and $35,000 to $50,000 worth of official inventory takes managerial talent, discipline, and intelligence.

Developing a Drug Formulary

Another supply category that needs immediate attention is the standardization of drugs. In many hospitals, drug inventory represents a larger dollar volume than does the total supply inventory, and materiel managers have been reluctant to tackle this area because of their lack of knowledge of drugs. To be effective, however, materiel managers must treat drugs as they would other supply categories. All drug expenditures and quantities should be questioned. A formulary should be developed and the number of drugs kept in inventory reduced to a minimum. Exotic and infrequently used drugs should be purchased in the smallest quantities possible and be dispensed directly to the patient without an inventory buildup. The formulary should also allow for recognized and approved substitutes. The materiel manager can look to the Product Standardization Committee, if it is well represented by physicians, to make these decisions.

Reducing the Frequency of Linen Changes

Cost per processed pound of linen has become an accepted indicator for measuring the effectiveness of the laundry production. In most hospitals in the U.S., the cost will be somewhere between 15¢ and 25¢ per pound, with the figure rising as labor and indirect expenses increase. In an attempt to reduce this figure, many hospitals have given up their laundries and contracted with commercial laundries or centralized hospital laundries, but the cost per pound still will gradually increase because it is payment for labor.

It could be that they have been attacking the problem from the wrong perspective. The cost reduction methods should involve linen use, not linen production. It may not be in the patient's best interest to change his or her bed linen every day, and in fact, a few hospitals that have found that their new policy of linen changing every other day is totally acceptable to both the patients and the nursing staff. Of course, if the patient's condition warrants more frequent changes, these are made on an as-needed basis. This recommendation has great cost-saving potential for hospitals. For example, a hospital that has two million pounds of processed linen per year at 20¢ per pound pays a $400,000 laundry bill. If that hospital cut its production pounds by one-third, it would reduce its laundry costs by approximately $133,000.

Prime Supplier Concept

The prime supplier technique can be effective as a cost containment measure. It can bring savings to the hospital through good prices regardless of quantities purchased, less paperwork, much less time spent interviewing vendors and less back orders. This technique is most effective when practiced on a group basis.

Group Purchasing

There has been a renewed interest among hospitals in group purchasing over the past five years. Of course, the benefits of the group efforts must be equal to or greater than the concessions made by the member hospitals. Certainly the tendency on the part of the suppliers to give a price to the group that is very advantageous to the smaller hospitals, fair to the medium-sized hospitals, and mediocre to the larger hospitals will not be tolerated very long by the larger institutions. This information points up the fact that group purchasing is just one method of getting better prices through negotiation, but is not the panacea for all purchasing problems. Sometimes a combination of the different purchasing techniques can get the best results. The materiel manager needs the flexibility to choose the right purchasing maneuver to bring about the desired results in each individual situation.

Requesting Instant Credit on Overcharges by the Vendors

Any problem arising from overcharging or a supply shortage with an overcharge should be taken care of immediately by the sales representative through an instant credit. The hospital should take every opportunity possible to keep its cash moving or invested, never in use by someone else.

Centralizing Purchasing

The act of purchasing and negotiation can best be done by the professional materiel manager or purchasing director. Centralized purchasing can best achieve uniformity of quality, best prices, and procedural and policy standardization.

Hand Writing Purchase Orders

It has been estimated that the processing of a purchase order can cost approximately $35, mostly because of labor costs. Much of the cost can be saved simply by writing the orders in a legible manner, instead of typing them.

Using FAX Equipment for Purchase Data Transmission

The manner in which data are transferred to the supplier also can be a factor in cost reduction. FAX or facsimile equipment performs both data transmission and data receiving functions. To the user, the procedure is a matter of calling a telephone number at the receiving end, putting the telephone receiver on the FAX terminal, and then letting the two machines talk to each other. Transmission time for most purchase orders is about two minutes.

The machines can be leased for rates ranging from $29 to $60 each month; however, the responsive supplier will pay for the equipment. The advantages of using FAX equipment are as follows:

(a) Speed—There is no faster system available for the price.
(b) Efficiency—The documents are transmitted error free.
(c) Cost—The costs associated with the equipment can be included as a cost of doing business for the supplier.
(d) Convenience—Transmissions can be performed at any time as there is no need for a person to be at the receiving end.
(e) Flexibility—If necessary, the order can include a picture of the supply or equipment needed.

Consolidating Rebates, Discounts and Allowances into the Invoiced Price

If you negotiate for rebates or discounts, be certain that these are figured into the invoiced prices. In some states if a separate rebate check is received monthly or yearly as is common practice, third parties consider the rebated amount as a reduction in revenue. Also, with all rebates and discounts being included in the invoiced price, the hospital has the use of the money for a longer period of time.

Tough But Ethical Negotiation

The hospital purchasing agent or materiel manager should conduct tough negotiation sessions on an annual basis for all supply categories, and all major agreements on price and service should be effective for at least a year. Since the hospital suppliers have been in control so long, the materiel manager must be creative and innovative in his approach at the negotiation table. It must, however, be remembered that concern about prices can overshadow the more important actions such as inventory reduction. Let's put the supply price negotiations into perspective. The maximum reduction obtainable from the toughest, most stringent type of negotiations is only about two percent if the hospital is getting good prices to begin with. At this rate the hospital could possibly pick up another $20,000 per each million dollars worth of purchases, so the money saved through purchasing is miniscule compared to that saved through internal materiel practices. In fact, hospitals practicing prudent purchasing should already be at a point beyond which the supplier cannot give.

Industrial Engineering Applications

Even if the hospital cannot afford a staff industrial engineer, it would be advisable to seek the help and advice of such a person on a periodic basis. There are many situations in the materiel management function that the industrial engineer could assist. For instance, in many institutions there are intricate and confusing distribution patterns, including pack wrapping, tray makeup, soiled and clean material flow, and instrumentation set up, that could be greatly simplified by industrial engineering techniques. This is just one of the areas in which the hospital management could contain costs by reducing personnel time and paper work under the auspices of the industrial engineer.

Reviewing and Studying All Purchase Alternatives

Often there are many alternatives to purchasing a commodity or service. An important one is to make an item instead of to buy it. Presently, hospitals lean toward buying disposables, but this can be a very costly decision unless accompanied by a reduction in man-hours previously spent preparing that item. But, there are still some items, such as water for irrigation, that it would be more advantageous for the hospital to make than to buy.

Another decision is whether to buy or rent. One sees the need for this decision most when the hospital is running at a high occupancy and additional supplies and equipment are required for the period. It may not be necessary for the hospital to spend money for extra suction machines, for example, and the materiel manager must figure out at what usage level it½
example, and the materiel manager must figure out at what usage level it
would be better to buy or rent.

To buy or borrow is a third option that the materiel manager faces, and timing is of utmost importance with this decision. At midnight on a weekend, it may be easiest and quickest to borrow the needed equipment or supply from another hospital.

To buy or lease is a fourth question for the materiel manager. In most cases, leasing represents an expensive monthly payment. There are, however, a few applications for leasing that are justifiable. The foremost is the situation of obsolescence. If a piece of equipment is needed by the institution and has a short lifespan, it may be advantageous to lease it. Another is when the hospital needs a piece of equipment which it cannot afford outright. In most cases, however, the hospital will come out ahead if it buys supplies and equipment.

The materiel manager may also have to decide whether to buy something or get it free. This decision often comes up when a company has a product that has to be used in conjunction with another piece of equipment. For example, some of the companies that make anesthetics often will have a special offer that if the hospital buys their product at list price, the company will give the hospital the equipment needed for dispensing it. Oddly enough, this may not always be in the best interest of the hospital. Sometimes getting something free may be more expensive than buying it in the long run.

Supply Utilization Studies

Much emphasis is put on purchasing, processing, and distributing supplies, but hardly any attention is given to how that product is used in the institution. The materiel manager must set up standards and specifications for the efficient and effective use of all supplies and equipment. He or his agent should monitor this use in the actual setting on a periodic and planned basis. If abuse and misuses of the supplies and equipment are seen, he should plan an inservice program for the entire using staff. In most cases, hospital equipment is not worn out, it is abused and misused. It would be in the best interests of the hospitals for the materiel manager to pay more attention to this important aspect of materiel management.

Eliminating All Bulk Warehousing

In addition to central stores and central supply, many hospitals have added another duplicative effort by introducing warehousing into the supply picture. This warehousing space can be in an older part of the building or at an offsite location. In addition to rent or the per square footage charge and indirect expenses, there is that ever present cost of inventory buildup. In other words, warehousing should be eliminated in today's hospital supply market, especially since no supply is more than a day away.

Establishing Effective Limits for All Supplies Based on an Economic Order

Supply maximums and minimums actually represent good supply discipline since they indicate that the materiel manager has determined a limit above which he cannot go for economic reasons and below which he cannot go for supply service reasons. This maximum and minimum continuum should be reviewed on a periodic, seasonal basis to assure cost effectiveness and supply continuity of service. There has been much discussion about economic order quantities with complex mathematical ratios and complicated formulas, but in practice, these are more complicated than useful. If supply maximums and minimums are established realistically over a period of time, the economic order quantity is simply the difference between the maximum and the minimum.

Better Utilization of the Vendors

In the past, sales representatives have been noted for their hard sell and their marketing techniques. However, with the concept of materiel management evolving, the role of the salesman is changing. He should become a representative to a hospital from his company. In this role, the representative can be very beneficial to the hospital, performing the following functions for it.

(a) Advising the materiel manager or purchasing agent about quality products that may be less expensive than what the hospital is presently using.
(b) Assisting with annual physical inventory under the control and supervision of the materiel manager.
(c) Providing the hospital with information that can assist in establishing effective supply maximums and minimums.

(d) Informing the materiel manager or purchasing agent of price increases with enough notice that he does not feel pressure to take advantage of the offer.
(e) Providing the materiel manager with the monthly, quarterly, and annual reports on supply procurement and utilization.
(f) Obtaining supplies for the hospital from sources other than his own company when there is a definite need to do so. Such supply continuity is the responsibility of the prime supplier.
(g) Providing the materiel manager with future supply trends such as supply increases, supply stockouts, and product alterations.

Certainly the sales representative of the past should become the service representative of the future.

Evaluating New Products at the Vendor's Expense

If it is decided to evaluate a product, the supplier should provide the necessary material at his company's expense. This is merely a cost of doing business to the supplier, but is an unnecessary expense to the hospital. Also, it is advantageous for the hospital to request a reasonable evaluation period for most movable, capital equipment. This simple procedure can save the hospital thousands of dollars even in the short run.

Employee Orientation

If cost containment programs are going to be worthwhile, the hospital employees need to know about these efforts and how to achieve them. It is extremely important that the materiel manager get this point across to his or her employees and to all of the hospital employees on a timely and periodic basis. Therefore, employee orientation must be continuous. Informing employees about the materiel objectives for the institution is a key responsibility of materiel managers if they are to expect any results from their efforts.

Time and Motion Studies of All Supply Functions

It is imperative that the materiel manager review all functions of materiel management from acquisition to disposition on a timely basis and either make the necessary changes or evaluate a proposed change for a short period of time. If he does not have the time to perform this function, he should recommend to top management that time and motion studies be performed by an outside consultant on a limited basis. Most systems, procedures, programs, and plans can be improved, and it behooves the materiel manager to provide or seek assistance in this area from a professional source. For the materiel manager and his staff, time is money. If the time element of a procedure is improved, there should be an improvement in its cost effectiveness.

Continuous Patient Charge Review

In general, hospitals do not have the best record for establishing patient charge criteria. This entire area should be reviewed and made more effective by both the materiel and financial managers. Patient supply charges must be based upon many criteria, but one of the foremost is price. With the present trend of supply prices always in a state of flux, this fact alone should cause the patient supply charge to be reviewed and changed almost constantly. The materiel manager or key personnel on his staff must be in this purchase-charge loop, insuring that their hospital charges exceed costs and that the charges are indeed made.

Inhouse Biomedical Engineering Expertise

Hospitals have large quantities of complicated, sophisticated, and very expensive patient care equipment, which must be tended to by trained biomedical engineers. The cost of such expertise on an as-needed basis is very expensive, so it makes sense for one or a group of hospitals to hire such a person on a full-time basis.

Effective Preventive Maintenance Programs

For the most part, supply rooms are filled with expensive equipment and supplies. It is the responsibility of the materiel manager to see that the appropriate preventive maintenance is given to all equipment and supplies under his jurisdiction. Remember, it can either be cared for now or totally replaced later.

An Assets Management Program

Capital equipment is an important part of materiel management because generally it is through materiel management that the equipment is specified, ordered, received and distributed to the appropriate user. In addition, hospitals are reimbursed for capital equipment depreciation on a concise and factual schedule. It only makes good sense that there be a materiel management program which assures that equipment is properly received, priced, distributed to the appropriate area, inventoried and accounted for on a planned basis, and depreciated properly. This is commonly called an assets management program or property management. The better this function is executed, the more justification the hospital has for receiving dollars through depreciation.

Appropriate Product Substitution

Hospitals are fortunate in that there often are several products which will provide about the same results. In many cases, the hospital materiel manager is hard pressed to prove one superior or inferior to the other. The establishment of an effective product standardization process involves the ability to choose product substitutes. Therefore, for every standard item, there should be an acceptable backup. If this decision has been made before the need arises, the materiel manager has more flexibility with the purchasing function. It is suggested that by whatever process the hospital has for accepting standard items, there should be equal consideration given at that time for finding an appropriate and acceptable substitute.

Value Analysis

Value analysis is a technique that can be used very effectively by the Product Standardization Committee. The essence of value analysis is the questioning and challenging of the need for the function of each product or piece of equipment. Next, consideration should be given to alternate ways or methods to perform the product's function. Last, comparison studies must be performed. If acceptable methods are found to accomplish the same end more efficiently or inexpensively, then a change should be proposed.

Results-Oriented Product Inservice Programs

No product or piece of equipment should ever gain entrance into the hospital without proper and thorough inservice programs. Both the hospital and supplier have major responsibilities in this area. The supplier's major responsibility lies in the initial inservice, and the hospital should provide the necessary followup. The sales representative and hospital inservice coordinator should meet with all applicable personnel in small groups and provide practical instructions and then allow each employee to use the product or equipment under trained supervision. This training should be repeated in three months to review the actual use of the product by hospital personnel. If possible, written examinations should be given to determine the amount of information retained by the trainees. Participation in such inservice training should be a prerequisite for using the new product.

Pay for Capital Equipment Purchases Only After Installation and Hospital Approval

Most hospital equipment manufacturers and suppliers stipulate that the hospital make term payments on purchases, a policy heavily weighted in favor of the supplier. Hospital materiel managers should formulate a payment schedule that would give the hospital the upper hand. For example, all major capital purchases should be negotiated on the premise that no payment will be made until the installation has been approved by the necessary hospital authorities. This will result in faster installations, as well as allow the hospital to keep its money invested longer. Hospitals should take such return on investment into consideration when purchasing equipment, especially major large dollar volume capital items.

Simplifying the Purchase Process

Much time, effort, and expense can go into the purchase process. The tendency is omnipresent to complicate this function by much paper work, computerization keypunching, producing multiple copies, and holding time-consuming sales interviews. Take a hard look at your purchasing function and establish realistic purchase simplification objectives. For instance, try to decrease the number of vendors with whom the hospital is doing small amounts of business. This will mean that the materiel manager, purchasing agent, or buyer spends less time with sales representatives and writes fewer purchase orders and checks. Also make an effort to limit the purchase document to only one original piece of paper. Schedule all major negotiations on a two-year basis and monitor your prices on a periodic basis to determine the cost effectiveness of your prices. In summary, make a personal determination to see how simple you can make the purchase process.

Questioning All Computer Applications in the Materiel Areas for Cost Effectiveness

Certainly there are possible applications for computerization in the purchase and inventory functions, but only after much thought and deliberation. The more reasonable approach lies in simplification not computerization, since computer time and computer operators' salaries are costly. To begin with, the materiel manager should reduce the number of supplies in inventory to a workable, manual level. Next, a time study should be performed to determine how much time and effort and expense are involved in the inventory process. Then request that a parallel study be performed using the computer. It is very likely that the use of the computer in this area will be more expensive than the manual operations. Do not be lured by the "prestige" of having your inventories on a computer program. The main objective is to find out what items must be reordered, and one of the best ways to do this is by the "eyeball method." It is simple and does not have to be rechecked for accuracy.

Sharing Services

Hospitals can certainly contain costs by shared programs. These programs do not always have to concern group purchasing or collections, but can involve simply sharing ideas, prices, and drug and product information systems. Hospital materiel managers should make a list of all of their functions and programs and get together on a local or regional basis and discuss the pros and cons of sharing any and all programs, being careful not to duplicate costs for which they are getting no value. The whole idea behind sharing of services is that higher volumes mean lower costs for all institutions. If this is not the case, then the entire idea should be questioned on an individual basis. Be careful, too, to guard against developing antagonisms with the management of hospitals with which you are sharing services. Before entering such a relationship, have a good understanding of all ramifications and costs. In some cases, it may be better and less expensive to go it alone.

Questioning All Automated Efforts in the Materiel Areas for Cost Effectiveness

Most functions in the materiel areas must be people processed, and any time there is a disproportionate mix of automation and people, costs soar. Automation usually breeds high installation costs, system inflexibility, costly repair, and expensive operational costs. In addition, people are still necessary to process the supplies that go on the system. Consequently, in the materiel management arena, vigorously question and contest all automated efforts in the name of cost containment and practicality.

Negotiating for Longer Equipment Warranties

Never settle for less than a 12-month warranty on all parts and service on all major capital purchases, despite the trend for manufacturers to decrease the warranty to 6 months or even 90 days. The terms and length of the warranty are negotiable, and hospitals should start negotiating longer warranties for parts and service. In many cases, hospitals can get at least a two-year warranty if their negotiations are strong, and extended warranties at the manufacturer's expense can be at least as attractive as a very sizeable discount off the list price. The materiel manager should try for both, but when all negotiations over price break down, he has the warranty over which to bargain.

Supply Cost Emphasis and Awareness Program

In most cases, the personnel who use the supplies and equipment, including the physicians, have no awareness of its costs. The materiel manager could address this by featuring a different supply display each week in a prominent place where all personnel would see it. In the display, the cost of the item should be made known with the percentage of cost increase over the past five years. It could also point up the cost of the item to the patient with a short summary of the factors which make up the cost, as well as the total number of the items used on an annual basis. Last, it should include some plea for containing costs by proper use of the item. The format of the cost awareness program could be flexible but continuous, because the number of items used and abused by the hospital is infinite.

Return for Credit Policy

A hospital cannot afford to have its capital tied up in supplies that do not turn over at a constant rate and bring a fairly good rate of return. Therefore, the materiel manager should formulate a minimum turnover rate for all supplies kept in inventory, especially the more expensive ones. For instance, it could be the policy of the institution to return all supplies for credit after 90 or 120 days of inactivity. This policy will also prevent obsolescence and pilferage.

Using Hot Air Hand Dryers Instead of Paper Towels

In some high use areas such as public toilets and rest rooms, there is much waste of paper towels. The materiel manager in coordination with the executive housekeeper should perform studies on these areas to determine the cost of paper towels on an annual basis, then compare these figures with the cost of installing hot air hand dryers.

Using All of a Product Before Replacing It

Many times new items are introduced into the hospital without considering the quantity of the old product in stock. As a result, the new product comes in and the old product is never used again. This is especially true of forms. The materiel manager should formulate a policy that a new product cannot be purchased unless all quantities of the old product are used first. If this is not feasible, the supplier of the new product should be required to reimburse the hospital for the total amount of the old product on hand. Remember, the time to negotiate all terms with the supplier is before the new product gains access to the hospital.

In Some Cases, Lower the Standards of Quality

There are some instances in which the product does not have to be of the best quality. For example, some nursing policies stipulate that underpads used for an incontinent patient be changed every two to four hours. The highest quality, most absorbent, larger underpad would be wasted in such cases, and the lesser quality, less expensive, smaller underpad would be quite acceptable. Try to match up the quality of the product with the situation. There are times when reusable items such as wash cloths and abdominal pads are treated as though they were disposable. Determine what these situations are and purchase the quality of product to match the need.

Question All Patient Convenience Products

Since hospitals are put in the unenviable position of being the patients' keeper, decisions are made that can raise the cost of their care in behalf of their best interests. For example, most hospitals use and charge for patient admission kits. The average cost to the patient for this item is between three and four dollars. Unfortunately, the patient has no say in this decision. The patient may already have a toothbrush, toothpaste, mouthwash, and everything else in the kit, but he gets it whether he needs it or not. There are many more items that fall into this category, and the materiel manager and the Product Standardization Committee should review each to determine whether or not it is necessary.

There are many more cost containment ideas that must be considered by the prudent materiel manager. It is amazing what hospitals will do in the name of cost containment and in many cases will come out paying more in the long run. In reference to cost containment and materiel management in hospitals, one is reminded of the following story:

> A group of former hospital employees decided to go into business for themselves. They began a trucking company with a small fleet of heavy trucks. One of their feats was to take a three ton truck over a two ton load limit bridge to service a customer. They reasoned among themselves that rules were made to be broken, so they decided to take the three ton truck over the two ton load limit bridge. Well, of course, the inevitable happened; the bridge collapsed, and the truck went into the ravine. They rented a crane, got the truck out, fixed the truck and fixed the bridge. They again reasoned that since the new bridge was built of new material, they could run their truck over the bridge even though its load capacity was still two tons. The second time, the bridge collapsed, and the truck went into the ravine. They rented a crane, got the truck out, fixed the truck, and fixed the bridge. This time, they reasoned that the third time would be the charm. So on the third try, the bridge collapsed, and the truck again went into the ravine. They rented a crane, got the truck out, fixed the truck, and fixed the bridge. They went through this routine six times, until one of them stated that they must make a management decision since they weren't making any progress. Their decision, BUY THE CRANE!

Hospitals should operate their materiel management functions just as though they were in business for a profit. Definitely, good materiel practices are imperative for cost avoidance, cost containment, and cost effectiveness. Our patients expect us to give them the best buy for their health care dollars. It is a challenge that hospitals can ill afford not to meet!

Pertinent Points to Ponder

1. What is the difference between cost containment and cost avoidance?
2. Why is there so much interest lately in cost containment for hospitals?
3. What is meant by voluntary cost containment?
4. How can cost containment be forced upon hospitals? Explain.
5. Where must the cost containment efforts begin? Why?
6. Are there any hospital departments that cannot participate in cost containment programs? Explain.

7. What department probably holds the greatest potential for cost containment? Why?
8. Is a hospital cost containment committee really necessary? Why or why not?
9. Why haven't hospitals formed cost containment committees in the past?
10. How can the hospital actually document the results of cost containment?
11. Is it possible that cost containment programs can actually increase costs? Explain.
12. In addition to the cost containment ideas set forth in this chapter, list six more that you have implemented in your hospital.

Chapter 22

Excuses, Excuses, Excuses

Having been both a materiel manager and an administrator, I have heard nearly all the excuses ever invented as to why materiel management won't work or why it can't be implemented. Over the years, I have collected and cataloged a great number of these, which I would like to share with my readers.

Excuse Number 1—Materiel Management Is Too Expensive

This reason is often given by administrators. They will indicate that their hospital hasn't implemented materiel management because it is too costly. This statement indicates that they do not fully understand the concept. It must be reiterated that materiel management is as individualized as are the different hospitals. Its very essence is administrative support and cost containment, and one cannot implement a strong materiel management thrust without administrative backing. By the same token, materiel management will save costs, not increase them. If implemented effectively, materiel management will provide the hospital with total supply service at a better level of quality, an increased mode of service, and a reduced cost.

Excuse Number 2—My Administrator Won't Support Me

In a recent survey of 500 U.S. hospitals, this excuse was given by over 50 percent of the respondents. This indicates a lack of credibility somewhere. The philosophy of materiel management is such that it can be implemented from the line level to the board level, so there are some concepts that the materiel manager or purchasing agent can implement without administrative approval. For example, the reduction of inventories can be performed without asking anyone. After it has been successfully done, the administrator can be told. Show me an administrator who would get upset over a reduction in staff! When a materiel manager or purchasing agent gives me this excuse, I usually caution him that his administrator may think he has already implemented materiel management principles. Your administrator, too, may expect that you have already initiated this sure thing.

Excuse Number 3—Materiel Management Means More Personnel

If there is anything that a hospital doesn't need, it is more personnel. Actually, with the amalgamation of the functions of supply, process and distribution, there most surely will be a reduction in the number of personnel. However, it takes managerial effort to reap these benefits. One cannot expect the very words "materiel management" to possess the power to reduce automatically personnel. The concept will, however, provide the impetus to combine functions, amalgamate supervision, and provide more service with fewer people.

Excuse Number 4—My Hospital Is Too Small For Materiel Management

A large proportion of the nation's hospitals are in the small hospital category. In most cases, they need as much assistance in the area of materiel management as do the larger ones. In fact, a very small savings can make the difference in operating at a profit or operating at a loss, and small hospitals can greatly benefit from the implementation of materiel management principles.

Excuse Number 5—Materiel Management Is a Fad That Will Soon Pass

To the contrary, hospital materiel management is here to stay. It has been around for many years, especially in industry and it is picking up momentum. More than likely, the materiel manager of today will be the assistant administrator of tomorrow. Materiel management offers vertical mobility to the purchasing agent, the C.S.R. supervisor, the pharmacist, and others. It also offers a definite career ladder for the young graduates of programs in hospital administration. Simply stated, it represents the application of good management principles to the materiel process.

Excuse Number 6—Materiel Management Is Too Complex

Actually, materiel management emphasizes the simple management principles of planning, organizing, directing, staffing, and controlling. Moreover, it represents a return to the basics and fundamentals of good materiel practices. Materiel management creates an atmosphere whereby simple principles are used to conquer complex issues.

Excuse Number 7—My Hospital Is Too Large and Complicated

Being too large and complicated is an excellent reason to initiate materiel management. It will turn the fragmented chaos into an integrated system. A hospital does not get too large or too small for the application of good materiel management practices.

Excuse Number 8—My Hospital Is Too Old for This New Concept

Older hospitals usually have a lack of space and difficult distribution patterns. These are two good reasons to implement the philosophy of materiel management. A hospital never gets too old for the application of good materiel management practices.

Excuse Number 9—Materiel Management Takes Too Long To Implement

Of course, if you never get started, it will take too long! However, while you are using this excuse, you could begin the implementation of materiel management. The opponents of the principle who indicate it takes five to ten years to implement materiel management are confused between actual application and total implementation. The philosophy of materiel management is so broad and encompassing, that it may never be totally implemented. However, this is what makes the concept so promising. Any hospital can be on its way with materiel management applications within three to six months. The whole idea is to begin somewhere and stop offering excuses!

Excuse Number 10—My Hospital Is Different

Regardless of size, mission, ownership, location, age, management expertise, objective, or specialty, materiel management can help you. Whatever your materiel objectives, they can be implemented through effective materiel management.

Excuse Number 11—Materiel Management Takes Specially Trained Personnel

It is true that the initiation of materiel management takes leadership and a management perspective. However, the personnel who are now working at the hospital can be directed to accomplish the goals and objectives of materiel management. Again, it must be stressed that materiel management for the most part is an individual hospital concept. The results of the hospital's materiel efforts will determine if it is effective materiel management or not!

Excuse Number 12—I've Got Bigger Problems, Materiel Management Is the Least of My Worries

I still hear administrators downplay the materiel management function by stating that supplies only constitute around 10 percent of the total hospital expense budget, whereas the personnel component makes up 65 to 70 percent of the total expenses. This reasoning does not, however, take into account that there are people associated with the supplies. Some authorities estimate that as much as 46 percent of the hospital expense budget centers around the area of materiel management. In addition, over the past five to ten years, the cost of supplies has risen half again as much as payroll costs. While cost containment is the hospitals' last salvation from government controls, much of it can be realized in the materiel areas. Finally, capital equipment, which is not thought of as an operating expense, is considered to be under the materiel management umbrella and can balloon into millions of dollars in some hospitals on an annual basis.

None of our excuses really make that much sense when brought into perspective. Materiel management for hospitals is here to stay and must be handled by trained and competent managers. It is a dynamic and intriguing concept which can have far-reaching consequences to the manager as well as the patient. To practice materiel management will not always be easy. In fact, the determined materiel manager is a marked person who dares to be different in a status quo society.

Chapter 23

Case Reports of Materiel Management Implementation

Case Report 1

Development of the Materiel Management Concept

Seemor Smith, F.A.C.H.A., became the administrator of Southeast Memorial Hospital, a 350-bed N.P.A. institution, only six months ago. Southeast Memorial operates at about 93 percent occupancy and has an average length of stay of seven days. It has an annual operating budget of $22 million and operates without a deficit. Mr. Smith has three assistants—one in charge of personnel and service departments, one in charge of finance, admitting, and the business office, and the other in charge of the professional departments. Southeast Memorial is a general medical/surgical hospital with departments of obstetrics and psychiatry.

Mr. Smith has a master's degree in business administration and considerable experience in the area of materiel management at the three other hospitals he has administered. However, he finds that Southeast Memorial is very weak in this area. Purchasing presently reports to the Department of Finance. Furthermore, Southeast Memorial is now without a purchasing agent since the former one, Mr. Stormor, left with the former administrator. In the interim, the purchasing is being performed by the comptroller.

Mr. Smith realizes that he has many problems in this area and decides to hire a consultant to perform an analytical study before he delineates and restructures the job description and hires a new purchasing agent. The consultant is to research every aspect of the materiel function and report the findings to Mr. Smith.

The consultant firm sent three representatives into Southeast Memorial with the authority to look over the entire institution. Within 120 days they scheduled a conference with Mr. Smith and presented him with the following findings:

- The purchasing function was extremely decentralized and fragmented, and purchase orders were not uniformly utilized. The purchasing agent mainly purchased for central stores. The chief dietitian purchased all staples, fresh meats, and vegetables without the use of purchase orders. The invoices were received and approved by the dietitian and sent to accounting for payment. All pharmaceuticals, intravenous solutions, and sets were purchased by the chief pharmacist with the aid of her "want book." The chief technologists in both radiology and pathology also performed their own purchasing without purchase orders, received the supplies themselves, approved the invoices, and directed them to Accounting for approval. They took pride in the fact that they did a "super" job in the area of purchasing. The chief of maintenance indicated that one of the most important aspects of his job was purchasing, and he intended to perform this task as long as he was the department director. He did use purchase orders and sent a copy to purchasing for the files. Surgery, emergency room, intensive and coronary care, and central supply, all of which are under the supervision of nursing, interviewed sales representatives and could order emergency supplies directly without the use of a purchase order. All other nursing units had to requisition their supplies from central stores. Any new items for the nursing units were sent to the Standards Committee for approval before they could be purchased. The administrative secretary seemed to order all printed matter and office supplies directly without any documentation. The librarian indicated that only she could or should order books and magazines. All department heads indicated they could order any piece of equipment without prior approval as long as it was approved in their annual budget. All other supplies were ordered through the central purchasing office.
- In reference to inventories, both official and unofficial, the consultants engaged a private firm of inventory specialists to take an accounting. The results were as follows.

Central stores	$ 185,600
Warehouse (bulk stores)	300,000
Surgery	100,500
Central sterile supply	86,300
Dietary stores (including frozen)	50,000
Pharmacy	115,000
Nursing units (10–35 bed units)	100,000
Emergency room	20,000
ICU-CCU	62,300
Radiology	87,000
Laboratory	62,000
Maintenance	87,000
Respiratory therapy	10,000
P.T.—O.T.	26,000
Clinics	16,000
Office areas	51,600
TOTAL	$1,359,300

It was interesting to note that when the department directors were asked by the consultants how much inventory was in their departments, almost all indicated they had no inventory.

- In reference to personnel, the consultants found the following components:

Purchasing administration	6 full-time equivalents (F.T.E.s)
Central stores	15 F.T.E.s
Warehouse	8 F.T.E.s
Central sterile supply	22 F.T.E.s
Pharmacy	25 F.T.E.s

- In reference to space, the consultants found the following allocations:

Central stores	6,000 sq. ft.
Warehouse	15,000 sq. ft.
Central sterile supply	5,000 sq. ft.
Pharmacy	3,000 sq. ft.
Surgery	5,000 sq. ft.
Each nursing unit (approximately)	300 sq. ft.

At the conclusion of the survey, the consultants recommended that they be retained to develop and implement a complete materiel management concept. They indicated that they could do this in approximately six to eight months.

Pertinent Points to Ponder

1. What will be Mr. Smith's decision? Why?
2. If you had this decision to make, what would be yours and why?
3. Is there other information that you need to know in order to make responsible implementation planning?
4. Delineate an organizational chart depicting the authority relationships as you see them in this situation.
5. If you were interviewed and asked to take the job of materiel manager, would you, and under what conditions?
6. Do you feel that the situation portrayed in this case is typical or atypical of the average hospital purchasing and supply functions?
7. Why do you think the department heads indicated that they had no inventory?
8. What are the construction costs of hospitals per square foot in your area?
9. If you were interviewing for the position of materiel manager of this hospital, would you want to know the results of the consultants' report?
10. Would the results of the report make a difference to you either way? Why?
11. Why would Mr. Smith decide to hire the consultant first rather than a materiel manager?
12. How much do you think you could cut expenses in the first year and in what areas would these savings be realized?

Case Report 2

The Total Supply Cart Exchange Program

Fred Smith, materiel manager for Midwest Memorial Hospital, has been in this position for three years. Midwest Hospital is a general medical-surgical hospital consisting of 500 beds. There are 14 nursing units with 32 beds each, a medical intensive care unit of 26 beds and a surgical intensive care unit of 26 beds. The hospital has a very large emergency room which gives care to approximately 50,000 patients per year. The operating suite consists of 16 rooms and does about 45 operations a day in a five and a half day work week.

In reference to supplies, all nursing units, operating suites, and the emergency room have ample storerooms and are on a weekly requisition system of supply procurement. All supplies are requisitioned and received directly from central stores.

Mr. Smith, having come from a hospital with an excellent total supply cart exchange program, has been trying for two years to implement the same kind of program at Midwest Memorial. He was given the necessary administrative approval to begin a pilot cart system on at least two units. He and his central stores personnel conferred at great length on the topic, and after much deliberation decided to implement a cart exchange system for chargeable supplies only in the emergency room and for nonchargeable supplies only in the operating suites.

To date, the pilot study has been disastrous. There seems to be an increase of inventory in both areas where the study is being performed. Charges have not been improved from the emergency room, and they are frequently running out of chargeable items. Supervisors of both the emergency room and the operating room have voiced their dissatisfaction with the pilot program and want it discontinued. Mr. Smith has requested that the pilot program be phased out of the operating and emergency rooms and be tried on other nursing units. However, administration feels that until the cart exchange program has proven beneficial and is working well in the two test areas, there will be no expansion of the project. On the other hand, word is out among all of the other nursing units that the cart exchange program is very problematical, and the nurses are being encouraged by their counterparts in the emergency and operating rooms not to participate in this "fly by night" project.

Mr. Smith and his central stores associates are wondering what happened and where they went wrong.

Pertinent Points to Ponder

1. In your opinion, what did happen?
2. What was Mr. Smith's first mistake?
3. This case study seems like a comedy of errors. How many mistakes can you enumerate?
4. What should be the first step in the successful implementation of a total supply cart exchange program?

5. Who should be involved in this decision?
6. In your opinion, are pilot studies or test cases generally successful?
7. What are the essential components of a total supply cart exchange program?
8. Before the cart system implementation, how can you determine that there are lost charges and how many?
9. How can you test an automated cart distribution system before purchasing it?
10. Delineate a plan to bring order to this chaos so that it will have credibility in the eyes of nursing and administration.
11. Since all supplies were requisitioned from central stores, what would be your estimate of Mr. Smith's total central stores inventory?
12. Can a total supply cart exchange program be effective in departments such as radiology and laboratory?

Case Report 3

A Group Purchasing Dilemma

Jack Moore became the group purchasing coordinator for the Central Counties Shared Services Corporation about two years ago. Previously he had been the purchasing agent for a 400-bed hospital. The board of trustees of the shared services corporation was made up of the chief executive officers of each of the 15 hospitals in a three-county area. His boss was supposed to be the president of the corporation, who was elected from the 15 chief executive officers for a one-year term, but all of the other board members called him almost daily and gave him instructions. His second boss was a shared service committee made up of the materiel managers or directors of purchasing of each of the 15 hospitals. This committee met every two weeks and explored items or services to add to their group purchasing or shared service efforts. The materiel managers and purchasing agents also called Mr. Moore almost daily with their needs and suggestions.

The corporation, in conjunction with the shared services committee, had been fairly successful in negotiating group purchasing programs, even though only eight of the hospitals agreed to participate. Mr. Moore estimates a meager $2,000 savings per month for the entire group.

One of the group purchasing contracts that Mr. Moore is pleased with was just negotiated with a national television manufacturer. The terms are that if the hospitals buy at least 100 televisions during the one-year contract period, the discount will be 50 percent off the retail price of any of the company's catalog items. If the hospitals reach a collective $25,000 purchase volume for the contract period, they will receive another five percent discount. In addition, the hospitals are exempt from a four percent sales tax.

One of the leading products of the company is a television with a large projection screen and a recorder to tape programs for delayed playback. News of this contract travels fast since the holiday season is approaching. Many of the chief executive officers, materiel managers, and purchasing agents have called Mr. Moore and asked him to order several of the televisions and other products for their personal use. One material manager indicated that several of his friends had asked that he also place an order for them. He reasoned that this would help the hospitals reach the volume discount and would greatly reduce the price to him and his friends. He further indicated that the hospital could keep the additional five percent discount and that he and his friends would not have to pay the sales tax.

Mr. Moore was perplexed by this situation and was undecided as to what to do.

Pertinent Points to Ponder

1. Does this constitute a conflict of interest situation?
2. Should Mr. Moore inform his board of trustees and get a board policy decision?
3. If the board approves of this situation, should Mr. Moore contact the company representatives and inform them of this policy decision?
4. If there is approval, who should be able to purchase at this discount price? Only members of the board and shared services committee? Employees of all the hospitals? Relatives of the hospital employees?
5. Should hospital purchase orders be used with an explanation that the goods are being bought for employees of the hospital?
6. If television sets or other products are purchased by employees and others, how is the sales tax handled?
7. How are the service contracts handled in this situation? Are the products brought back to the hospital for service?
8. As the coordinator for group purchasing, would you feel comfortable in this situation?

9. Have any laws been broken?
10. What would prevent one of the purchasing agents from buying in quantities through the hospital contract and reselling at a profit?
11. What should be Mr. Moore's answer to inquiries such as these?
12. Does this situation constitute a breach in purchasing ethics?

Case Report 4

Board of Trustees and Potential Conflict of Interest

Robert Greene has been the materiel manager for Medical Memorial Hospital for the past five years. He is performing his duties admirably and has much respect from administration for his talents and expertise in managing materiel. Medical Memorial Hospital is a 250-bed not-for-profit hospital governed by a 20-member community board of trustees. Medical Memorial is in the midst of a building program which will increase its size to 500 beds. The administrator has asked Mr. Greene to coordinate all of the purchasing and negotiation of contracts for the entire building project. Accordingly, for the last four months Mr. Greene has delegated all of his regular materiel duties to the director of purchasing and has spent all of his time "fast tracking" and coordinating the construction project.

Many of the board members are also in business in the city of 500,000 people. One of the members of the board is a general contractor. Mr. Greene had hoped to get at least three bids on all major contracts, all from union contractors. William Jones, the board member who is president of a local general contractor firm, called Mr. Greene and informed him that he wanted to bid as a general contractor. It is estimated that the general contract will be approximately $8 million. Mr. Greene sends Mr. Jones necessary bid documents and requirements, then immediately informs the administrator of this action. The administrator decides to wait and see what happens.

The day for opening the bids arrives and the president of the board along with members of the medical staff, administration, and various community leaders, announces the entire bid process along with the lowest bidder for each contract. Sure enough, the lowest bidder for the general construction contract by a margin of $150,000 was William Jones, Incorporated.

The next day, Mr. Greene received telephone calls from both of the other general contractors indicating that they were having the bid procedure investigated. They both claimed that they were victims of foul play. The next morning, the newspaper headlines read, "Hospital Construction Contract Goes to Board Member." The president asked the administrator and Mr. Greene to join him and the executive committee in a conference on this matter. As Mr. Greene prepared for the discussion, he wondered if his job was on the line.

Pertinent Points to Ponder

1. Is a hospital board member exempt from contracts involving that hospital?
2. Was Mr. Greene right to notify the administrator?
3. Did the administrator act in a responsible manner?
4. Should the president of the board of trustees and the other members of the board have been informed of Mr. Jones' contract bid?
5. Does this constitute a conflict of interest?
6. Should members of the board of trustees do business with their hospital under any circumstances?
7. If the difference between Mr. Jones' bid and the next lowest bidder was a matter of less than $100, would this fact make any difference in the decision?
8. Can the hospital keep Mr. Jones from submitting a bid? Why or why not?
9. Can the hospital accept the next highest bid instead of Mr. Jones' bid? Would this be prudent?
10. Who was at fault in this situation?
11. Did Mr. Greene prudently carry out his duties as the coordinator of the construction project?
12. What should be the board of trustees decision and why?
13. If the board decided to exclude Mr. Jones' bid and give the contract to the next lowest bidder, would Mr. Jones have reason for legal action against the hospital?
14. Is it possible that Mr. Jones had information that helped him get the bid?

Case Report 5

The Small Hospital Situation

Williams County Hospital is a 65-bed not-for-profit hospital located in the northwest United States. The hospital is located in a town of about 2,500 people, but serves a population of almost 12,000. There are five family practitioners and one general surgeon on the staff of the hospital. The hospital operates at about 95 percent occupancy on an annual basis and manages to break at least even.

Evelyn Hill has been the purchasing agent for six years. Prior to that she was the executive housekeeper. In her position as purchasing agent, she also has the responsibilities for laundry, linen, central supply, and housekeeping. The pharmacy is directed by a part-time pharmacist who owns the only retail drug store in town. In most cases, the drugs are purchased, prepared, and unit-dosed from his store. Mrs. Hill has been told that this practice saves the hospital many thousands of dollars because the hospital does not have to carry a large inventory. Mrs. Hill reports directly to the comptroller.

The hospital has two nursing stations with 32 and 33 beds. Central stores has approximately 10,000 sq. ft. and contains about $125,000 worth of inventory. The reason for the large inventory is that the hospital is located about 150 miles from the major suppliers. The pharmacy inventory is around $25,000 and the dietary stores about $35,000. The nursing units and the departments have ample inventories. Mrs. Hill takes pride in the fact that the hospital hardly ever runs out of items. The central supply room is open 16 hours per day, seven days per week and is staffed by four F.T.E.s (Full-Time-Equivalents).

Mrs. Hill gets to attend one or two educational seminars each year. She hears that a total materiel management program can provide excellent service at a very minimal cost. After discussing these new ideas with her supervisor, she is told that the hospital is too small for the application of the materiel management philosophy. Besides, initiation of the materiel management concept will cost thousands of dollars. Her supervisor indicates that things are just fine the way they are. She leaves his office with mixed emotions. She wonders if there is a size restriction to hospital materiel management.

Pertinent Points to Ponder

1. Could Williams County Hospital benefit from good materiel management?
2. Is there a size below which or above which materiel management principles are not effective?

3. Why do some administrators have the erroneous impression that the development of the materiel management concept will result in a large initial capital outlay?
4. Why do you feel that Mrs. Hill's supervisor indicated that "things are just fine the way they are"?
5. What should be Mrs. Hill's first step to initiate materiel management in Williams County Hospital?
6. What signs are there that the hospital could use principles of materiel management?
7. Would the use of a materiel management consultant be helpful in this case?
8. Do you feel Mrs. Hill will ever get the title of "materiel manager?"
9. Would it help her to have the title of materiel manager?
10. What should be the dollar volume of the official inventories of this hospital per bed?
11. How do per bed inventory figures of small hospitals compare with those of larger hospitals?
12. Did you notice any potential conflicts of interest? If so, what were they?

Case Report 6

The Standardization Committee

Allan Roy, the materiel manager of Community Hospital, has been asked by the administrator to develop a product standardization committee. Community Hospital is a 600-bed not-for-profit hospital serving a population of 350,000. By most standards, it is operated efficiently, always ending the fiscal year with an earned surplus.

Mr. Roy has had some experience with a standardization committee in his last hospital of 250 beds. However, the standardization efforts there had not been too rewarding. On the other hand, Community Hospital has had several unsuccessful attempts at product standardization. In one case, the physicians requested that none of the patient supply items be standardized. They wanted free rein to order and stock any product for their patients. After all, that's what store rooms are for. In another case, the nurses felt that they were the only ones coming under the standardization procedure and asked that they be left out or that every other department be included in the process. Since there was some union activity in the area, administration again abandoned the standardization process.

With all of the current cost containment pressures, the administrator thinks that the timing may now be right. He has delegated the responsibility of standardization to Mr. Roy, who feels he must get more information about how other hospitals are handling this problem. He sends out a questionnaire to 25 hospitals in the surrounding three counties to gather data. The two who answer indicate that product standardization was performed rather haphazardly and no real helpful data were received from the survey.

Mr. Roy decides to begin by appointing a committee. He feels that one reason for the lack of success of most committees is that there are too many members, so he sets up a three-member committee comprised of the director of nursing, the comptroller, and himself. He thinks that with only three members there will not be too much dissension and decisions will be unanimous. Mr. Roy also adds one of the local supply representatives as an ex-officio member. The committee meets on call no more frequently than every two months. There are no minutes of the meetings and the decisions are not published to the various departments and nursing units.

The committee decides to exclude the following items from the agenda: drugs, forms, office supplies, laboratory supplies, radiology supplies, linen, housekeeping items, and capital equipment. Nurses and department heads find it hard to get items on the agenda and feel they get the run around when they want a supply considered as a standard item. The committee tries to keep the meeting agenda limited to six items and the meeting usually lasts only a half an hour. The committee members feel they run a tight ship!

After six months, the administrator asks for a report of the committee's progress. Mr. Roy meets with the other two members and they develop an administrative report. It was short and not so sweet. After six months of operating a tight ship, the committee has managed to increase the hospital's costs for supplies and materiel. The committee members are surprised and undecided as to whether to forward the report to the administrator.

Pertinent Points to Ponder

1. Who should appoint members to the product standardization committee?
2. How many members should be on the committee for it to be most effective?
3. Should sales representatives be allowed to attend standardization committee meetings? Why or why not?
4. How often should the committee meet?

5. What should be the composition of the membership of the committee?
6. Do physicians make effective members of the product standardization committee? Why or why not?
7. How should physicians be appointed to the committee?
8. Should an attending physician ever be appointed as chairman of the committee? Why or why not?
9. Would you consider the product standardization committee to be a cost containment effort? Why or why not?
10. How should product specifications be written?
11. What does "standardization" really mean?
12. How does one measure the effectiveness of a product standardization committee?

Case Report 7

Central Sterile Supply

Doris Summers, director of nursing of Summervale Hospital, a 262-bed not-for-profit institution, has asked the administrator to put the central sterile supply under her supervision. She states in her proposal that central sterile supply is open only 16 hours per day, seven days a week. Often her nursing supervisors have to go to the central supply after regular hours for items that are not on the total supply cart exchange system. She further indicates that staffing is tight in the area and many times the 3 to 11 shift is left uncovered, and as a result, her evening supervisor has to function as the central supply supervisor. In addition, she believes that this area should be staffed around the clock with professional registered nurses, which it is not at present. She further justifies her position by stating that she could always provide backup staffing for the area from her pool of professional nurses.

The administrator is perplexed and concerned with this turn of events and requests a conference with Mr. Adams, the director of pharmacy, who is responsible for the central sterile supply. The administrator makes Mr. Adams fully aware of Mrs. Summers' proposal. He replies that things are not as bad as Mrs. Summers indicates, and states that since materiel management has initiated the total supply cart exchange program, there is little need to staff the central sterile supply more than eight hours per day. He further feels that Mrs. Summers is from the old school and will not be content until central supply is back under her wing. Mr. Adams just levels with the administrator and states that he feels that central sterile supply should not be under nursing or pharmacy, but under materiel management. The administrator indicates he will give this idea some thought.

The administrator schedules a conference with the director of materiel management, Jim Buyers. The administrator relates the entire problem to Mr. Buyers, who states very directly that he wants no part of central sterile supply. He feels that if the professionals cannot manage it, neither can he. He indicates that with the influx of sterile disposable supplies, the central sterile supply eventually will be a thing of the past anyway. It is his contention that there are many problems with quality control in this area and he feels that all sterile products should be purchased from manufacturers, who will assume all of the liability. The administrator, surprised by this reply, asks Mr. Buyers where he feels central sterile supply belongs organizationally. Mr. Buyers states that he feels central sterile supply should be phased out as soon as possible, but should be the responsibility of surgery until that time.

The administrator is now more confused than ever. Should he just ignore the entire situation in hopes that it will go away?

Pertinent Points to Ponder

1. How did central supply areas first get started?
2. Who should be responsible for this area?
3. Are professional nurses required in the central sterile area?
4. What do you think about Mr. Buyers' comment that the central sterile supply should be phased out?
5. In your opinion, what should be the role of a central sterile supply?
6. What do the abbreviations "CSR", "CSS", and "CSD" stand for?
7. Of the three departments discussed–nursing, pharmacy and materiel management–which do you think should manage central sterile supply?
8. What is the basic difference between central supply and central stores?
9. Who dropped the ball in this situation?
10. Who should have submitted the proposal to take over central supply?
11. What should be the qualifications of a central supply supervisor?
12. What should be the staffing pattern for the central supply in a hospital of this size?

Case Report 8

Internal Control

Fred Turner, materiel manager of Wayside Hospital, a 275-bed, not-for-profit hospital, has been in this position for two years. Prior to that, he was the purchasing agent and was in charge of establishing the department. Then with the trend toward materiel management in hospitals, the administrator promoted Fred to his present position, but did not hire another purchasing agent. Fred has been heard to say that there is no difference between a purchasing agent and a materiel manager—just a fancier title. In his present position, he is in charge of all procurement, receiving, and delivery.

At the closing of each fiscal year, Fred spends about 15 minutes with the representatives of the hospital's auditing team. They spot check about 15 items on the physical inventory and ask him a few questions about internal control. Fred is not sure he knows enough about internal control and initiates some independent study on his own to upgrade his knowledge in this area. In summary, he finds that it is bad practice to have the same person buy, receive, and make payment approvals. In fact, it would be prudent practice to have different people in each of the three steps. Presently, he purchases, has ultimate approval of the receipt of the items, and signs his approval on the original invoice that the items indeed were received. He begins to see where his internal control might not be that good. In fact, he sees himself as being in triple jeopardy if there are problems of receiving and payment credibility. He decides to immediately initiate a new procedure of internal control for his peace of mind.

He continues to purchase all supplies and equipment, sending the original purchase order to the vendor. At the same time, the first copy is sent to data processing and then forwarded to accounting. The second copy is sent to receiving to be checked at the time of receipt. All approved vendors are responsible for sending the original payment invoice with the shipment. The receiving clerk matches the receiving copy with the original invoice and indicates by his signature and date that the appropriate supplies have been received. The receiving copy and invoice are sent to accounting. If there are no discrepancies in the three documents, then payment is made. No back orders are permitted. If, for example, one item is to be back ordered from a list of 25 items, a separate purchase order is originated for it. Fred feels that this gives him an orderly and tight control system.

In fact, Fred tests his internal control procedure periodically and documents the findings. For example, he will change the quantity on the first copy of a certain item to see if someone notices the discrepancy and refuses payment. He has checked his internal control procedure 12 times in the last year and has found that in 50 percent of the test cases, payment was made in spite of the discrepancy. In the other 50 percent, payment was held and there was much bragging that the accounting department was saving the hospital from bankruptcy.

One day as Fred is remotely supervising the receiving process, he notices a maneuver that stimulates his further interest. It is early morning and the dietary shipments are being received. He sees that his receiving clerk checks in the hospital dietary supplies from the receiving copy of the invoice, then proceeds to receive ten large-size country hams on a separate invoice and pays the driver in cash. Fred waits until the driver is gone and then questions his clerk about this behavior. The clerk is nervous and immediately states that he is doing nothing wrong.

Fred further investigates the situation and finds that his receiving clerk has a business going on the side. After the hospital sends in a purchase order, the receiving clerk calls and asks the company to add to that order, but add to it on a separate invoice which will be paid in cash. The receiving clerk gets the hospital best quantity prices for all of his items and then sells them to members of administration, department heads, other "special" employees, and friends at a reasonable mark-up. This way, everybody comes out ahead. The receiving clerk admits to doing this with about all of the hospital vendors for all kinds of supplies and equipment. He repeatedly says that he has done no wrong.

Fred immediately suspends the receiving clerk for six days and indicates to him that his job just may be on the line. Fred debates in his mind whether to and how to communicate this "criminal act" to his superiors.

Pertinent Points to Ponder

1. What exactly is internal control?
2. Why is it important?
3. Outline an organizational process for good internal control.
4. Did Fred have a good system for internal control?
5. Do you feel that Fred was right in creating problematical situations to test his control measures?
6. In the 50 percent of the test cases that went without being observed, who was at fault in not recognizing the discrepancies?
7. Why do you think the auditors were interested in internal control procedures?
8. How do you think they test for internal control?
9. Was the receiving clerk's actions a flagrant act of fraud and cover-up?

10. Do you feel the vendors knew of the clerk's side business? Why didn't they notify the hospital materiel manager?
11. Are the vendors partly to blame in this case? If so, what should be done to them?
12. Were Fred's actions toward the receiving clerk justified? Will he tell his superiors? Do you think the clerk will be fired? Why or why not?

Case Report 9

Selecting The Materiel Manager

Hamilton Community Hospital is a 487-bed not-for-profit institution located in a mid-Atlantic state. John Stephens, the chief executive officer, has been with the hospital for the past five years. The hospital has not gone the so called "materiel management route." However, Mr. Stephens is very interested in the concept of total materiel management and will give it his support. He has gone to a few conferences dealing with the subject, one of which was sponsored by the American College of Hospital Administrators. He is impressed with the idea and puts together an organizational profile for the function which he submits to his board of trustees for their recommendations and approval.

The board, never having heard of the concept, asked for full explanation. He fully informed them of the new department's function, authority, and responsibilities, comparing the idea with the industrial materiel concepts. The board accepted the idea enthusiastically, asked the administrator to initiate the program with their blessings, and approved a new position budget salary range of $30,000 to $37,000. They also asked for periodic progress reports as to the effects the new department was having on hospital revenues, cost containment, and overall costs. Mr. Stephens immediately meets with his administrative staff consisting of the vice president of patient care services, the vice president of personnel, and the vice president of financial operations. Their basic consideration is the selection of the materiel manager. They begin the review of potential candidates for the position. One of the first persons to be considered is the present purchasing agent. He has been in this position for the past 14 years and is an easy-going person who tries to stay out of the political mainstream. He has not been enthusiastic about centralized purchasing and some of the other concepts of materiel planning, but on the other hand, no one has encouraged him either. The purchasing agent is presently making use of the hospital's education tuition reimbursement program by attending a local university to work on his bachelor's degree in business administration.

The vice president of patient care services suggests the director of pharmacy as a good strong candidate. The director is a woman who has been with the hospital for approximately five years. Under her direction, many aggressive, innovative programs have been initiated, such as total unit-dose systems, I.V. admixture programs, and clinical pharmacy projects. She has a bachelor's degree in pharmacy and is currently preparing for her master's degree in hospital pharmacy. It is pointed out that the pharmacist already has a professional status by training and would be technically acceptable to all departments. The director of pharmacy presently reports to the vice president of patient services.

The vice president of personnel reminds the group that the director of the central supply department is highly qualified. He has a B.S.N. and has been with the hospital for three years. He is very knowledgeable of the supply, process, and distribution functions. Product sterility and quality control are his specialties. He has an excellent track record in reference to supervision and "people" development.

The vice president of financial operations states that she would like to see someone in this position with a good financial background since this area is becoming highly involved with the revenue and cost pictures. She suggests the comptroller and the business manager as possible candidates. The comptroller is a C.P.A. who has been with the hospital seven years. The business manager is working on his degree in marketing and has been with the hospital approximately two years. Other suggestions for candidates are the industrial engineer, the dietary manager and the executive housekeeper.

The chief executive officer states that perhaps the search should be expanded to industry. He suggests that an industrial purchasing agent or an experienced materiel manager from another hospital should be given serious consideration. After all, they have the experience and will fit into the position with very little training or orientation. He stresses the fact that the candidate must demonstrate that he or she has been able to obtain desirable results in his or her last position. He further indicates that some of the recent graduates from the programs in hospital and health care administration might be excellent candidates.

After a few hours of deliberation, the group exhausts their potential candidate lists. Someone asks, "What's the next move?"

Pertinent Points to Ponder

1. Do you feel that the chief executive officer is going about the selection process in the right way? Why or why not?

2. If you were ranking the candidates mentioned for the position from most to least acceptable, what would be your preference listing? Why?
3. What do you consider their next step?
4. Should this position be advertised on the local and national levels? Why?
5. Do you think the salary range is appropriate for the position in an institution of this size?
6. The chief executive officer could save much time, effort, disgruntlement, and money by promoting the purchasing agent to this position. What would be the pros and cons of this move?
7. Should potential candidates from within the hospital have preference over outside candidates? Why or why not?
8. Can you think of other potential candidates that were not mentioned?
9. Who should structure the final job description for this position?
10. In your opinion, what should be the title for the position? Why?
11. Do you think the materiel manager should be specialty or generally qualified?
12. Who do you think will get the position and why?

Case Report 10

Product and Equipment Specifications

Mountain Medical Center is a 400-bed not-for-profit hospital located in a city of just over a million population. There are nine other hospitals which serve the city and surrounding communities.

Charles Doyle has been the materiel manager of Mountain Medical Center for only ten months. He was selected for the position primarily to develop the total materiel management concept. Previously, he was the assistant administrator for materiel management at a 250-bed institution where he was quite successful in developing the concept. Mr. Doyle has approximately six years experience in materiel management and holds a degree in industrial engineering.

So far in his tenure at Mountain Medical Center, he has been very successful in the implementation of the first two projects. A total supply cart exchange program has been operational for at least three months and is receiving praise from nursing service. Also, the purchasing function is now completely centralized. When he arrived, pharmacy, dietary, laboratory, and maintenance were involved in the purchasing function. However, after five months under centralized purchasing, those departments have found that the procurement is being performed better and at lower costs.

He has defined his next objective as the development of product and equipment specifications so that the ordering process can be more precise. Being an industrial engineer by trade, he has always been exposed to definite product specifications. The first step of this project was to ask the purchasing director for a list of all approved products and their specifications. The purchasing director delivered to him a storeroom catalog that had been published two years ago and not updated since. Mr. Doyle explained that he wanted a detailed description of each product and piece of equipment ordered by the hospital. The purchasing director stated that no such list existed. "How do you order for this hospital?" quipped Mr. Doyle. The reply was short but sad. "By trade names only," replied the director of purchasing. From his further questioning, Mr. Doyle found that substitutions were not made except in acts of God or dire emergencies. Most of the staff physicians had been trained in the university located in the city and were accustomed to ordering specifically by the trade names of the products that were used there. They did not use the generic names at all. It was rumored that many companies would almost give their products away to the university hospital so that they would be assured of getting all of the business from the other hospitals in town. Also, Mountain Medical Center is a big teaching hospital affiliated with the university and tne residents pose a big problem by insisting on the same products and equipment as are used at the university. Furthermore, all of the department heads are accustomed to specifying brand names and numbers on all their supply requisitions. In other words, they have usually met with all of the manufacturers or suppliers and have selected, objectively or subjectively, the product they wanted. For example, if a paper copier is needed, the brand name, product number, and usually price are specified on the requisition with a byline which states, "No substitutions will be accepted." Therefore, the art of negotiation has been taken from the purchasing process and it is a mere rubber stamp function.

In his discussions with the chief pharmacist, Mr. Doyle finds that here again the physicians will not accept other than brand names. The pharmacy formulary committee should be entitled the "brand name" committee. If the pharmacist does not have the specific drug that was ordered but does have a generic equivalent, he is instructed not to call the physician to ask to substitute, but get the item ordered at all costs. In conversations with the chief radiology technologist, the technologist relates the same kind of story. Requisitions are sent to purchasing with brand names and manufacturer's numbers for film and chemicals. No substitutes are allowed. Mr. Doyle even sees this phenomenon present in the meager group purchasing efforts of the shared services committee. No specifications are written, but brand names are stated.

From his conference with the director of plant and maintenance, he gets a different insight into the problem. The director reviews and approves all requisitions for equipment. He states that equipment specifications are very difficult to write, and in many cases, would require consultation with an electrical or mechanical engineer. Therefore, equipment specifications are expensive. Also, in addition, any piece of equipment completely specified by the hospital usually is a new piece of equipment that is not manufactured. In most cases, the companies who will bid on such a piece of equipment pass all of the charges on to the hospital. The director of maintenance relates that in many cases his ideas for equipment were much more practical for hospital use, but since they were termed "experimental," all costs and liability connected with use were passed on to the hospital. He states he quit fighting the battle and gave up on pertinent equipment specifications long ago. Manufacturers build what they want to regardless of what the hospital needs.

Mr. Doyle sees that he is definitely going to have difficulty with meeting his objective in reference to product and equipment specifications. After much deliberation, he decides to present this subject to the product standardization committee for their review and assistance. After all, isn't this what the standards committee is supposed to be doing?

Pertinent Points to Ponder

1. Why are product and equipment specifications important to the hospital?
2. In reference to product specifications, is there a difference between hospitals and industry?
3. Why are hospitals hesitant to write product and equipment specifications?
4. Whose task is this?
5. What factors should be considered in the writing of such specifications?
6. How do the manufacturers of hospital products and equipment arrive at their specifications?

7. Should all products and equipment used by hospitals have complete specifications? Why or why not?
8. How will hospital specifications differ from manufacturer specifications for the same item?
9. If a hospital does not have product specifications, how is the competitive bid procedure handled?
10. How are product or equipment equivalencies handled in the bid procedure?
11. In what ways do product equivalencies differ from product substitutions?
12. Should the medical staff be involved in the development of product specifications? If so, in what ways?

Case Report 11

Problems with Group Purchasing

Joe West is the materiel manager for Park Mountain Memorial Hospital, a 950-bed not-for-profit institution. He has been in this position for the past five years and takes pride in his cost reduction efforts. One of the first things he did after coming to the hospital was to take a total physical inventory of all official and unofficial supplies. He and his staff took the official inventories in central stores, central supply, pharmacy, and dietary. However, the hospital acquired the services of a company whose primary business was taking inventories to count all unofficial inventories. The official inventory was $1 million; the unofficial inventory $2.5 million. He has since been able to reduce the official inventory to $500,000 and the unofficial inventory to $1 million. The administration is very pleased with this progress and Mr. West feels that he can reduce the official inventory to about $300,000 and the unofficial inventory to about $500,000.

Mr. West uses stockless purchasing and the prime supplier concept to assist in keeping the physical inventories at manageable levels. Furthermore, physical inventories are taken quarterly and each department gets an itemized listing of all supplies with a dollar range as to what the inventory should be. Therefore, the department head can help the materiel manager in the reduction of inventory. Since the department heads know that administration, which gets a quarterly report, supports low supply inventories, all of them enthusiastically try to make each physical count a new all-time low.

Mr. West has two purchasing agents who do all of the buying. He feels that since the hospital has the supply volume of a 950-bed institution, they can always negotiate excellent prices. In fact, he feels that at this size, the hospital should be able to get prices that equal or better bid prices. In comparing prices with the university hospital which must bid almost all large volume items, he finds that his hospital's prices are much better.

Recently, however, he has received much pressure from his administrator and the materiel managers of the other 15 hospitals in the city to participate in group purchasing efforts. It seems that the state director of insurance is forcing the insurance companies to insist that the hospitals participate in group purchasing endeavors. Of the sixteen hospitals in the area, six are under 250 beds, seven are between 300 and 450 beds, one is 750 beds, one is 950 beds, and the university hospital is around 1,200 beds. The group has received several single-category supply quotations, such as on sutures, underpads, paper goods, etc. In each case, the prices are higher than what Park Mountain Memorial Hospital is presently paying for the same items. In each case, the suppliers insist on an all-or-nothing contract. In these group purchasing efforts, the smaller hospitals receive better prices than before, the average size hospitals pay about the same, and the larger hospitals pay higher prices. The group purchasing committee feels that all of the hospitals should participate for the sake of the group and to fulfill the state's requirements.

Mr. West feels that this kind of thinking is nonsense and refuses to participate in the group efforts unless his hospital pays less or the same as before. He and his staff have extrapolated the volumes and savings or losses in each of the 16 hospitals and have concluded that the suppliers, not the hospitals, are coming out ahead. In many cases, the suppliers under these agreements ask the hospitals to order in larger quantities than they normally would. In fact, the supplies are often drop-shipped from the manufacturer instead of being kept in the local warehouses. Mr. West pointed out to his colleagues that it looks as though the suppliers are benefiting more than the hospitals from group purchasing.

He encouraged the group purchasing committee to get tougher and negotiate better prices or his hospital would not participate in the group contracts. He even jokingly remarked that he would be glad to order for all of the other hospitals.

Mr. West met with his administrator and explained the situation. The administrator supported Mr. West's position and immediately issued a hospital policy statement on the subject of group purchasing to all concerned.

Pertinent Points to Ponder

1. What do you feel was the substance of the hospital's policy statement?

2. Do you think it was wise to issue such a statement at this time?
3. To whom do you think the policy statement was distributed?
4. Are there advantages to group purchasing other than price?
5. Even with the advantage of better prices, are there disadvantages which legitimately would keep a hospital from participating in group purchasing?
6. In your opinion, why hasn't group purchasing caught on with the majority of hospitals.
7. If a supplier is getting a large percentage of the hospital's business already, why would the supplier give a better price because of the group participation?
8. Is it possible to increase supply costs through group purchasing?
9. Are there higher administrative costs associated with group purchasing efforts?
10. Can hospitals that are located 200 or 300 miles apart really benefit from group purchasing?
11. What are the differences between group purchasing and the prime supplier approach?
12. Why are hospital purchasing agents usually turned off by organized group purchasing efforts?

Case Report 12

The Perpetual Inventory

John Marshall is the materiel manager of River City Hospital, a 375-bed not-for-profit hospital. He has been in this position for two years and is doing a good job of developing the materiel management concept. He has the total support of the administration in his efforts and tries to document his successes to measure the progress made from year to year. When he came to River City Hospital, there was a $325,000 inventory in central stores. This included medical-surgical supplies, intravenous solutions and sets, linens, sterile supplies, forms, dressings, and office supplies. The inventory has remained about the same because he has been putting emphasis on other phases of materiel management and did not want to rock the boat in too many places at the same time.

Ruth Wilson is the central stores manager and reports directly to Mr. Marshall. She has been with the hospital for five years and has developed a perpetual inventory that is her pride and joy. There are 3,000 different supplies on the system and she cannot wait until central stores merges with central supply so she can add another 500 items. Miss Wilson's perpetual system consists of two cards per item. One card names the item, its description, price, vendors, maximums, and minimums; the second gives the issues, receipts, balance on hand, unit cost, total cost, and a history of usage by date. The equivalent work of one and two-fifths clerk typists is required to keep it current. Whenever an item reaches the minimum, the clerk places a red tag on the card where it can be readily seen. Once a day, the clerk wheels the card file up to the purchasing director's office. When the purchasing director orders the item, he records on the proper card the date and amount and replaces the red tag with a green one. At the end of the day, the entire file is again wheeled down to central stores, where issues and receipts are continuously recorded. Whenever the supplies that were ordered are received, the green tags are removed to indicate that the item has been returned to an acceptable level.

Miss Wilson feels that she has ultimate control over the entire central stores domain through her perpetual inventory system. The hospital has computer capabilities, but the inventory system is not on the computer system. Miss Wilson has indicated that the computerized inventory system is not as fast as her perpetual system and certainly not as accessible. She claims she cannot justify the expense of computerized inventories and that the performance does not measure up to her manual system.

Mr. Marshall, on the other hand, does not believe that either system is justified in terms of time or costs. He and Miss Wilson have had a disagreement as to the effectiveness of her manual system. He claims that the only predictable characteristic of the perpetual inventory system is that it is perpetually incorrect. She sets out to prove that her system is effective. They go into the central stores area and spot check the shelf counts with the perpetual balance for 25 items, and in 15 cases the two figures do not correspond. In addition, he finds a balance of minus five for one item. The clerk who keeps the system states that this balance represents a case in which they distributed 15 items of an article of which only ten were indicated on the cards. Mr. Marshall then asked the clerk what would happen when fifteen more are received, and Miss Wilson replied that the hospital will then again have ten. Miss Wilson, embarrassed by this series of events, concedes that the system is not as reliable as she had once believed it to be.

Mr. Marshall knows how bad Miss Wilson feels and he does not dwell on the subject. He gently points out that if the perpetual inventory system was so great, the auditors would accept it instead of asking for a physical count annually. He explains to her that the main problem does not lie in the perpetual system, but in the fact that there are too many items in stock. He suggests that an inventory reduction program be started that would eliminate all inventory items except the 450 or so needed on a daily basis by the nursing units. He tells her of the new "eyeball" method of inventory keeping that he recently heard about in a materiel management seminar. Since there would be only a few items in stock, the purchasing director could review the minimums and maximums (printed right on the shelf) and could make out the order documents in one step in less than an hour per day. Miss Wilson was intrigued by the possibility of the new system and indicated that she could reduce her staff by at least two full-time equivalents. She was happy that there would be no more typing of the perpetual inventory cards.

The next day, Miss Wilson is attending a materiel and financial seminar and the speaker mentions the fact that the auditors require that a perpetual inventory system be operational in each hospital. She cannot wait to relay this important information to her boss.

Pertinent Points to Ponder

1. What exactly is a perpetual inventory system?
2. In your opinion, why did the perpetual inventory concept get started?
3. Have you ever heard of a perpetual system for the pharmacy?
4. Why do you feel Miss Wilson was pleased with her perpetual inventory system?
5. What makes it virtually impossible for a perpetual system to be correct most of the time?
6. Do you really think that Miss Wilson wanted to do away with her perpetual system? Why or why not?
7. Explain how the eyeball method works in actual practice.
8. Do you think it could work for you? Why or why not?
9. Why do you feel Miss Wilson could not wait to inform Mr. Marshall of her discovery?
10. Was the news correct?
11. If your auditors made such a demand at your hospital would you have to do it?
12. What is the purpose of the annual audit and how does it apply to materiel management?

Case Report 13

Organizational Structure

While being interviewed for the new position of director of materiel management at Highland Hospital, a 390-bed institution, Alex Brown made it clear to the administrator that one of the prerequisites for his taking the position was his approval of the organizational structure of the new department. He was especially interested in the reporting and supervisory structure of the materiel manager. The administrator assured Mr. Brown that if he was selected for the position, he could have this privilege.

After a month the administrator calls and informs Mr. Brown that he has been selected for the position. The administrator and Mr. Brown arrange a mutually acceptable date for their initial orientation conference. The administrator states that he is happy to have Mr. Brown join the staff and pledges his support for the development of the total materiel management concept. Before Mr. Brown can ask, the administrator says that he has given much thought to the structuring of the new department within the organization. He further states that there seems to be some flexibility in the selection of organizational roles and he presents Alex with the following organizational models from which to choose.

Model A

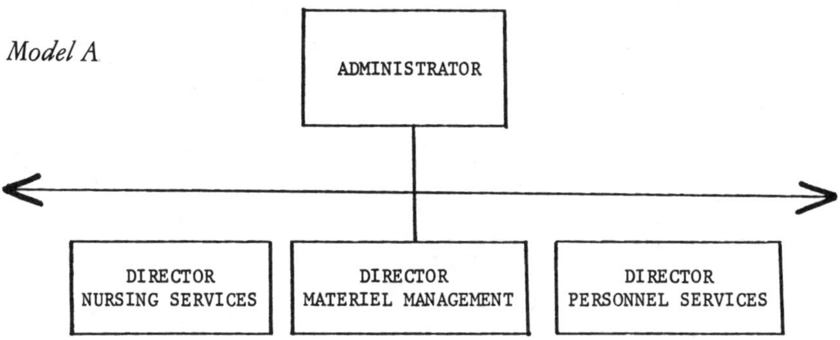

Model B

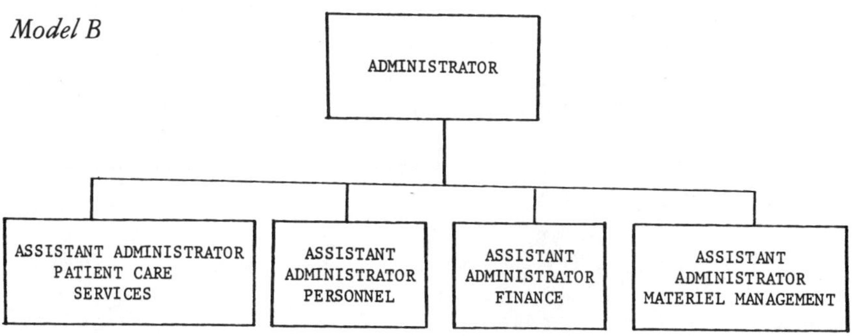

Model C

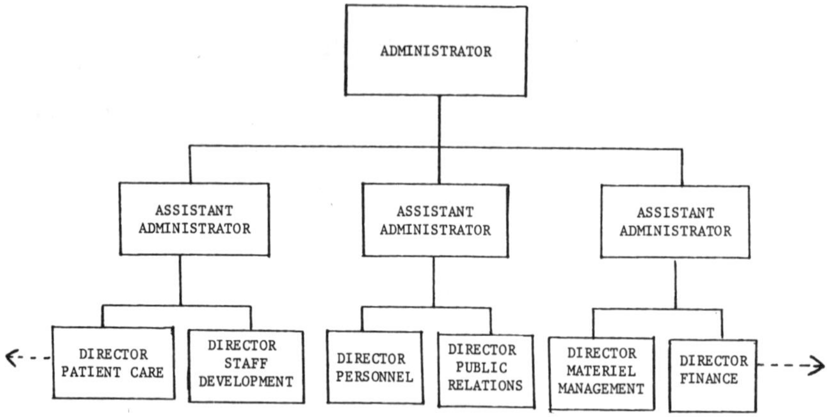

Model D

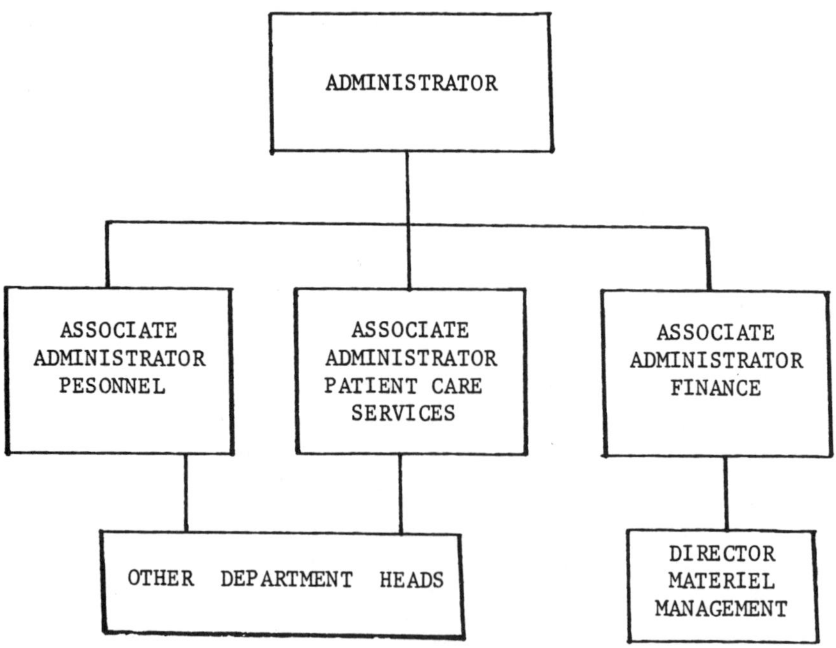

Model E

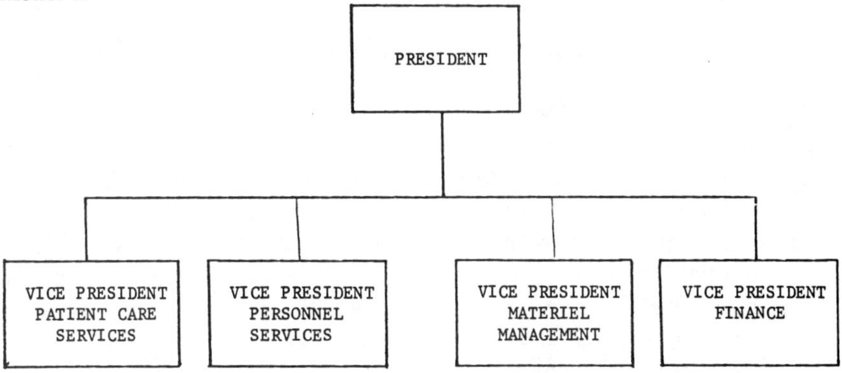

After careful consideration of each of the organizational models, Mr. Brown makes his selection.

Pertinent Points to Ponder

1. In most cases, can the materiel manager select his organizational role? Why or why not?
2. What are the advantages and disadvantages of being able to choose your reporting position within the organization.
3. Upon what one criterion do you feel Mr. Brown made his decision?
4. If you are looking for a certain reporting role, when is the proper time to make this fact known?
5. Are there certain risks in being bold about how you want to report? Why?
6. Mr. Brown did not request that certain areas report to him. Why not?
7. Do you feel he would have been in a good position to delineate what departments or areas report to him?
8. Which model do you feel Mr. Brown selected and why?
9. Which model do you think the administrator preferred and why?
10. What are the differences between models B and E?
11. Do you think that there is a salary difference between the models and why?
12. Which model was the least acceptable to Mr. Brown and why?

Case Report 14

Centralization of Purchasing

Campbell Memorial Hospital is a 450-bed municipal hospital located in a southeastern city of 200,000 people. There are three other hospitals serving the area. Joe Williams was hired by the hospital about two and a half years ago as the director of purchasing. However, a year ago he was given the title of materiel manager. At the time, the administrator, who has been with the institution for 20 years, spent almost a half day orienting Joe to his new duties and objectives as the materiel manager. He indicates to Mr. Williams that the government and third party payers are becoming more involved and interested in the purchasing function, mentions the concept of prudent purchasing, and asks Mr. Williams to see that the hospital complies with the principle in every respect. He states that the hospital must tighten up on its purchasing practices and he sees no alternative to centralizing the purchasing function into the materiel management department. The administrator then inquires how far the hospital has advanced toward purchasing centralization.

Mr. Williams informs him that the purchasing function is badly fragmented. The radiologist and pathologist insist on seeing sales representatives and placing orders with them. He has tried to work with the chief dietitian but she tells him that only a qualified dietitian can purchase for her department. She indicates that quality and portion control are very important to her menu planning, and she does not see the purchasing of dietary products ever being performed by anyone else. The pharmacist states that it is a state law that he must order and receive all drugs, so purchasing can never legally be involved in the procurement of pharmaceuticals. The director of maintenance is very aggressive about his purchasing responsibilities, and informs Mr. Williams that no one but an engineer can specify and purchase complex machine parts and highly technical items. In addition, other departments and attending physicians order supplies and equipment from time to time, and the purchasing department must track down who ordered them when they are received.

The administrator is appalled by this news and pledges his support to Mr. Williams in developing centralized purchasing. Mr. Williams asks the administrator to put his support in the form of a memorandum to all department heads and members of the medical staff. The administrator indicates that this would not be a good move politically, but agrees to meet with the department heads and convey this understanding. At the very next department head meeting, the administrator announces that Mr. Williams will become the director of materiel management and that one of his primary objectives will be to centralize the entire purchasing process. The department heads are perplexed by this announcement and there is much discussion on why centralized purchasing should be implemented. The administrator and Mr. Williams each give several reasons, among which is the prudent buyer principle. The department heads, minus the radiologist and pathologist who are not present, indicate their concern and disagreement with this edict.

Mr. Williams spends the next few days wondering how to approach the problem. He is approached first by the chief pharmacist who indicates that there are ways to get around the legal ramifications of drug purchasing and states that he would like to give centralized purchasing a try. Presently, Mr. Williams is purchasing all intravenous solutions and sets. Over the next few weeks, he and the pharmacist work out a very effective system of ordering and the pharmacist is relieved to have this responsibility off his shoulders. The dietitian resigns, and the hospital hires a dietary manager who wants nothing to do with purchasing. The director of maintenance asks to be excepted from the procedure for a six-month period because of pressing personnel problems in his department. Mr. Williams agrees to this, but schedules an appointment for six months hence. The heads of the departments of radiology and pathology are still performing their own purchasing. Mr. Williams schedules a meeting with both physicians. They indicate to him that their products are of a very technical nature and only a physician specialist can order their supplies and equipment. Furthermore, they indicate that their hospital contracts indicate they can specify and purchase their supplies and equipment and state that they intend to abide by the letter of the contract. Mr. Williams explains to them that the prudent buyer principle is being used to review the hospital's purchasing practices and that the auditors will find their purchasing practice to be a flagrant violation of this principle. Both physicians pass this off by saying that physicians are exempt from the prudent buyer principle, and that they are getting good deals for the hospital.

After almost a year of bickering and negotiating with the various departments, the only exceptions to the centralized purchasing policy are radiology, pathology, and maintenance. No one has been around to apply the prudent buyer principle, and the department heads who have complied state that the centralized purchasing policy should be applied uniformly or not at all. Mr. Williams is preparing for his annual evaluation with the administrator. He has several recommendations in reference to centralized purchasing, among which is a materiel management policy that no supplies or equipment will be received unless there is a purchase order number. He plans to enforce centralized purchasing by putting the onus on the suppliers to see that all orders are processed through materiel management. Mr. Williams thinks he now has the solution to his problem.

Pertinent Points to Ponder

1. What are the apparent advantages of centralized purchasing for the hospital? The departments? The materiel management department?
2. Why wouldn't a department head support centralized purchasing?
3. Why would a department want to be involved in the actual purchasing process?
4. In your opinion, why didn't the administrator put this policy in writing?
5. What did the administrator have in mind when he spoke of purchasing?
6. Do you feel that the administrator is really behind centralized purchasing?
7. Could Mr. Williams be more aggressive in carrying out his objective of complete centralized purchasing? In what ways?
8. Why do you suppose the pharmacist was the first to begin the policy implementation?
9. Do you think the chief dietitian quit because of this policy? If she did, do you think it was in the best interest of the hospital?
10. Was it a mistake on the part of Mr. Williams to confer with the pathologist and radiologist at the same time? Why or why not?
11. Do you think the pathologist and radiologist were right when they said that their contracts with the hospital gave them the authority to purchase? Why would such a clause be written into a hospital specialist contract?
12. What is your opinion of putting pressure on the suppliers to get control of the departments which are exceptions to centralized purchasing? Do you think it will be successful? What will the administrator think of this departmental policy? Does he have to approve it?

Case Report 15

Decentralized Materiel Management

Western Memorial Medical Center is a 500-bed not-for-profit institution located in a large metropolis. The Medical Center has all of the medical and subspecialty services and is considered a major teaching and research institution. The operating budget for the current fiscal year is $55 million. In the most recently completed fiscal year, the Medical Center delivered 155,000 inpatient days and 300,000 outpatient visits, and the emergency room treated over 125,000 patients. It spent approximately $1.5 million for pharmaceuticals, $1.75 million for medical-surgical items, and $500,000 for food items. The Medical Center is presently in the middle of a 250-bed approved expansion program which will be completed in 18 months.

Gordon Turner, the materiel manager for the Medical Center for the past six years, has just resigned to become the assistant administrator for materiel management in a hospital in another state. The chief executive officer of the Medical Center appoints the purchasing agent as the acting head of materiel management until a suitable replacement can be found. The department heads have always wanted to get into purchasing and materiel management, so they request that they be granted permission to try decentralized materiel management for a period of one year before a materiel manager is hired. Under the plan, all department heads would be given authority to purchase and control the supplies and equipment under their own budgetary guidelines. The director of central supply would purchase all medical-surgical supplies, the pharmacist all pharmaceuticals, and the dietary manager all related items. The present purchasing agent and his staff would purchase miscellaneous items and process all receipts of supplies and equipment. The administrator was intrigued by the experiment and agreed to a 12-month evaluation period, after which he would make the decision as to whether to continue the program.

The experiment begins. The purchasing agent who was appointed acting head of materiel management quits in disgust, and the central stores manager becomes the new purchasing agent. Supplies are expensed to the applicable departments as soon as they are received. Many of the department heads find that they do not have enough space for storage, and they begin putting their supplies in sequestered areas of the central stores. Therefore, the central stores becomes an area of both official and unofficial inventory. Every nook and cranny of the hospital has been taken over by some department head for storage space. Many of the departments request and receive added personnel to take over their materiel functions. Sales representatives have a field day visiting and selling to all of the various department heads. Many departments buy in quantity lots to receive the best quantity price. Shipments come in at all times since there is no scheduling with the purchasing department. Some departments use purchase orders and some do not. There are frequent stockouts, and since the department heads do not know what items are commonly used by the other departments, there is no attempt to use their inventory during a shortage. Every department becomes a total supply island! The evaluation period ends with a request from the department heads that the hospital purchase or rent warehouse space.

At the end of the trial period the administrator schedules a critique of the study with all department directors present. He asks each of them what has been his or her experience with the decentralized program. Almost all of the department heads indicate that they have learned more about supply management and feel they have control over their total departments,including personnel, supplies, and equipment. For the most part, they are pleased with the program and want it continued. They even hint that they want to take on the personnel and financial administrations of their departments! However, 2 of the 27 department heads express their disgust and unhappiness with the program and want no more to do with it. They state that if they wanted to be materiel managers they would have prepared for supply procurement in college rather than their chosen fields of endeavor. They indicate that their resignations will be forthcoming if the program is not discontinued immediately. The administrator thanks the group for their participation and input into the program and states that he has obtained the services of the hospital's auditing firm to evaluate the program from an objective viewpoint.

The auditing firm conducts the survey and compares it with their past baseline data. The results are very revealing. During the experiment, hospital inventories have more then tripled. There have been 15 extra personnel hired because of the program, and the central stores inventory is off by a plus $350,000. There is virtually no internal control maintained, and invoices are sometimes paid twice. Prices for the same items purchased by different departments vary as much as 50 percent. There are no policies and procedures for purchasing by the individual departments since some 75 people are purchasing supplies and equipment without regard for a uniform purchase order system. The product standardization committee has become defunct. The auditing firm issues a special confidential report of its findings directly to the administrator, who immediately meets with the department heads and delineates a plan of action to be completed in exactly 90 days. The department heads listen intently as if their jobs depend on it.

Pertinent Points to Ponder

1. Why do you think the administrator agreed to the evaluation of a decentralized materiel program?

2. In your opinion, why did the purchasing agent quit?
3. What conditions prompted the department heads' request for central warehousing?
4. If you could interview the sales representatives servicing this hospital, what do you think would be their opinion of the evaluation?
5. From your experience, who do you think were the two objecting department heads? Why them?
6. What two department heads led the crusade to keep the program and why?
7. Why did the department heads' evaluation and the auditing firm's survey vary so greatly?
8. Why do you think the inventory more than tripled?
9. Do you feel that any of the departments actually operated more effectively under decentralized materiel management? If so, which ones and why?
10. Do you think that the auditing firm's report will get to the board of trustees? Why or why not?
11. Did the administrator actually solve some problems by permitting the experiment? Why?
12. The administrator immediately met with the department heads and delineated a plan of action to be completed in exactly 90 days. Provide this plan of action with the necessary details.

Case Report 16

Stockless Purchasing

The Tri-County Hospital is a 300-bed N.P.A. institution located in a southeastern state. The hospital has 150 physicians on staff and operates at about 85 percent occupancy. The administrator boasts of the fact that the hospital has an operating surplus each year.

Bob Allen has been the director of materiel management for three years. He has an excellent record of cost containment in the area of materiel management, and is supported in his efforts by the hospital administration. The hospital presently has about $350,000 inventory between central stores and central supply. There are approximately 3,000 different items in stock, excluding pharmacy and dietary stores. Mr. Allen has maintained a watchful eye on the inventory level over the past three years and given much thought to inventory reduction programs. Last year, he implemented a total supply cart exchange program for all of the nursing units including the emergency room. The ten-room operating suite is also on a case cart program. The cart program has been operating surprisingly well for the past eight months after its total implementation. Mr. Allen sees this program primarily as a forecasting system since he will know if there is a shortage of an item for the units at least 24 hours in advance. This will give him plenty of time to correct any stockouts or get acceptable substitute items.

In conjunction with the cart exchange program for the units, he develops a program he refers to as ''stockless purchasing'' in order to reduce inventory in the departments and the central stores. From his semiannual surveys of the unofficial inventory in the various departments, he approximates that each department has a two-month supply. He hopes to accomplish at least three objectives from his stockless purchasing project. First, he wants to reduce the number of items in the central stores to around 500. The remaining 500 items would be the supplies which are kept on the exchange carts. He intends to reduce the inventory to about $50,000 and turn it over at least 24 times per year. Second, he would like to reduce the inventory in each department to a one-month supply. Third, Mr. Allen hopes to put the central supply operation in the space freed-up in central stores by the inventory reduction. The central supply is presently in prime space on the third floor of the hospital. The hospital then proposes to develop an occupational therapy department, a revenue producing area, in that space. Mr. Allen reduces the three objectives into a written proposal for administrative approval, in which he states his feeling that the total project will net the hospital at least $1 million the first year.

Administration discusses this proposal with all of the department heads and decides to approve the project without exceptions. Mr. Allen begins to work with the radiology department first. He and his staff prepare a departmental purchase order-requisition form based on preprinted quotas of each item for a 30 day period. The plan is to receive the goods on the first day of each month and reorder on the last, taking into consideration the appropriate lead times. In this manner, the expense, cost, and revenue of each item will be accounted for in the same period. It was found that for the department of radiology, all items could be ordered from one prime vendor and one secondary vendor, as opposed to the eight suppliers previously used. By giving the entire order to two vendors, a 10 percent overall discount was realized, and paperwork, purchase orders, and checks were reduced to an absolute minimum. After a successful two-month pilot project of stockless purchasing in radiology, all radiology supplies (worth about $52,000) were phased out of central stores. The chief technologist in radiology was so pleased by his entire inventory management being taken over by materiel management that he wrote a memo to all other department heads praising the system. This same procedure was used in all departments, including laboratory, physical medical, respiratory therapy, administration, and surgery. The last department to be included was the laboratory.

After nine months, Mr. Allen and his staff had successfully implemented stockless purchasing in all of the departments. He figured the inventory reduction to be $650,000 from the departments alone. Surgery, being the highest inventory accumulation area, had almost $300,000 of inventory, which was reduced to a very workable $60,000. Central stores inventory went from $350,000 to $45,000.

Then the necessary renovations were made in the central stores, and the central sterile supply was moved into that area. By this move the staff was reduced from nineteen employees to five and all supply functions were available around the clock. Nursing was so pleased with this change that they sent a memo to administration expressing their appreciation that another department also was going to be giving full service.

Mr. Allen then gives the director of physical medicine the approval to start developing a renovation program for the area vacated by central supply. Naturally, he is pleased with how much progress can be made simply by knowing what to do, when to do it, and through what channels to proceed. He now starts to take the wraps off of another proposed project.

Pertinent Points to Ponder

1. By definition, what is stockless purchasing?
2. Why do you suppose it has not been implemented by more hospitals?
3. What are the advantages, as you see them, of stockless purchasing?
4. Should you get administrative approval before implementing stockless purchasing? Why or why not?
5. What conditions must be present for its implementation?
6. What disadvantages, if any, do you see to its implementation?
7. What was the main reason for Mr. Allen's success?
8. Why did he begin with radiology?
9. Why did he indicate that the laboratory was the last department to start the program?
10. Do you think that the inventory figures quoted for surgery are realistic? Why or why not?

11. What advantages can you delineate for combining central stores with central supply?
12. What do you think Mr. Allen's next project is and why?

Case Report 17

Patient Charges

Adams Memorial Hospital is a 650-bed not-for-profit institution located in a midwestern city with a population of 750,000. It has a good reputation and is noted for its fairly low patient per diem rates. Jeff Sharp has been the materiel manager for approximately five years.

Mr. Sharp is concerned about the way patient charges are established in the institution, so he decides to confer with the administrator, to whom he relates directly, about the matter. The administrator asks that the comptroller and the assistant administrator for finance join them in the conference. Mr. Sharp relates the entire concern in detail, stating that there is no uniformity or commonality to the patient charge system. The various department heads are responsible for developing their patient charge rates which they do by calling their counterparts in the other hospitals and establishing a comparable charge. In other words, if it was found that a certain item was priced at $3.00 at one institution and $4.00 at another institution, most likely, Adams Memorial Hospital's price to the patient would be $3.50. The department heads usually establish patient charges by the rule of thumb that they do not want to be the highest or the lowest. He further relates that the same supply item with identical costs dispensed from two different revenue centers will probably have different patient charges. For instance, an individual roll of four-inch rubber elastic bandage charged to the patient is $4 from the central stores, $4.50 from the emergency room, $3.50 from central supply, and $5 from the cast room.

Mr. Sharp says that basically there are three distinct charge classifications being used at the hospital: one for items that are totally used by the patient, like dressings and drugs; one for items such as trays that may be made up of both disposable and reusable supplies; and one for patient procedures such as a chest X-ray. He states that the latter two categories are somewhat directed and uniform. For example, trays are based on the cost of the supplies plus a personnel time cost factor, and procedure charges are based on time and motion studies concerning time involved and equipment used. However, supplies, which represent the largest dollar volumes of time, are sometimes marked up to varying degrees. Furthermore, whether the patient is charged at all depends solely on the department head or the employee using the supply. Mr. Sharp points out that on some units, the nurses will not charge the patient for expensive supplies if they know he or she does not have insurance. He estimates that the hospital loses at least $20,000 per month in "lost" charges for supplies from the nursing units alone.

Mr. Sharp relates that his efforts in putting charge tickets on the stock items in the nursing units have ended in frustration for him and his staff. Sometimes charges are made out but then kept on the units for weeks after the patients have been discharged. One day while making rounds, he found approximately $10,000 worth of such charges. Also, he says that to get patient charges from the emergency room is next to impossible. They are too busy caring for the emergency patients to be concerned with the charges, and no records are kept of what was used on which patients. Surgery is almost as bad. He states that he could continue with this story of woe, but at least these accounts relate a large proportion of the problem.

The administrator shakes his head in disbelief and inquires of his other two associates if they concur with Mr. Sharp's observations. They both nod agreement. He asks, "Why hasn't something been done before now? No wonder we have the lowest per diem in the city." The administrator calms down and asks what can be done about the situation. The assistant administrator in charge of finance states that he feels a multidisciplined, patient charge review committee should be appointed to deal with the matter. The comptroller asks that a new position of a cost and charge analyst be created to establish all patient charges in a responsible and uniform matter. There is a sudden silence, and the administrator asks if Mr. Sharp has any suggestions since he delineated the problems in the first place. Mr. Sharp states that he feels the hospital should use an all-inclusive rate for patient charges. In this manner, the patient would be charged a certain per diem for all supplies and pharmaceuticals. It would be less expensive in the long run, since no one would have to take the time to establish individual charges or spend precious time looking for lost charges.

All of Mr. Sharp's associates were stunned by his recommendation!

Pertinent Points to Ponder

1. Is this a typical situation in most hospitals? Why or why not?
2. Is there a scientific, easy way to establish patient charges on an a la carte basis? How?
3. Do you think that the administrator knew all along the hospital was having patient charge trouble? Why?
4. Who in the organization should have the responsibility of establishing patient charges?

5. How should the materiel management department be involved in patient charging?
6. What should be the basis for all patient charges?
7. Did the patient charge problems have anything to do with the hospital's low per diem? Why or why not?
8. Of the three suggestions for solving the problem, which did you like best and why?
9. Of the three suggestions for solving the problem, which did you like least and why?
10. The administrator did not give a suggestion for solving the patient charge problem. In your opinion, why didn't he?
11. What exactly is an all-inclusive rate for supplies?
12. What would be the third party payers' reactions to the concept of an all-inclusive supply rate?

Case Report 18

The Prime Supplier Concept

Rockland Medical Center is a 425-bed not-for-profit institution located in a northeastern city of 350,000. Rockland has a good patient care reputation, but is known for its high per diem rates in comparison to the other three institutions in the city. When questioned about the high costs, the administrator states that the Medical Center is a teaching institution and as a consequence, gets sicker patients. As of yet, no one has refuted his argument.

Robert Higby has been the materiel manager for six years. He feels he is doing a fair job in developing the total materiel management concept. He has lost the battle of centralized purchasing thus far with the exceptions of pharmacy, maintenance, and dietary, but he has been successful in instituting a total cart exchange program and amalgamating central supply into the central stores. Mr. Higby is well thought of by his colleagues and has been unsuccessfully approached with job offers from other hospitals. He openly states that he would like to get more materiel successes under his belt before he leaves the Medical Center.

Mr. Higby has set as his next goal the development of the prime supplier concept. He has done much research on the subject and has visited several other hospitals that have gone this route. He sincerely feels that this concept will assist him in achieving two more of his objectives—inventory reduction and simpler methods of procurement. Presently, he is concerned with a high central stores inventory which approximates $800,000. This includes intravenous solutions and sets, office supplies, processed goods, forms, and medical-surgical supplies. He is purchasing these supplies from about 50 different dealers and considers this to be an anathema to good materiel management. After he does some initial research, he decides to experiment with one or two small supply categories before going to the administrator and asking for approval to move into the large categories of medical-surgical, laboratory, and staple foods.

His first endeavor into the prime supplier world was in the area of forms, in which the inventory was at least $150,000 at all times. He defines the proposal in writing and asks five companies to bid on it. The terms of the proposal are that the printer gives the hospital the best volume price, but only delivers and bills for a two-week supply. This is repeated until the entire original order is used. In this manner, the hospital does not have to keep any forms in inventory and the appropriate departments or units are charged accordingly. Of the five companies, four return quotations. Mr. Higby selects the lowest and within six months reduces his forms inventory to a zero balance. He carefully documents the savings.

In another area, he works with the chief pharmacist using the prime supplier technique. The pharmacist was utilizing all three of the local drug wholesalers to supply the hospital's indirect pharmaceuticals, amounting to about $400,000 per year. Simply by getting them to bid against each other for the total business, Mr. Higby saves the hospital another $40,000. The pharmacist is grateful and Mr. Higby documents this success for the prime supplier approach.

He now begins to prepare his most important case in favor of the prime supplier approach in the area of medical-surgical supplies. The hospital is presently purchasing about $2 million worth of medical supplies annually from about 25 different vendors. Therefore, he draws up the following proposal.

a. The hospital is to receive the best volume price regardless of the quantity ordered. (This would allow Mr. Higby to reduce his inventory and still get the best prices.)
b. The prime supplier will give an across-the-board 12 percent discount off all items purchased.
c. The prime supplier agrees to stock at least a 60-day reserve inventory for all specified stock items.
d. The prime supplier will provide transportation and free deliveries will be made to the hospital twice a week.
e. If the prime supplier ever has a shortage or back order on the hospital stock items, the hospital will receive a 10 percent rebate on the total quantity of the items.

f. The prime supplier will provide the hospital with purchase orders at no expense
g. The hospital will receive at least 60 days prior protection on all stock items.
h. The term of the agreement is two years.

Mr. Higby conservatively estimates that in volume discounts and inventory reduction, this prime supplier contract will save the hospital $250,000 the first year and $50,000 the second year. Besides, it will reduce the number of purchase orders and checks, the number of suppliers will be reduced to two, and the purchasing agent will be saved much time and many headaches. Mr. Higby feels he has an airtight case and is ready for his presentation to the administrator.

Mr. Higby begins his presentation by revealing the tremendous savings in the areas of printed matter and indirect pharmaceuticals. The administrator studies carefully the handouts that Mr. Higby has prepared on both cases. After a short period of concentration, the administrator proclaims with a smile that this is what materiel management is all about. It is finally beginning to bring substantial dividends. He congratulates Mr. Higby and reiterates his support for the total materiel management concept. Mr. Higby accepts the accolades, and then presents him the third case proposal. He reads the entire documentation and begins to ask several questions. Mr. Higby gives good reasoned answers to all of his questions, but, the administrator tells him to table this proposal indefinitely, stating that this prime supplier concept for medical-surgical supplies represents "putting all of your eggs in one basket." The administrator feels that this action may cause some of the smaller supply houses in the city to close their doors. Besides, many of these companies gave substantial amounts to the hospital building fund. He asks Mr. Higby to direct his energies into some of the other more important areas of materiel management.

As Mr. Higby leaves the administrator's offices, he thinks to himself that those other job offers are looking much better than ever.

Pertinent Points to Ponder

1. What is the prime supplier concept?
2. What are the advantages and disadvantages of this approach?
3. Do you feel that it is a form of group purchasing? Why or why not?
4. Why didn't Mr. Higby get the administrator's approval for the prime supplier contracts for forms printing and indirect drugs?

5. In your opinion, why did he decide to ask the administrator's approval for the medical-surgical contract?
6. Do you feel he should have gone ahead with his plans without telling the administrator? Why or why not?
7. Was Mr. Higby's approach to the administrator well planned? Why?
8. Do you think it was hard for the administrator to reject the proposal? Why?
9. Do you think that the administrator knew all along of Mr. Higby's investigations into this major supply category? Why?
10. Were the administrator's reasons for disapproving the contract valid? Why or why not?
11. What did he mean when he stated that the prime supplier approach represented "putting all of your eggs in one basket?" Did you ever gather eggs? How many baskets did you use?
12. Who won in this situation? Who lost?

Case Report 19

Evaluation of the Materiel Efforts

Upton General Hospital is a 325-bed not-for-profit institution located in the suburb of a city with a population of 150,000. It is a 2-year-old modern complex which replaced a 100-year-old institution located in the inner city. The new structure meets all of the requirements of the various planning and governmental agencies.

Ken White, the materiel manager, has been with the institution for ten years. He is proud to be associated with Upton General Hospital and his materiel efforts are strongly supported by top management. His hospital is an example of the ultimate in materiel management systems and planning. Many visitors come to review and work in the department. Mr. White very modestly tells everyone that a good materiel department comes through years of planning and lots of hard work. His dreams have finally come true, but only after ten years of failures, surveys, proposals, and successes. He indicates that the key to materiel management success is discipline and commitment. One must set one's sights high and not compromise.

As a key member of the management team, Mr. White was in on the planning of the new hospital from beginning to end. As a result, the materiel management department is very effective. It is located on the ground level, and all materiel functions, including central stores, central processing, materiel administration, pharmacy, centralized receiving, and distribution, are located together. A total supply cart exchange program is functioning beautifully for all nursing units and departments. Centralized purchasing is religiously practiced and inventories are kept to absolute minimums, including $35,000 in central stores, $40,000 in pharmacy, and $20,000 in dietary items and staple foods. Each nursing unit of 35 beds has a total inventory of $350. The departments, including surgery, have a maximum of three weeks stock of supplies.

The prime supplier concept is practiced on a group basis with three other hospitals. Stockless purchasing is performed for all departments and supply duplication is at an absolute minimum. The entire central stores has only 425 stock items and they are for the cart exchange program. These stock items only are on a computerized perpetual inventory. A product standardization committee approves all supplies including drugs before they are purchased, establishes the patient charge for all applicable items, sees that product procedures are written, and performs followup reviews on all approved items. It has been a lifesaver for Mr. White. Good orientation programs exist for both the hospital and materiel management employees. Finally, to put the icing on the cake, Upton General's materiel costs per bed were found to be the lowest by a wide margin according to a recent state-wide survey of 250 hospitals.

Mr. White wonders if it is time to move on to bigger and better things. However, he decides to stay and develop other programs for the hospital. Accordingly, he decides to have an all day conference with key members of his staff to explore other possibilities for improving service or reducing costs. After much discussion and deliberation, they decide to ask the supply consumers what they feel about the present materiel efforts and what they propose for the future. Some supervisors feel that asking the head nurses about the materiel efforts is asking for trouble; after all, they reasoned, no other department including nursing has asked us to evaluate them. Mr. White states that the department of materiel management is taking the initiative to improve its service by asking for the candid opinions of the consumers. He convinces his staff to develop the survey and distribute it to some 50 consumers of materiel services, including all department heads, head nurses, and some selected supervisors. The survey is in two parts, one evaluating the present service and the other dealing with areas of future improvement. Respondents are given two weeks to complete it.

All surveys are returned before the due date, with about 85 percent signed by the persons completing them. The results are collated into one disappointing report. For instance, there is a summary question regarding whether total present services are considered poor, fair, good, or excellent. The results show that of the 50 participants, 10 thought the total present services to be poor, 38 thought fair, and only 2 felt them to be good.

In reference to future plans, the following recommendations are made:

1. Put more supplies back on the units and in the departments.
2. Establish a telephone hot line for requesting supplies not on the cart which are needed right away.
3. Do away with the standardization committee and let us have anything we need.
4. Keep the central stores area open twenty-four hours a day seven days a week like all other responsible departments.
5. Provide inservice sessions to answer all our supply questions.
6. Develop a centralized patient escort service which can also be responsible for delivering supplies.
7. Do away with patient charges.
8. Let us see sales representatives at any time.
9. Allow department heads and head nurses to request items and equipment for evaluation without going through the purchase process.
10. Have your employees be nice to us when we call for an item.

After reviewing the summary of the survey results, Mr. White debates whether or not he will share the results with his supervisors and employees.

Pertinent Points to Ponder

1. Would you agree that on the surface, Mr. White's materiel management department looks outstanding?
2. Would you still agree after seeing the summary of the survey results? Why or why not?
3. For a service department such as materiel management, is a performance survey appropriate? Why?
4. Should the other departments get to evaluate the materiel efforts? Why?
5. What are the likely pitfalls of such a survey?
6. What are the advantages of such a survey?
7. Why do you suppose the department heads and head nurses saw the materiel efforts differently than Mr. White and his employees?

8. Should Mr. White share the survey results with his supervisors and employees? Why?
9. What will happen if he doesn't?
10. What do you personally think about the consumers' list of ten recommendations?
11. Do you feel they were justified? Why?
12. Will the survey be repeated ever again? Why or why not?

Case Report 20

Supply Cost Reimbursement

The Regional Medical Center is a 400-bed not-for-profit institution located in a city of approximately 1 million people. There are ten other hospitals in and around the metropolitan area which have about 5,000 beds for general acute medical care.

The administrators' council for the area, which is made up of each of the administrators from the 11 hospitals, is committed to the idea of cost containment through group purchasing and shared services. Three years ago, the council established a separate corporation just for shared services and group purchasing endeavors called Hospital Group Endeavors, Ltd. Its six-person staff includes the executive director, an assistant director, a group purchasing coordinator, a shared services coordinator, and two secretaries and its personnel budget is $124,000 per year.

H.G.E., supported and encouraged all along by the third party payers and the state insurance commissioner, has formulated fairly aggressive plans for both group purchasing and shared services. The hospitals are presently participating in centralized laundry services, laboratory reference work, supervisory training programs, medical education, biomedical engineering services, legal services, nursing pools, C.A.T. scanning, and cobalt therapy services. It should be noted that the shared laundry and linen project actually raised the cost of processed pounds of linen over what each hospital was previously paying and has been hampered by unionization attempts. The hospitals also have combined their efforts in purchasing such supply items as medical gases, sutures, beverages, underpads, paper products, office supplies, bread, meats, milk, X-ray film, laboratory reagents, and intravenous fluids.

Tom Dodd is the departmental director of purchasing for Regional Medical Center. There has been some talk about making him the materiel manager, but nothing has materialized yet and the center has not initiated materiel management. Mr. Dodd has not been active in promoting the total materiel management philosophy, mainly because it will be more work for him. He has participated in all the group purchasing projects, but has not been overly enthusiastic about its success. He mainly participates to keep the administrator off his back, because he has stated on many occasions that he can match or beat the group prices after they have been negotiated.

Mr. Dodd is asked by the group purchasing coordinator of H.G.E. to document the apparent savings from group purchasing that have been realized by Regional Medical Center over the past year and to project future savings for the next year. The coordinator explains that this is for a year-end report that he must present to the administrators' council. So Mr. Dodd reluctantly goes over all of the group purchases for his hospital and seriously doubts in his mind that savings have been realized, but knows he should state something. After two days of thinking and documenting, he decides to indicate that his hospital has saved approximately $10,000 for the past year and projects a potential savings for next year of $20,000. After he submits his report, he learns from the coordinator of group purchasing that some hospitals indicated they saved at least a $100,000 and projected next year's saving to be around $250,000. Mr. Dodd knows all of the other purchasing agents and materiel managers and he is certain that these figures have been grossly overstated. Now he wonders if he should have been more enterprising with his statistics.

That afternoon, he is in a conference with the hospital's comptroller who is a C.P.A. and is well respected in the hospital field. Mr. Dodd tells him of the group purchasing efforts and what is projected for the future, expecting his guest to be very enthusiastic about group purchasing. However, the comptroller explains another facet of supply costs of which Mr. Dodd was not aware. The comptroller states that the insurance companies in the area reimburse the hospitals for patient charge supplies using a certain formula based on the costs of the items. For central supply and central stores items, the hospitals get two and one-half times the purchase cost of the items. Therefore, if the hospitals decrease the cost of the supplies, they also decrease their revenues from those items. So, in reality, supply savings could result in lost revenues for the hospital.

After the conference, Mr. Dodd is more confused than ever. He wonders now if he saved the hospital money or caused it to lose revenue. He reasons that it actually doesn't matter that much because his savings were not as large as he had stated. But what about those other hospitals?

Pertinent Points to Ponder

1. Is H.G.E. fairly representative of a typical shared services corporation? Why?

2. How does a separate corporation such as H.G.E. get its operating funds?
3. Is the staff of H.G.E. top heavy and expensive? Why?
4. In your opinion, to whom does the executive director report and why?
5. Is Mr. Dodd's behavior toward group purchasing efforts fairly typical of most purchasing agents? Why?
6. How does the hospital actually document its savings through group purchasing? Does it actually mean that the hospital was losing all of this money up to now?
7. Why do many purchasing agents feel that group purchasing gives them a bad image?
8. Are Mr. Dodd's concerns about the savings to his hospital from group purchasing programs well founded? Who would know, if he doesn't?
9. Would you select Mr. Dodd as your materiel manager? Why or why not?
10. Do you agree with the comptroller's explanation of the reimbursement of costs? In your opinion, should he have explained this to Mr. Dodd at this time?
11. Can a hospital actually lose money by reducing costs? Why or why not?
12. What reimbursement policy exists in the area in which your hospital is located? Get to know it!

Case Report 21

Administrative Reports

Robinson Memorial Hospital is a 575-bed not-for-profit general-acute institution located in a city with a population of 500,000. The hospital is presently involved with a 200-bed expansion which will be completed in approximately two years. Joe Harris, the materiel manager for the past six years, is a very capable person who is presently working toward his degree in industrial engineering. He is well respected by his hospital colleagues as well as the other materiel managers from the seven other area hospitals. He is only 37, but is considered to be the dean of the local materiel managers. He has had the unquestioned support of the past administrator, but recently there has been a change in the top management leadership. Mr. Harris was offered a good position with his former boss, but Mr. Harris' family did not want to leave the state so he decided to stay at Robinson Memorial.

The new administrator, Charles Green, has been on the job only three months. Mr. Green has a masters degree in hospital administration and much experience in the management of a corporation involving several hospitals run for profit. He has a very keen business sense and is known as an operations expert. Mr. Harris has talked to Mr. Green briefly about the effective materiel management department at Robinson Memorial. Mr. Green relates that he has never heard of the materiel efforts of Robinson Memorial before and is interested in becoming more informed.

One Monday morning, Mr. Green's secretary calls Mr. Harris and schedules a four-hour briefing session with Mr. Green for the following Friday. She informs Mr. Harris to be prepared to discuss the entire materiel management thrust with Mr. Green using reports, slides, charts and anything else he has available. Mr. Harris is overwhelmed with this request and begins preparation for his presentation. He has a few slides of the operation, but not nearly enough to discuss thoroughly the entire operation. He begins to draw flow charts of the various phases of the organization and even delineates an organizational chart for the first time. Mr. Harris finds that he has little written documentation to show for his fine efforts, and starts a search for the folder that has the materiel management policies and procedures. When he finally finds it, he feels for the first time, the need for good policies and procedures. He reads each of the ten policies and procedures in the folder and remembers that they were written hastily for a Joint Commission survey. He is not happy with them and decides to make the development of a policy and procedure manual one of his future short-term objectives. He finally gathers all of the information he has and puts it into a presentable format.

On Friday morning, Mr. Green begins by telling Mr. Harris something about his past administrative experience. In fact, Mr. Green was once a purchasing agent in a 250-bed institution. Mr. Harris find the new administrator to be extremely conversant in the areas of purchasing and materiel management. After a rather lengthy introduction, Mr. Harris is asked to present his program. He begins by going back to when he first came to the hospital, recapping each of the problems one by one. He discusses the services available from materiel management and submits a list of objectives for the future.

After an hour's presentation, Mr. Harris runs out of things to say, so he opens the meeting for discussion. Mr. Green comments that he had felt the presentation would take longer and has several unanswered questions. One was how many and what kinds of administrative reports are generated from the materiel management areas. Mr. Harris answers by saying that the former administrator did not request any reports, so he had not developed any for administrative review. Mr. Green finds this to be very strange and asks how did the former administrator know what was going on in the materiel management department. Mr. Harris replies that the former administrator trusted him. Mr. Green indicates that trust has nothing to do with a definite need to know what was going on in the materiel areas. Mr. Harris asks what reports he would like to see generated, and Mr. Green says that Mr. Harris should be the judge of that. However, Mr. Harris confesses that he has never developed an administrative report and does not even know the format to use. Mr. Green gives him a list of subjects about which he would like information, and tells Mr. Harris to develop an appropriate format. Mr. Green lists the following topics:

a. Monthly budget figures.
b. A monthly activity report from the central stores area.
c. A monthly activity report from the pharmacy.
d. A monthly profit or loss report from the standardization committee.
e. A monthly linen usage report by department and unit.
f. A quarterly physical inventory report for all official and unofficial inventories.
g. A periodic report concerning group purchasing and shared service efforts.
h. A monthly lost charge report from all of the units.
i. A monthly report on anything out of the ordinary that he feels administration should know.
j. An annual operational summary.

Mr. Green states that this list will be good for starters, but that more reports may be added. He further states his disbelief that there were no administrative reports generated from such an important area.

As Mr. Harris leaves the conference, he feels that the only reason Mr. Green wants these cumbersome reports is that he distrusts and wants to check up on him.

Pertinent Points to Ponder

1. In your present position, do you make monthly administrative reports? Why?
2. How did the former administrator know whether Mr. Harris was doing a good job or not?
3. Is it just a matter of trust? Why?

4. If the administrator has never asked for reports, should the materiel manager develop them anyway? Why?
5. Is there certain information in reference to materiel management that the administrator should know on a monthly basis? What for instance?
6. How does one develop a format for reports?
7. Why didn't Mr. Green request a certain format or any specific information?
8. Do you feel that Mr. Green's background in profit-making hospitals was responsible for his wanting materiel reports? Why or why not?
9. Is Mr. Green asking for too much information from Mr. Harris for starters? Why?
10. Is it possible that this information is already coming to Mr. Green from other sources? Why or why not?
11. Is it possible that good administrative reports could strengthen Mr. Harris' materiel management efforts? Why?
12. What would you do if you were Mr. Harris?

Case Report 22

Centralized Warehousing

Hillvale Hospital is a 200-bed not-for-profit institution located in a city with a population of 750,000. There are 15 other hospitals located within a 25-mile radius of the city ranging in size from 75 to 800 beds. There is a very active group purchasing program among the hospitals.

William Loy, the materiel manager for Hillvale for the past five years, is well respected as a materiel manager and has the strong support of his administrator. It has even been rumored that when the present administrator retires or leaves, Mr. Loy will take his place. Mr. Loy is working on his degree in business administration by going to night school. He has been upgrading the materiel management department at Hillvale and is responsible for developing a very active and results-oriented standardization committee. The total supply cart exchange program, which he implemented, has been well accepted by all those who use it.

Since his hospital is one of the smaller in the group, Mr. Loy has tried to work every angle to see that Hillvale Hospital gets the lowest prices possible for all supplies and equipment. He was the first to implement the prime supplier concept for medical-surgical supplies, which all the hospitals in the area now use on a group purchasing basis. Mr. Loy swears by this method. He feels that all hospitals get excellent prices on all medical-surgical supplies across-the-board without having to purchase in large quantities. Also, he stresses that the hospitals do not even have to standardize on the supplies, just order them from the same vendor. According to a recent state price comparison survey of 150 supplies, the hospitals in Mr. Loy's area are getting among the lowest prices in the state.

Since the hospitals have had excellent results from group purchasing programs, some administrators have asked the group purchasing coordinator to research the idea of centralized warehousing and purchasing directly from the manufacturers. The group purchasing coordinator informs each of the materiel managers about the proposal and requests them to meet and discuss the pros and cons of such an endeavor. Mr. Loy confers with his administrator in reference to the proposal and states that this is an absurd idea since there are three surgical houses with at least a million square feet of warehousing space located just minutes from all of the hospitals. He feels the hospitals should utilize the suppliers' warehousing capabilities, especially since the cost of every supply includes a small percentage for warehousing. He further argues that if the hospitals get into the act, they will be paying twice for storage. Mr. Loy says that from his initial research of the proposal, it will cost the hospitals an additional $250,000 a year, which includes costs such as rent, salaries of at least ten additional employees, purchase costs of two trucks, insurance, utilities, and initial inventory. He explains further that many supplies and drugs are already purchased directly from the manufacturer and absolutely no savings will accrue from the purchase of these items. Even if the hospitals could save $25,000 per year by purchasing directly from the manufacturers, they would have to buy in such quantities that the savings would be more than offset by the holding costs of the inventory. He summarizes his argument by saying that the hospitals should continue their present program of utilizing the suppliers to the fullest degree and not become their competitors.

The administrator has been taking notes all along. He smiles and says that Mr. Loy presents a very convincing story, and confesses that he was one of the six administrators that proposed central warehousing. The additional facts however, persuade him to discourage such an endeavor.

Mr. Loy attends the group purchasing committee the next day and gives the same presentation against central warehousing. The materiel managers are unanimous in their decision to recommend that the central warehousing proposal be dropped from consideration. Mr. Loy is pleased with his colleagues' faith in him.

Pertinent Points to Ponder

1. What are the advantages and disadvantages of centralized supply warehousing for hospitals?
2. Why do you think this proposal came from the administrators and not the materiel managers?
3. If the materiel managers had proposed such a program to the administrators' council, do you think they would have approved it?
4. The views of the group purchasing coordinator were never presented. What do you think his vote would have been and why?
5. Will all manufacturers of hospital supplies and equipment sell directly to the hospitals at a discount price? Why or why not?
6. Do you think the administrators' council accepts the recommendation of the group purchasing committee? Why or why not?
7. Do you think the various sales representatives knew of this proposal? Why?
8. In your opinion, why didn't they openly come out against it?
9. What percentage of supply costs does warehousing represent?
10. What is basically wrong with hospitals setting up a common warehouse?
11. In your opinion, who will get the praise or blame for defeating the proposal? Why?
12. Is central warehousing ever advantageous for hospitals? If so, under what conditions?

Case Report 23

Cost Containment Efforts

Madison Memorial Hospital is a 398-bed not-for-profit institution located in a southern city with a population of 285,000 people. The hospital enjoys a good reputation within the community it serves, and ends each fiscal year with an earned surplus. There is talk of adding a 100-bed wing to the complex, but the planning has not yet begun. John Smith is the executive director, and has the reputation of running a tight ship.

Dick Simmons, the materiel manager for the past eight years, came directly from industry and has established a good reputation in hospital materiel management. However, he admits that the key to his success has been the excellent support he has received from Mr. Smith. Mr. Smith does not like to see waste of any type. He supports near-zero inventories, very tight staffing patterns, and a strict standardization committee. He has encouraged Mr. Simmons to get a charge for every patient charge item that is used. He deplores lost patient charges.

One day, Mr. Smith gets a call from the executive director of the state hospital association asking for assistance in documenting cost containment efforts in the hospitals all over the state. He asks Mr. Smith to put in writing programs that have resulted in cost containment over the past year at Madison Memorial and to list programs for the next year that will also result in cost containment. In both cases, Mr. Smith should indicate the total savings for each year. He states that this information is needed to present evidence of cost reduction programs brought about by the hospitals and the third party payers. Data from all the hospitals throughout the state will be correlated and presented to the state insurance commissioner. Mr. Smith enthusiastically agrees to participate.

Mr. Smith asks all of the department heads to present in writing all cost containment programs initiated in their departments last year and to list cost containment programs expected to be initiated for the coming year. Mr. Simmons feels that many or most of these efforts can be realized in the materiel management areas. To prove his point, he lists the following cost containment or reduction programs initiated in the past year:

PROGRAM	*SAVINGS*
a. Reduced official inventories in central stores and pharmacy.	$150,000
b. Amalgamated the central supply with central stores. Reduced inventory and ten personnel.	inventory-50,000 personnel-65,000
c. Reduced the departmental unofficial inventories by at least 30 days.	100,000
d. Negotiated prime supplier contracts for food, indirect pharmaceuticals, medical-surgical supplies, and forms.	110,000
e. Renegotiated the elevator maintenance contracts from full to term service.	28,000
f. Group purchasing contracts.	75,000
TOTAL SAVINGS	$578,000

He lists the following proposed cost containment or reduction programs for the next year:

PROGRAM	*PROJECTED SAVINGS*
a. Change patient linen only three times per week instead of every day.	$100,000
b. Negotiate additional group purchasing contracts.	50,000
c. Further reduce staff by two employees.	18,000
TOTAL PROJECTED SAVINGS	$168,000

Mr. Simmons proudly submits his programs and documented savings to Mr. Smith. Mr. Smith was stunned by the figures since all of the other departments together only submitted approximately $175,000 savings for last year and $185,000 projected savings for the next year. He asks Mr. Simmons to double check his figures. Mr. Simmons indicates that he has done so several times and that they represent a rather conservative total. He is both positive and proud of the figures!

Pertinent Points to Ponder

1. What exactly is cost containment?
2. What is the difference between cost containment and cost reduction?
3. If a hospital realizes a cost containment of $100,000 for a certain period, does this mean that the patient costs can be adjusted accordingly? Explain.
4. If a hospital realizes a cost reduction of $100,000 for a certain period, does this mean that the patient costs can be adjusted accordingly? Explain.
5. Do you feel comfortable with Mr. Simmons' figures? Why or why not?
6. Why do you feel that all the other departments projected such a meager amount?
7. With which figures do you feel more comfortable, the other departments' or Mr. Simmons'?
8. What are your comments about Mr. Simmons' proposed plans

of changing linen only three times per week unless the patients need it done more often?

9. Is it a realistic and practical program? Explain.
10. Do you feel Mr. Smith will give his approval to it? Explain.
11. If a hospital actually reduces its official inventory by $100,000, does this same savings carry over to succeeding years? Why or why not?
12. Should interest from savings on monies freed up by cost reduction programs be counted as part of the total savings? Explain.

Case Report 24

Prudent Purchaser Considerations

Coastal Medical Complex is a 410-bed not-for-profit institution located in a northwestern city with a population of 810,000. There are six other hospitals serving the area. Coastal is a teaching hospital affiliated with a large medical school. However, it is funded strictly through operations. Coastal Medical Complex enjoys a good reputation within the community it serves, but it is known to have the highest patient per diem costs in the area. It has all major medical and surgical specialties and subspecialties. By all standards, the hospital is full service.

Tom Sidney has been the director of purchasing for the Coastal Medical Complex for six years. In this position, he has departmental director status and can relate to all of the other department heads on an equal basis. Mr. Sidney is about thirty-nine years old and is working on his undergraduate degree at the state university in business administration. He hopes to continue his education and become a hospital administrator because he feels that is the only way he will ever get things done. He has tried several times to get his title changed to materiel manager, but each time the administrator has asked for an overall materiel master plan before any title change is made. He has requested that Mr. Sidney develop a total materiel management concept, but Mr. Sidney has not responded with any enthusiasm. Mr. Sidney seems to have the philosophy that if the system works don't try to change it. The administrator's attempts to have the materiel efforts upgraded have been in vain because of the lack of interest on the part of Mr. Sidney. Mr. Sidney's ideas of upgrading materiel efforts involve computerization and automation. In other words, his answer to inventory problems is to provide computer capabilities directly for all central stores items. In addition, he proposes a $1.5 million automated cart system to assist in supply distribution. He has often said that the only way to go is to go first class, and all other efforts are not worth considering. Therefore, with this philosophy, he has not been able to make much materiel progress at Coastal Medical Complex.

One day, the assistant administrator for finance asks to meet with the administrator and the director of purchasing. He briefly summarizes his concerns by stating that the Medicare auditors have indicated that they will be performing a prudent purchasing audit at the hospital in about four weeks. The financial administrator states that he and his staff would like to perform a trial run of the audit and see if there are any major problems that need immediate attention. He further indicates that he has gained access to a prudent purchaser checklist and knows what the auditors will be looking for. He thinks he and his staff can provide the results of the trial run in about five concentrated working days. Mr. Sidney objects violently to the proposal, stating that this is just an excuse for the financial director to take over the purchasing function. Mr. Sidney relates that he and the financial administrator have had problems for sometime over materiel management practices and this will give him a chance to get his foot in the door. Furthermore, his department operates efficiently and that there is no need for a trial audit. After hearing from both parties, the administrator states that he thinks the prudent purchases preview is an excellent idea and asks the financial administrator to begin immediately. If things are as Mr. Sidney states, the trial audit will just prove his point.

The trial audit is conducted and a week later the results are presented to the administrator and the director of purchasing. Much interesting data are exposed. For instance, the purchasing function is presently being performed by at least 36 different people. There are no uniform or approved prices. Purchase orders are issued for only 50 percent of the purchases and they do not show terms or prices and are not prenumbered and controlled in a numbered sequence. The prices paid for a high volume sampling of supplies are the highest in the area. Discounts, allowances, and rebates are taken at the end of the year, are not shown on the purchase order or price list, and are not double checked by the purchasing department. Sometimes "in-kind" supplies are substituted for rebates and discounts, but no record is kept. There is no record of a list of personnel authorized to initiate requisitions and purchase orders or of competitive bids being obtained on all purchases of materials, supplies, services, and/or construction contracts over a certain minimum amount. When prices which are higher than customary, there is absolutely no documentation of the explanations. There is no list of approved vendors, suppliers, and contractors. Minimums and maximums for each supply have not been established and purchasing policies and procedures have not been delineated. Finally, there is evidence that some of the vendors have rented storage space from the hospital and in essence are using the hospital as a shipping point. In summary, there is no materiel management plan at Coastal Medical Complex.

The financial administrator states that the hospital is in trouble in reference to the prudent purchasing policy and that he would like to request a delay of the audit. The administrator is very concerned and perplexed by the information he has just heard, and he asks Mr. Sidney if he has anything to say. Mr. Sidney states "Yes, I hereby resign my position as director of purchasing at Coastal Medical Complex."

Pertinent Points to Ponder

1. What is your opinion of Mr. Sidney's attitudes toward materiel management?
2. Why do you suppose he has such attitudes?
3. Did you get the impression that the administrator was supportive or nonsupportive of the materiel management concept? Why?
4. Why is it that many materiel managers and purchasing agents feel that a system must be complicated or sophisticated to be effective?
5. Should there be a close relationship between financial management and materiel management? Why or why not?
6. In your opinion, why did the financial administrator request a trial audit?
7. What did you think of Mr. Sidney's reaction to the trial audit?
8. Do you think the financial administrator was out to get Mr. Sidney or to take over materiel management? Why?
9. Does Coastal Medical Complex have prudent purchasing problems as was stated by the financial administrator? Why?
10. What are the penalties for nonprudent purchasing?
11. Are you familiar with the prudent purchasing guidelines? What are they? Have you seen a prudent purchaser checklist?
12. Do you approve of Mr. Sidney's resignation? Why? Was it timely? Do you think the administrator accepted his resignation gladly? If Mr. Sidney had not resigned, do you think he would have been fired, suspended, reprimanded, cautioned, or congratulated? Why?

Case Report 25

The Profit-Making Hospital

Bethel General Hospital was a 285-bed, religiously affiliated, not-for-profit institution located in a community of 35,000. It had been operating in the red for the past five years, and last year the operations deficit was $500,000. The sponsoring body decided to close the hospital, which concerned the community because there is not another hospital within 50 miles. The city mayor requested and was granted an emergency meeting with the members of the sponsoring body, during which he and his commissioners asked that the hospital not be closed. The city would make up any deficit in operating funds, mainly because the hospital was a major community employer with a staff of 1,000 full-time employees. The members stated that the decision had been made and it was final. The mayor threatened court action but that did not concern the sponsoring body; however, they did offer to sell the hospital and all supporting equipment to the city for $3.5 million. The mayor and the commissioners asked for 30 days in which to make a decision.

The mayor called an emergency session of city council and discussed the matter. The council turned down the proposal that the city purchase the hospital, but did give the mayor approval to approach a hospital management firm to see if a firm would be interested in buying the hospital. The first one he called indicated interest in purchasing the hospital and asked the mayor to set up an appointment for them with the sponsoring body. The next day, an agreement for purchase was made which included the following terms:

a. Purchase the hospital and equipment for a price of $3 million.
b. Change the name of the hospital.
c. Keep the administrator, if he wants to stay, for at least two years at his present salary.
d. Provide optimum patient care to the community.
e. Continue to meet all accreditation standards.

The hospital management firm did not request any financial assistance from the city government. The hospital administrator agreed to stay and the name of the hospital was changed to Peoples Hospital, Inc., a profit-making institution. The administrator was sent to the firm's headquarters for three months for an indepth orientation to their philosophy of management. The hospital has now been under the new management for the past 15 months.

The Peoples Hospital, Inc., now operating with a good profit margin had reduced the staff to 570 and eliminated some infrequently used services.

The firm has recruited two new surgeons and two general practitioners. In addition, the hospital has a new assistant administrator, Jack Strong, who is in charge of purchasing, central stores, central supply, print shop, supply distribution, property management, and pharmacy. Mr. Strong is very experienced in the area of materiel management and has been with the firm for the past ten years. He has made several changes. The central stores and central supply have been combined, resulting in a net reduction of seven people. The inventory has been reduced from $712,500 to $100,000 with more reduction contemplated. Purchasing has been centralized and all supplies and equipment must be purchased from the firm's approved prime suppliers. There is no standardization committee, but the hospital uses the firm's centralized standard items and formulary drugs. In other words, all 25 hospitals owned and operated by the firm use the same supplies and drugs. No other item or substitutes are purchased. They truly rely on volume buying and large-scale negotiations. The hospital's materiel policy and procedure manual were developed and approved in the firm's central office.

Mr. Strong has just received the latest monthly operations statement and sees that the hospital has had another good month especially in the materiel areas. He is very pleased with his progress because he receives a bonus for supply cost reduction and containment. He feels he has just scratched the surface and begins to delineate other cost reduction programs.

Pertinent Points to Ponder

1. What is meant by the term "nonprofit hospital"?
2. How does it differ from the profit-making hospital?
3. What are the advantages of each?
4. Why do you feel the management firm did not request financial assistance from the city?
5. In your opinion, what services were eliminated from the hospital initially?
6. Why do you think the firm selected the name Peoples Hospital?
7. In your opinion, why has the same hospital administrator been apparently successful with operating the Peoples Hospital, whereas he was unsuccessful in the other situation?
8. Did the administrator hire Mr. Strong? Why or why not?
9. How long do you feel Mr. Strong will stay at Peoples Hospital? Why?
10. When Mr. Strong stated that he received a bonus, what do you think he meant?

11. What other cost reduction programs do you think he has in mind?
12. Why can't a not-for-profit hospital be operated like a profit-making institution?

Glossary

Accounts Payable—The unpaid liability due to suppliers, manufacturers, and others for supplies, equipment, and service purchased from them.

Assets Management Program—A joint responsibility of materiel management and financial management whereby capital equipment is ordered, received, depreciated, and recorded on a systematic basis. The program can be maintained either manually or by computer.

Automated Cart System—This commonly used phrase is a misnomer because there is no such thing as an automated cart system. The phrase more properly refers to an automated distribution system for supply carts.

Back Door Buying—A term commonly used to describe decentralized purchasing whereby the departments can order from any and all vendors.

Back Door Selling—A term commonly used to describe the sales tactics in a hospital with a decentralized purchasing function.

Back Order—An item or items that are not shipped with the other supplies ordered at the same time or not shipped when expected.

Budgeting—A process by which revenues and expenses are forecasted over a specified period of time.

Bulk Stores—A supply holding area where supplies are stored in their manufactured quantity state. These quantities are requisitioned and broken down into usable quantities to be distributed from central stores and central supply.

Business Motivation Percentage—An incentive offered by the supplier to increase business over a certain specified volume. This term is usually characteristic of the prime supplier contract. For example, the supplier may offer the hospital a one percent discount on all purchases up to and over a million dollars.

Buyer—An employee in the materiel management organizational structure who is solely in charge of procuring supplies of a certain category. This position is usually a line responsibility and has no supervisory obligation.

Capital Equipment—Equipment of a certain value, usually over $100, with a life expectancy of more than a year, which is controlled and depreciated through a property management program. This type of equipment is not included in the annual operating expense budget.

Cart Exchange System—A type of supply distribution whereby supplies for a unit or department are depleted and replenished via a mobile cart.

Centralized Purchasing—A type of purchasing whereby the authority and responsibility for the procurement of all supplies and equipment is vested in one department or with one position.

Conflict of Interest—According to the AHA *Guidelines on Resolution of Conflicts of Interest in Health Care Institutions,* a potential conflict of interest may arise out of a duality of interest when the personal interests of institutional officials come in conflict with the interests of the institution.

Corporate Prime Supplier Agreement—A type of purchasing whereby the hospital can buy entire categories of applicable supplies from a parent company and all of its subsidiaries, branches, franchises, etc. at the same negotiated levels of price, quality, and service. The total corporate purchases are combined for volume price and service considerations.

Cost Containment—According to the AHA manual *Organizing A Cost Containment Committee In The Hospital,* "Cost containment involves the utilization of human resources and physical assets in a way that ensures economical delivery of high-quality health care. The true goals of a cost containment effort in a hospital are to evaluate whether the institution is obtaining optimum quality and quantity of goods and services for its money and to seek improved ways of acquiring those goods and services—all within the parameters of the institution's established standards of patient care."

C.P.D.—An acronym for Central Processing Department, where most of the hospital's processing and reprocessing is performed.

Discount—Represents a decrease in the listed price of supplies and equipment by the supplier for reasons such as volume buying and group purchasing.

Disposable—A product designed for one-time use.

Disposition—A materiel management function whereby the unusable remains of supplies and equipment are disposed.

Distribution—A materiel management function whereby supplies and equipment are delivered from receiving and/or storage to their point of utilization by either manual or automated means.

E.O.Q.—An acronym for economic order quantity. Simply stated, the E.O.Q. is the difference between a realistically established supply maximum and minimum taking into consideration lead times, holding costs, and available space.

FAX Copier—A piece of electronic equipment which receives and transmits a facsimile of a document over the telephone lines.

F.O.B.—An acronym for free on board, a term which represents how supply delivery or transportation is to be paid. "F.O.B. hospital" means that the cost of the item includes transportation to the hospital.

Forecasting—A materiel management function in which the quantities and supply usage patterns are fairly accurately predicted over a specified period of time.

Group Purchasing—A type of purchasing whereby hospitals combine their volumes of certain categories of supplies to receive better prices or supply service or both.

In-and-Out—A term used by suppliers to represent a batching or accumulation of hospitals' orders until a manufacturer's minimum reorder quantity is met.

Internal Control—A procedure of checks and balances to ensure that a product is purchased, received, and paid for in an ethical and prudent manner.

Inventory—As a noun, supplies or stock on hand. As a verb, to take a physical count of supplies on hand.

Inventory Reduction—A planned process through which supply quantities are decreased to adequate quantities to more appropriately reflect the inventory turnover rate and usage patterns. It is an achievable cost containment objective.

Invoice—A request on the part of the supplier for payment of goods and services rendered.

Lead Time—The number of days between supply order and supply receipt.

Line Authority—The authority to make a decision and act on it.

Logistics—A term, commonly used by the armed services, which refers to the management of materiel in general.

M.A.C.—An acronym for maximum allowable cost. The term refers to a proposal by the Department of Health, Education and Welfare (HEW) to limit federal reimbursement for multiple-source drugs to the cost of the least expensive among generally available and acceptable therapeutic equivalents. The M.A.C. proposal was first published in the Federal Register of November 15, 1974. This concept will probably be expanded to include hospital supplies and equipment in the near future.

Management—The function of getting things done through and with people and directing the efforts of these individuals toward a common goal or objective.

Manual Exchange—This materiel management term is commonly used to refer to the distribution of supply carts by people instead of automation.

Materiel Management—The management (handling) and control of supplies, equipment, and their related activities from acquisition to disposition. It represents a continuum along which many similar supply functions take place under the disciplined supervision of the materiel manager. Among those functions are supply specification, purchasing, receiving, supply processing, distribution, inventory control, supply utilization, standardization, value analysis, cost analysis, and forecasting.

Materiel Manager—The title given to a trained and experienced professional who has both line and staff authority over the management and control of supplies and equipment in a hospital or health facility.

Maximum—A volume ceiling established on individual supply items based on lead times, usage, holding costs, and space availability.

Minimum—A volume low point established on individual supply items based on careful consideration of lead times, usage, and holding costs.

Negotiation—An act that should occur during the purchasing function and entails bargaining for better prices, quality, and service.

Objective—A goal which is usually accompanied by an achievable timetable.

Official Inventory—A classification of supplies or inventory that is brought into a storage space or unit, counted, and controlled until dispensed to a using department of the hospital. It is assigned to an official inventory account number and when it is dispensed, the inventory account is relieved of the amount, which is charged off to the receiving department. This type of inventory is found most often in central stores, central sterile supply, dietary, and pharmacy.

Par Level—A maximum supply volume, usually applicable to unofficial inventory in the nursing units and departments, based on predetermined quotas which are established from previous use for that particular supply in that area for a specific time interval.

Patient Charge—A supply item which has been properly reviewed and determined to be one that should be individually charged to the patient. This supply item is appropriately marked up to reflect the direct and indirect costs and is considered to be under controlled conditions in most supply systems.

Penalty Clause—A negotiable aspect of the prime supplier contract in which the hospital receives a predetermined percentage of the total cost of a supply item that is back ordered by the prime supplier.

Perpetual Inventory System—A procedure for continual maintenance of a written or computerized record for supply orders, receipts, issues, and balances, usually with total cost extensions.

Policy—A statement of intent.

Price Protection—The freezing of a supply price by the supplier or manufacturer for a certain period of time.

Prime Supplier Agreement—A type of purchasing in which entire categories of supplies are bought from a single vendor. This term is synonymous with prime vendor, contract purchasing, systems contracting, and solo vendor.

Procedure—A detailed plan for action. The procedure takes the intent spelled out in the policy and details it for action.

Processing—A materiel management function whereby supplies and equipment are manufactured and/or made available for reuse by the hospital.

Prudent Buyer Concept—A section of the Medicare regulations which stipulates "the prudent and cost-conscious buyer not only refuses to pay more than the going price for an item or service, but seeks to economize by minimizing cost. This is especially so when the buyer is an institution or organization which makes bulk purchases and can, therefore, often gain discounts because of the size of its purchases. In addition, bulk purchase of items or services often gives the buyer leverage in bargaining with suppliers for other items or services. Any alert and cost-conscious buyer seeks such advantages, and it is expected that Medicare providers of services will also seek them."

Purchasing—A materiel management function whereby all hospital supplies and equipment are bought and acquired using standardized specifications.

Purchasing Agent—A position in the materiel management organizational structure that has responsibility for supply and equipment procurement. This position usually has managerial and supervisory obligations and often is filled by the director of the department of purchasing.

Purchase Order—A document that represents a commitment to purchase goods and services under certain specified terms of quality, quantity, and price.

Quality Control—A process through which supplies and equipment are rendered worthy and acceptable for their proper use.

Rebate—A return of a percentage of the payment for the supplies and equipment after a certain period of time by the supplier usually after certain terms have been met (i.e., projected volumes).

Receiving—A materiel management function whereby supplies and equipment which have been properly ordered are received from the transportation source, appropriately recorded, and taken to a supply area.

Requisition—A written or verbal means of requesting supplies and equipment from the supply areas.

Reverse Distribution—A form of distribution in which the user or consumer of the supply has the burden of obtaining the supply from the provider (the supply areas).

R.O.P.—An acronym for reorder point. It basically represents a supply minimum at which point the supply should be reordered.

Safety Stock—Represents the difference between reorder point quantities and dependable lead time quantities which are based on variable supply use patterns.

Shared Services—The combination of efforts of two or more hospitals for functions or services in order to receive better cost considerations or better service or both.

S.P.D.—An acronym for three important materiel management functions: supply, process, and distribution.

Staff Authority—A position characterized by an advisory relationship.

Standardization—A materiel management function whereby a product review is conducted to establish a purchasing standard for a supply, after which this standard is used to purchase an item to meet that specification with consideration given to quality, price, service, and availability.

Statement of Services—A listing of supply services available from the Department of Materiel Management.

Stockless Purchasing—This form of purchasing represents buying supplies for direct utilization by the respective departments without a duplication or accumulation in the central stores.

Stock-Out—A term most commonly used by hospitals to indicate a supply outage from a source such as central stores or central supply.

Supervision—The process of directing and managing subordinates to proper task performance.

Supply—A materiel management function whereby supplies and certain equipment are stocked for reasonable periods of time with consideration given to usage, lead times, holding costs, and available storage space.

T-Order—A term most commonly used by suppliers to indicate that the order is being transferred and shipped from another warehouse or branch operated by the same supplier.

Uncomplicated Purchase Order—A purchase order that has been processed without back orders.

Unofficial Inventory—Those supplies that have been expensed and dispensed to the various departments and units where they are temporarily stored until used.

Value Added—A process whereby a supply is made more usable for the consumer, such as bulk stock being broken down into units of use which renders the product more convenient (valuable) for use.

Warehousing—A form of inventory buildup which is usually located off-site and in bulk quantities.

Index

A

Administrative Reports, 71–72
  annual, 226
  monthly, 223–225
  quarterly, 225
  semi-Annual, 226
Administrative Support, 10
Ammer, Dean S., 21, 23
Assets Management, 274, 275
Automation, 167, 168, 277

B

Backdoor Buying, 116
Backdoor Selling, 116
Back Orders, 77–78
Biomedical Engineering, 274
Blue Cross, 24
Budgeting, 235–240
Budgets, 27
Buyer's Market, 203

C

Canadian Hospital Association, 1
Capital Equipment Acquisition
  hospital policy for, 217–218
  negotiation for, 219–221
Cart Attendant
  job description for, 52–55
Cart Quotas, 49, 50, 51
Centralized Purchasing, 91–94, 115–117
Committees
  impact upon materiel management, 229–233
Computer Applications, 276–277
Consignment, 262
Continuing Education, 26, 27
Continuum of Supply Functions, 3
Contract Purchasing
  advantages of, 207, 208
  methodology for, 207
  See also Prime Supplier
Contracts and Agreements, 72–74
Convenience Products, 279, 280
Cost Analysis, 3
Cost Containment
  committee for, 232
  policies and procedures for, 63–67
  ways to achieve, 259–281

Cost In use, 151–153
C.S.R., 1, 2

D

Delivery of Supplies, 95–96
Department Conferences, 26
Disaster Plan, 27
Distribution, 3
  supply, 163–186
Drug Formulary, 83–85, 267

E

Economic Order Quantity, 272
Equal Employment Opportunity
  Act, 22
Exchange Cart Coordinator
  job description for, 46–52
Excuses, 283–286

F

Facsimile Equipment, 269
Feedback Techniques, 142, 143
Forms
  printed, 264, 265, 266

G

Governmental Controls, 153–154
Group Purchasing, 268
  See also Prime Supplier and
    Contract Purchasing

H

Hospital Expenses
  distribution of, 6

I

Industrial Engineering Application,
  270
Infection Control, 146, 148
Inservice Training, 155, 156
Instant Credit, 268
Inventory
  definition of, 188–191
  official, 24, 259, 260
  reduction of, 187–195
  unofficial, 24, 260, 261
Isolation Cart
  processing of, 97–99

J

Job Descriptions, 26, 31–61
Joint Commission on Accreditation of
  Hospitals, 22, 28

L

Lending of Supplies, 88–90
Linen Changes
  reducing the frequency of,
    267, 268
Linen Processing, 78–79

M

Materiel Management
  administrative understanding
    of, 10
  consumer evaluation of, 245–249
  definition of, 1, 2
  establishment of objectives of, 12
  major functions of, 7
  organizational format for, 13
  organization of, 5
  planning and implementation of,
    9, 14, 15, 16, 17
  telling the story of, 251–257

Materiel Manager
  definition of, 23, 24
  hospital trained, 241–242
  industry trained, 242
  job description for, 32–36
  managerial profile of, 24, 25
  salary of, 11
  schedule of tasks of, 29
  selection of, 10, 11
  the pharmacist as, 243, 244
Medicaid, 22
Medical Staff, 254–255
Medicare, 22

N

Negotiation, 270

O

Occupational Safety and Health Act, 22
Organizational Chart, 5, 25
Orientation Programs, 27
Outdated Supplies, 85–86

P

Par Levels, 165, 166
Patient Charges, 3, 80, 81, 274
Performance Evaluations, 26, 86–88
Pharmacist
  job description for, 40–43
Policies and Procedures, 26, 63–108
Preventive Maintenance, 27, 274
Prime Supplier
  advantages of, 209, 210
  anatomy of, 208, 209
  definition of, 208
Processing Supervisor
  job description for, 57–60
Product Substitution, 99–100, 275
Prudent Buyer Principle, 103–105
Purchasing
  fundamentals of, 113–115
  See also Centralized Purchasing
  policies of, 203–207
  See also Contract Purchasing
  the act of, 109–112
Purchasing Agent
  job description for, 37–40
Purchasing Alternatives, 270, 271

R

Radioisotopes
  receiving of, 81–83
Rebates, 269, 270
Receiving, 3
Receiving Clerk
  job description for, 55–57
Requisitioning, 164, 165
Returned Goods
  policy and procedure for, 67–69

S

Sales Representatives
  departmental visitation of, 74–76
  orientation for, 157–158
  telling the story to, 255–256
Shared Services, 277
Sharing of Prices, 117–119
S.P.D. Area
  amalgamation of, 261
  general sanitation of, 96–97
S.P.D. Supervisor
  job description for, 44–46
Specifications
  supply and equipment, 3
Standardization, 3
Standardization Committee, 122
  administrative support for, 122

interface with other committees, 135, 136
ojectives of, 129–130
policies and guidelines for, 130, 135
representation of, 126, 128
Standardization of Products, 102, 103, 121–161
Statement of Services, 69–71, 246
Stockless Purchasing, 100–101, 197–201
Suppliers, 213–216
Supply Carts
automated vs. manual, 167–168
distribution of, 94–95
functions of, 181–184
Supply Locator List, 90–91
Supply Utilization Studies, 271

T

Taft Hartley Act, 22
Time and Motion Studies, 273, 274
Transfer of Equipment, 76–77

V

Value Analysis, 3, 149, 150, 275
Vendors, 272

W

Warehousing, 272
Warranties
equipment, 277, 278
Wholesaler, 263

About the Author

Charles E. Housley, M.B.A., F.A.C.H.A., is presently the associate administrator of Saint Anthony Hospital, Columbus, Ohio, and adjunct instructor in the program of hospital and health services administration at Ohio State University. He began his career in the health field as a hospital purchasing agent while still in high school. He graduated from the University of Tennessee in 1964. Mr. Housley became the assistant administrator of East Tennessee Children's Hospital, Knoxville, Tennessee, where purchasing and materiel management were his key responsibilities.

In 1965 he entered Xavier University, and in 1967 received his master's degree in business administration with a major in hospital administration after serving an administrative residency at Saint Anthony Hospital.

Mr. Housley was instrumental in founding the Young Administrators Colloquium of Central Ohio and became its first president. He became the first chairman of the Materiel Management Committee of the Ohio Hospital Association in 1975. This committee is an amalgamation of the former Purchasing Committee and the Central Services Committee. Mr. Housley is on the editorial advisory boards of *Hospital Purchasing Management,* DIMENSIONS *in Health Service,* and *Hospital Topics,* and is a frequent contributor to these magazines. The Canadian Hospital Association features his monthly column, "Materielly Speaking," in its magazine DIMENSIONS *in Health Service.*

In 1975 Mr. Housley received the Monsignor Griffin Award for literature from the Ohio Hospital Association for his article, "Provocative Approaches to Materiel Management," and in 1976 he received the Health Industry Manufacturers' Association award for his extensive work in materiel management. He is a consultant and frequent lecturer on the topic of hospital materiel management throughout the United States, Canada, and Mexico.